The Medical Interview

Mastering Skills for Clinical Practice

The Medical Interview
Mastering Skills for Clinical Practice

FIFTH EDITION

John L. Coulehan, MD, MPH, FACP

Head, Division of Medicine in Society
Health Science Center L-3-086
SUNY at Stony Brook
Stony Brook, NY

Marian L. Block, MD, ABFP

Chief Quality Officer
Western Pennsylvania Hospital
Pittsburgh, PA

F. A. Davis Company • Philadelphia

F. A. Davis Company
1915 Arch Street
Philadelphia, PA 19103
www.fadavis.com

Printed in the United States of America

Last digit indicates print number: 10 9 8 7 6 5 4 3 2 1

Acquisitions Editor: Andy McPhee
Developmental Editor: Melissa Reed
Art and Design Manager: Carolyn O'Brien

As new scientific information becomes available through basic and clinical research, recommended treatments and drug therapies undergo changes. The author(s) and publisher have done everything possible to make this book accurate, up to date, and in accord with accepted standards at the time of publication. The author(s), editors, and publisher are not responsible for errors or omissions or for consequences from application of the book, and make no warranty, expressed or implied, in regard to the contents of the book. Any practice described in this book should be applied by the reader in accordance with professional standards of care used in regard to the unique circumstances that may apply in each situation. The reader is advised always to check product information (package inserts) for changes and new information regarding dose and contraindications before administering any drug. Caution is especially urged when using new or infrequently ordered drugs.

Library of Congress Cataloging-in-Publication Data

Coulehan, John L., 1943-
   The medical interview : mastering skills for clinical practice / John L. Coulehan, Marian L. Block. — 5th ed.
      p. ; cm.
   Includes bibliographical references and index.
   ISBN 0-8036-1246-X (pbk.)
   1. Medical history taking. 2. Physical diagnosis. 3. Narrative medicine.
I. Block, Marian R., 1947- . II. Title.
   [DNLM: 1. Medical History Taking. 2. Physician-Patient Relations.
WB 290 C855m 2006]
RC65.C68 2006
616.07′51—dc22   2005022383

To Our Families

ACKNOWLEDGEMENTS

The Medical Interview includes numerous examples of clinician-patient interactions. Most are abstracted from taped interviews, although in every case we have removed personal references that might serve to identify the clinician or patient. In some cases we have altered the transcripts in ways that serve to demonstrate specific points more compactly. We are grateful to the patients and clinicians who permitted us to tape and publish these conversations.

We wish also to acknowledge our debt to teachers and colleagues. Three outstanding physician-educators deserve special thanks. Eric J. Cassell, MD, taught us how to observe the clinician-patient interaction systematically and encouraged us in this work for many years. The late Alvan Feinstein, MD, taught us that the medical interview is a source of scientific data about the patient and inspired us to find the science in the art of history taking. The late Kenneth D. Rogers, MD, gave us the whole-hearted and sustained support we needed, first, to develop our course in medical interviewing and, later, to write this book.

In the years since the first edition of this book was published, we have continued to learn from our students, our patients, and our colleagues, as well as from the burgeoning literature on the analysis of clinician-patient interactions. Although each of us had primary responsibilities for writing certain chapters, this book is a joint product; in a very special sense it is truly a collaborative effort, and we are both responsible for the entire text.

John L. Coulehan, MD, FACP
Marian R. Block, MD, ABFP

FOREWORD

Forewords are best brief and useful to the browsing or assigned reader. Like the classic Greek funeral oration a proper foreword is expected to bring praise upon the fallen (read: editors) in 20-plus prescribed ways.

Inherently and inevitably, daily work in medicine itself shares this conflict between brevity and fulfillment of task. On the one hand, you are being mightily socialized as learning-doctors to be brief, get to the heart of the matter, and present complex issues in few, succinct sentences. It is argued you must do all this in the names of busy-ness, business, being professional, and remaining objective.

On the other hand, gurus such as Coulehan and Block, sadly cursed with classic virtues, exhort you upon meeting each and every patient to listen, hear, understand, know with precision and completeness the disease and the illness, feel deeply and personally, show empathy but not sympathy, find respect for every patient from presidents to professors to corporate or other giants to the morally evil, spiritually bereft, foul and smelly, unmotivated, hostile, threatening patient your mother trained you to cross the street to avoid. Dear authors, come on, get real. Do you demand saintliness?

Such virtues are received so early in medical school they may feel handed down and therefore instinctively to be distrusted, especially when presented as commandments or charismatic invitations (medicine is an art, you therefore should become an artist, the easy way being to do exactly as I do, or even safer, become me; the narcissistic imperative, injected transformation). In fact, the approaches taught here have been blessed by robust science as *the critical elements of the best medicine.*

The best medicine is the sort you aspire to provide your patients and that you want for your loved ones. You will shortly be told to also meet institutional standards—to be satisfying to patients (who will hence come back and pay), efficient, and cost-effective, as we creep like Zeno's paradoxical tortoise racing Achilles ever more closely to rationing and capitation, with the result that institutional survival and the doctor's income rely on becoming faster or cheaper. You will also be advised that you must reduce risk (risk management departments are now almost universal in U.S. hospitals where "risk" refers to the hospital's, not the patient's, risk) and perform care of the highest quality, as defined by bureaucrats, department chairs, textbook writers (for example, Coulehan and Block and, mea culpa, myself as well), and medico-industrial complexes, such as big Pharma, big Imaging, and big Alternatives.

The behaviors, attitudes, knowledge, and principles Coulehan and Block teach in this book have, mostly, been scientifically demonstrated to result in higher quality, more efficient, more satisfying to you and your patients, and cheaper medical care than do the current norms of practice in communities and major medical schools and centers.

If you don't believe me, refer to the humanely sparse resources and Internet links herein or go to www.doc.com for access to the rich literature supporting my bald-faced assertions.

There will soon come a day when you will have mastered the commonly seen conditions in your practice to the level of your personal standards. Then the true joy and personal and intellectual satisfaction of your clinical work will come *most of all* from your deep encounters with patients as people. (It seems that some practitioners cannot find or have not been shown how to get on the road to such satisfaction and joy. As a result some skip the journey to their and their patients' peril.) Strong data show that the doctors most satisfied in their work, and thus least likely to burn out, exhibit high satisfaction with their psychosocial skills, a balanced approach to the biotechnical and psychosocial aspects of their cases, and personal life balance as well.

I was not initially inclined or skilled in listening (I was impatient), hearing (my mind was full of fascinating, new hypotheses I needed to test), feeling (no time, too painful), expressing emotions or talking about them (oh, please), and on down the list. What I did have were strong observational skills, the drive to be the best physician I could be, and an openness to learning and change. As an intern, I needed to master the big machine of the university hospital so I could spit out diagnoses and handle sick people. Even by that October, though, I was noticing we weren't helping even about a third of our patients. We often knew within 10 or 20 minutes of meeting the patient that the tests would be negative, and we did not know how to help the patients or ourselves in the terrible life situations we encountered: people dying with their eyes glued to ours, killing themselves through addiction or self-neglect, refusing rational chances to improve because of superstitious beliefs, our errors that killed or damaged, the persistence of our colleagues to ply their procedural wares that hurt or wounded many needlessly. You will no doubt write your own, personally salient list.

I set out to find who did know how to help these patients and in these situations. There was no Coulehan and Block then, and no meaningful, let alone effective, curriculum. So I made it a personal mission as a physician to discover empirically valid ways to be most helpful to patients and practitioners during the medical encounter, and also to find ways of teaching that allowed my learners to grasp the big things—to listen, hear, respect, show empathy, and acquire the Rogerian ways, so clearly noted in Chapter 2. Like a major league batter, I still know that I need regular, disciplined practice, such as listening to tapes of my interviews, monitoring patient's reactions, going to workshops to keep my edge and handle what my patients pitch to me.

Your good luck is that Coulehan and Block have distilled the current state of the art into highly readable, manageable, and practical chunks of interesting information. But like the new vintage wine drinker, don't believe that after one sip the wine will divulge to you its deepest pleasures. You need to open this book, sniff the outline and concepts, then drink slowly, returning again and again as it ages and your ability to understand deepens with experience and reflection.

Now, that was the peroration. This is the exhortation.

Take this book seriously to heart and mind, master what it teaches, and return to this or subsequent editions, or more advanced works as you deepen and grow. Buy many copies of this book to ennoble your friends and relatives (and also enrich the authors and publishers). The book presents foundational skills for you as a physician. As a mason of careers, I urge you to commit to building a rock-solid foundation and, later, to annually assessing and improving some part of it through self-review by videotape, through peer review, or by taking courses designed to help practitioners continue to grow as communicators and healers.

Mack Lipkin, MD

CONTENTS

PART THREE
Challenges in the Interactive Process

Introduction

The Poor Historian

History taking, the most clinically sophisticated procedure of medicine, is an extraordinary investigative technique: in few other forms of scientific research does the observed object talk.
Alvan Feinstein, *Clinical Judgment*

They cluster in the hall on rounds, eight of them—students, house officers, and attending physician—creating turbulence and obstructing flow. A nurse pushes a medication cabinet around them on the way down the hall, while the breakfast lorry closes in from the other direction. A medical student begins the presentation with "Mr. Blank is a 52-year-old man who presents with abdominal pain ... the patient is a poor historian."

Generations of physicians hearing a statement like this have had no problem understanding the speaker's intended meaning. In the culture of medicine, the term "poor historian" refers neither to the patient's occupation nor to his or her economic status. Rather, the term is usually used to blame the patient for an unsatisfactory outcome to a clinical interview. Despite the fact that the clinician performs the skilled professional work of the interview, we tend to assign an active role solely to the patient ("historian"), with the clinician presumably relegated to the status of passive observer.

The "poor historian" highlights a strange paradox in medicine. We teach entering students that the clinical history is the most important source of diagnostic information; in fact, perhaps 70% to 80% of all relevant data are derived from the medical interview. We also teach that the clinician-patient interaction is an important therapeutic tool. We reaffirm these beliefs in lectures, seminars, and clinical "pearls" throughout undergraduate and graduate medical education. Similarly, we teach a whole range of patient-centered practices and values, including fidelity, altruism, and compassion.

Yet at the same time our trainees learn a far different message from the medical culture they encounter in hospitals and clinics. In their day-to-day experience over many years of medical training, they encounter a tacit or hidden curriculum that presents a completely different perspective. The hidden curriculum says that *real* medicine is based only on "objective" data—numbers, graphs, and images—while "subjective" data—the patient's story—lacks value because it lacks quantification. In other words, what patients feel, the suffering they experience, and the disability that haunts them, all of which they describe through the medium of words, are secondary in importance to physiologic quantities that can be directly observed. Thus, most of the clinician's energy is devoted to tracking down and treating organ-based disease with little energy left over for the personal, social, cultural, or spiritual dimensions of illness. There is no need to pay attention to *who* the patient is. In fact, according to this view, patients often obstruct *real* medicine by introducing subjectivity into the clinical encounter; for example, they are "poor" historians, or they camouflage the needed data with unruly emotions and beliefs.

Clinical students soon learn to spend less time listening to the patient's story and more time among their peers agonizing over the meaning of laboratory values. Trainees learn to accept responsibility for how well (or how poorly) they perform a bone marrow aspiration, interpret an x-ray, or maneuver a colonoscope. After all, they recognize that these procedures require technical skills that must be learned, and it wouldn't make sense to blame the patient for an inadequately performed colonoscopy. Nonetheless, we commonly blame the patient for poor interview outcomes, stating with little room for doubt that, whether as a result of illness or education, anger or orneriness, the *patient* is a poor historian.

Stories of sickness and suffering—the kind of human stories that initially move us to enter a healing profession—gradually recede to the background as we become socialized into the technical culture of health care. Students and professionals preoccupy themselves with technical stories in which organs and instruments rather than people are the main protagonists. Sometimes, in fact, the patient's personal narrative is entirely forgotten.

Today it is common in clinical practice for investigations to bring unexpected results to light, and these, in turn, lead to more investigations along a sidetrack. After a while the clinical team is interested in, say, the incidental finding of a renal cyst on an abdominal MRI, while the cyst may have nothing to do with the patient's illness. The patient may have trouble getting anyone to pay attention to what he *feels* and *believes* and *experiences*. At some point, after multiple diagnostic tests and specialist consultations, the patient cries out, "*But you haven't done anything about my fatigue!*"

Yet this narrow, reductionistic way of thinking is not the only concept of medical practice available to us. At the same time, medical curricula and experienced clinicians continue to teach (and to model) a holistic, patient-centered brand of medicine in the tradition of the great clinician and educator William Osler, who wrote, "It is a safe rule to have no teaching without a patient for a text, and the best teaching is that taught by the patient himself."

The Oslerian tradition has gained ground in recent years for several reasons. Well-intentioned clinicians have discovered that highly specialized, machine-intensive medicine is not necessarily the best medicine. Patients often find themselves doing better by the numbers, but still feel dissatisfied and sick. Worse yet, they may experience iatrogenic morbidity, and even mortality, as a result of poorly coordinated care or medical mistakes. In today's culture people expect remarkable outcomes from medicine and frequently find themselves angry and confused when the system fails them. At the same time, studies have shown that good clinician-patient communication leads to better clinical outcomes and more satisfied patients, while poor communication leads to poor clinical outcomes, dissatisfaction, and malpractice litigation. In fact, when an adverse event occurs, clinician insensitivity is a major factor in a patient's decision to sue.

Clinicians have begun to understand that pain, suffering, and dysfunction must not only be *conceptualized* in broad human terms, but also it must be translated into *action* if we are to be effective healers. Effective clinical practice requires that health professionals, no matter what their specialties might be, develop core competencies in communication and clinician-patient interaction. In other words, the *culture* of teaching hospitals and clinics must be changed so that the conflict between the explicit (courses and formal teaching) and hidden (everyday clinical experience) curricula is lessened or eliminated.

In the graduate arena, the Accreditation Council for Graduate Medical Education (ACGME) has tackled this problem by adopting a requirement that specifies core clinical competencies be taught in all residency programs. In order to be accredited, residency training programs of all specialties must develop curricula to address core competencies in six domains: patient care, medical knowledge, practice-based learning, interpersonal and communication skills, professionalism, and systems-based practice. These broad categories include numerous intermediate level skill sets that relate to patient-centered medicine—for example, caring and respectful behaviors; clinical interviewing; informed decision making; listening skills; creation of therapeutic relationships; advocacy for patients within the health care system; and sensitivity to cultural, age, gender, and disability issues. The ACGME requires that residencies not only teach these competencies in a formal way, but also conduct performance-based evaluations of their residents.

The American Association of Medical Colleges (AAMC) has adopted a similar core curriculum project, as has the American Board of Medical Specialties. In the AAMC project, medical professionalism and communication in medicine are two of the five required domains; once again, interviewing skills are critical. In fact, the National Board of Medical Examiners has recently adopted a new examination (Step 2—Clinical Skills) to evaluate the student's ability to interact with patients, construct an accurate medical history, and engage in an effective clinical decision-making process. This examination, which utilizes a series of standardized patients, is predicated on the strong relationship between a student's interactive skills and the quality and quantity of data gathered in the interview.

This book is based on the premise that good clinician-patient communication is essential to good health care. Talking with patients is not a skill reserved for such specialists as psychiatrists, psychologists, and social workers. Medical interviewing is a basic clinical skill. It is essential for radiologists as well as internists, ophthalmologists as well as pediatricians, physical therapists as well as nurse practitioners. Interviewing skills are not a matter of common sense, nor do they necessarily develop with experience. These skills can be broken down into component parts, and they can be learned.

We contend that the medical history is a shared project, and the clinician bears a great deal of the "historian" responsibility. Too many times, "The patient is a poor historian" actually means "The clinical history is unclear because *I'm* a poor historian."

The book is divided into three parts. Part One, The Patient's Story, presents fundamentals of clinical interviewing (Chapters 1 and 2) and various components of the medical history (Chapters 3 through 8).

Part Two, Basic Skills in Practice, applies these interviewing skills to the clinical office setting (Chapter 9) and for use with children and adolescents (Chapter 10), older adults (Chapter 11), and persons from different cultures (Chapter 12).

Finally, Part Three, Challenges in the Interactive Process, considers difficult clinician-patient interactions (Chapter 13), telling bad news (Chapter 14), alternative and complementary approaches to health care (Chapter 15), ethics and professionalism in interviewing (Chapter 16), avoiding malpractice litigation (Chapter 17), patient education and negotiation (Chapter 18), and, finally, an example of the medical interview at work (Chapter 19).

In *The Medical Interview* we invite you to join in the exciting project of becoming a better historian and a more effective healer. This book is addressed primarily to students of medicine and other health professions who are just beginning their professional interaction with patients. However, it is also designed to serve as a resource for those who are further along in their education, including postgraduate trainees. Our particular emphasis is on microskills of the patient interview. Although we deal most extensively with basic history taking, we also illustrate how these same skills are building blocks for all types of clinician-patient interactions. They lie at the core of the art and science of medicine, where the patient's narrative is central.

PART ONE

THE PATIENT'S STORY

CHAPTER 1

Interviewing as a Clinical Skill

I Attach the Same Meaning

*A very good way to find out how another person
is thinking or feeling is to ask him.... At this point,
however, a difficulty arises. If I am to acquire
information in this way about another person's
experiences, I must understand what he says about
them. And this would seem to imply that I attach
the same meaning to his words as he does. But how,
it may be asked, can I ever be sure that this is so?*

A. J. Ayer, *The Problem of Knowledge*

OBSERVATION IN CLINICAL MEDICINE

Although medicine is based on a group of theoretical sciences, clinical
medicine itself is a practical science: it is the science of helping ill people
get well, rather than that of understanding disease. Like any other science, clinical medicine has basic units of observation, basic quantities of
measurement, and basic instruments for obtaining these measurements.
The units of observation are signs and symptoms, the quantities of measurement are words and sometimes numbers, and the most important
instrument is the medical practitioner. Like any other scientific instrument, the clinician must be objective, precise, sensitive, specific, and reliable when making observations about the patient's illness. (We explain
each of these terms in this chapter as they relate to understanding the
patient's symptoms.) In this text we examine interviewing and interac-
tional skills as fundamental to the science of medicine. As we will show,
interviewing skills are also at the core of the art of medicine. In fact,
in medicine, art and science are not only synergistic; they are often one
and the same.

Objectivity

What does it mean to be objective when interviewing a patient and taking a medical history? **Objectivity** means striving to remove one's own beliefs, prejudices, and preconceptions from observations; it involves eliminating bias or systematic distortion from one's observations. Other words for objectivity are **accuracy** and **validity.** The illness data should correspond to what the patient really felt and experienced. If, for example, you start with a preconceived notion of the illness and you discard or minimize ill-fitting items, you are not being objective. Consider the following interview (adapted from Platt and McMath, 1979), in which the clinician "knows" that the patient has lung disease and so is unable to hear the chief complaint:

Clinician	**Hello, I'm Dr. X. Are you Mrs. Y?**
Patient	Yes, thanks for seeing me, doctor.
	What sorts of troubles have you been having?
	I've been going downhill for years. Nothing seems to be working right.
	Tell me about the worst part.
	My legs. I have constant pain in my legs. I can't walk. It's gotten so bad I can't sleep.
	What about your breathing?
	Oh, that's all right. My breathing isn't so bad now. I just hurt all the time in my legs.
	Are you still smoking?
	Yes, I've gone back to cigarettes for relief. They calm my nerves. But I'm down to half a pack or so a day.
	Are you having pains in your chest? What about wheezing?
	No, I haven't needed to use my inhaler.
	Or cough?
	No, I hardly ever cough.
	How much are you actually able to do?
	Well, I could run around everywhere until about 2 years ago, but now I can hardly walk half a block.
	Why is that?
	My legs. They hurt. They get worse when I walk.
	Do they swell up?
	Well, they've been a bit swollen the last week or so, but the pain is there whether they swell or not.
	All right, let's talk a little more about your lung problem.

The clinician in this case seems to ignore the patient's leg pain; when she complains about it, the clinician replies with questions about chest and pulmonary symptoms. The clinician evidently undervalues patient reports that don't fit in with what he expects, while he overvalues data related to a diagnosis that he "knows," namely, the patient's chronic lung disease. Failure of objectivity is unscientific and could lead to a missed diagnosis; it is also likely to make the patient feel ignored. When patients feel ignored, they tend to say less, and opportunities to obtain other important data may be lost.

How might the same clinician respond on a better day? Consider this scenario:

Clinician	**Hello, I'm Dr. X. Are you Mrs. Y?**
Patient	Yes, thanks for seeing me, doctor.
	Well, I'm glad we could fit you in. What sorts of troubles have you been having?
	I've been going downhill for years. Nothing seems to be working right.
	Tell me about the worst part.
	My legs. I have constant pain in my legs. I can't walk. It's gotten so bad I can't sleep.
	Constant pain in your legs. Tell me more about that.
	Well, it's gotten so bad I can hardly walk half a block.
	You mean the pain forces you to stop?
	Yes, that's exactly it. And, well, it gets better when I stop, but never really goes away. Even at night when I'm lying still it wakes me up, it's so bad.

In her last statement, the patient gives a clear description of claudication, a symptom characteristic of severe peripheral vascular disease. The patient begins to volunteer important details about the leg pain that not only aid the diagnostic process but also help her feel understood.

 PRACTICE POINT
The first step in the process of active listening is to be objective, which requires putting aside your preconceived notions and focusing on what your patient is saying (see *Active Listening Skills,* below).

ACTIVE LISTENING SKILLS

You can connect with your patient through active listening. The following skills will help you to establish a therapeutic relationship:

- Choose a mutually comfortable setting.
- Remain quiet and attentive.

- Observe the patient respectfully as a whole person, and not just as a talker, or a diseased body, or a barrier to your lunch break.
- Allow the patient to tell the story with as few interruptions as possible.
- Listen for the primary symptom data, for example, "My head feels like it's caught in a vise."
- Assess the words the patient uses for accuracy and precision.
- Listen to the inflection and tone of words, and to the pauses between the words (paralanguage).
- Note discrepancies between *what* the patient says and *how* he or she says it, and the discrepancies in meaning between the words and gestures.
- Listen for the patient's interpretation, for example, "I think I have a brain tumor."
- Do not confuse the patient's *theory* with the patient's *symptoms.*
- Avoid forming your own theory about the patient's illness until you obtain a precise description of the symptoms and a coherent narrative.

INTERPRETATION VERSUS OBSERVATION

It is easy to confuse interpretation with observation. When you are talking with a patient, your observation is what the patient actually says or does; the patient's words are primary data. Preceptors sometimes encourage trainees to use terms that are really interpretations rather than descriptions. One example of such a term is "claudication," as in our example here; another is "angina," a certain kind of chest pain caused by coronary artery disease. These words are interpretations because they imply specific etiologies. The primary data of the symptom "angina" might be something like "midchest discomfort of a dull, pressing nature, lasting about 3 minutes, brought on by exertion, and relieved by rest." Interpretive terms are shorthand necessary for thinking and conversation in clinical practice; such terms are appropriate when the symptom has indeed been shown to be secondary to coronary artery disease. However, if you interpret the symptom prematurely, once you start using the word "angina," you may forget the patient's story and ignore data that point to the correct diagnosis.

◆ **PRACTICE POINT**
Be sure to observe what your patient says or does and don't prematurely interpret his or her symptoms. You run the risk of compromising your objectivity.

For example, a 68-year-old woman lived for several years with the diagnosis of angina—that is, coronary artery disease—because her clinician did not "hear" the primary data. Here is how she described her chest pain:

Clinician	**Tell me about this chest pain.**
Patient	It's soreness in here, right through here [pointing to midchest] a lot. Some pain in my arm and a feeling here. And a burning in the middle here and a burning in my throat.
	When does this pain seem to come on?
	Oh, it can be any time, doctor. Sometimes I even get it in the middle of the night.
	How about when you walk or are active in any way?
	No, I can just be sitting. Especially after I eat.

Despite the fact that the patient did not have and had never had exertional chest pain relieved by rest, the clinician ordered a complete cardiac workup, including coronary angiography. Even though the test results proved negative, she continued to carry a diagnosis of coronary artery disease and lived a confined and limited lifestyle because of fear. Finally, a new clinician listened more carefully to the story of burning and the nocturnal occurrence of pain and ordered an upper endoscopy, which revealed massive esophageal reflux with esophagitis and esophageal spasm. Perhaps it would have been more life threatening to overlook coronary artery disease, but for the patient much was lost. Frightened that she might die at any moment of a heart attack, she persisted in her belief that she had heart disease and was unable to be rehabilitated to an active life.

Patient Interpretation versus Primary Data

While objectivity means avoiding premature interpretation on your part, it also means distinguishing between the primary data and the patient's interpretation of what the data mean. This is important to remember when a patient tells you, "My ulcer is acting up," or "My heart is giving me a lot of trouble," or "I'm here for my Hodgkin's disease." In such instances, the patient is interpreting his or her symptoms as indicative of the presence of peptic ulcer or other known disease.

Here, for example, is the statement of a 78-year-old man who called his clinician with the following complaint:

> I don't know what's wrong. Somebody said I must have had the flu, but it's lasted so long and I've tried everything and I don't know what

to eat, so I just had to call and find out what you thought because it's been going on now 2 weeks and—you know me—I don't call unless I really have to. And someone said I must have appendicitis or what's that thing that old people get?

This patient, like many patients, focuses on the etiology of his problem and does not tell the story of his symptoms. All we know is that, whatever has been going on, it has lasted for about 2 weeks and is probably related to the gastrointestinal (GI) tract. The clinician's next response might be:

Clinician   Well, some people who get the flu do feel sick for quite some time.

Although this response shows that the clinician has heard the patient's theory, the clinician still would not know what is going on; worse, it shows acceptance of the patient's diagnosis without obtaining any primary data whatsoever. A better response might be:

Clinician   Well, some people who get the flu do feel sick for quite a while, but I'm not sure you have the flu. What exactly are your symptoms?

Patient   Well, I've been having severe diarrhea—just like water—for a few days and I hurt low down in my belly. And I'm weak, awful weak.

The clinician now has some primary data with which to start putting the diagnostic puzzle together.

Although the patient's interpretation should be considered separately from symptom data, the interpretation should not be ignored; it is important to acknowledge the patient's beliefs as legitimate, whether or not you agree with them. Such recognition of the patient's point of view is necessary in a therapeutic relationship and will maximize your opportunities for patient engagement and education (see Chapter 18, Education and Negotiation).

PRECISION

Precision is a characteristic of the scientific process that relates to the distribution of observations around the "real" value. Precise observations cluster around the mean, whereas imprecise observations are widely scattered. The basic units of measurement in a medical interview are words.

In a medical history, words describe sensations perceived by the patient and communicated to the clinician. As verbal measurements, words should be precise. They should be sufficiently detailed and unambiguous to contribute usefully to diagnostic reasoning by indicating the real data.

Getting the Details

In the issue of precision we are dealing not with a systematic bias that leads purposefully in one direction or another, but rather with random, unsystematic error introduced by vagueness, poor listening, or lack of attention to detail. For example, if a patient complains of being tired, does "tired" mean that the patient feels short of breath with activity, muscle weakness, lack of desire for activity, or sleepiness? Although the clinician may correctly register the patient's words, he or she may have no idea what is actually being described unless there is sufficient detail to distinguish among dyspnea on exertion, muscle weakness, lack of motivation, and somnolence. To make this distinction, the next question might go something like:

- "What do you mean by tired?"
- "Can you tell me more about this tiredness?"
- "How would you describe this feeling without using the word 'tired'?"

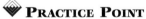 **PRACTICE POINT**
The good interviewer attempts to discover as precisely as possible what the patient is experiencing.

Here is an example of a clinician trying to get a precise history about a patient's chief complaint of headache:

Patient	See, I get these migraine headaches.
Clinician	**What do you mean by migraine headaches?**
	The last two headaches—I had two headaches last week, one on Monday and one on Thursday. Now they weren't real, real bad, but the ones that I had before that, I threw up. I got real, real cold.
	How often do you get these headaches?
	I had two real bad ones within 2 weeks' time; then I didn't have one for a few weeks. Now the ones that I had last week, I didn't throw up with them, but they were enough that I had to go to bed with them.

Are the headaches something that occur almost every week, almost every month, or every couple of months?
I get them all the time. It is just within the last few months that I have been getting them more frequently. But I have averaged maybe one or two a month.

When you get these headaches, where does it hurt?
They start here and they just go around [demonstrating on her head]. Sometimes they'll go on one side of my face, sometimes on the other side of my face. But they start in the back of my neck here.

Do you get any kind of problems with your eyes when these headaches are coming on?
Blurred vision. The light bothers me.

Both eyes or one eye?
I have to go, like, I go upstairs in my bedroom and like close everything up, and I just lie down with a blanket.

What kind of problem does the light give you when you have a headache?
It just bothers me, just the light itself, it's like a glare. The light itself bothers me.

What do these headaches keep you from doing?
Everything. I can't do a thing. When I get one, I have to go to bed. That's exactly what I do. Usually I throw up with them. I get real, real cold. It can be 90 degrees outside and I'm freezing. Mostly the throwing up is a light vomiting.

Is there anything you can think of that triggers these headaches?
Nothing, it just starts. I can get up with a headache. If I get up with it, I'm done for the whole day. I do nothing at all.

Do these headaches scare you?
No, I'm used to them.

Okay, so they don't frighten you, it's just a matter of trying to ...
To get rid of them.

There is no unambiguous test for the etiology of headache; only a careful and precise history can distinguish between migraine and other types of headache. By asking "What do you mean by migraine headache?" this clinician does not accept the patient's or previous provider's diagnosis of "migraine" (an interpretation) and goes on to get many details (precision) about frequency, location, visual symptoms, and other associated symptoms.

SENSITIVITY AND SPECIFICITY

Objectivity and precision are two criteria by which we judge medical data, including the medical history. Two additional criteria are **sensitivity** and **specificity.** The sensitivity of a test expresses its ability to "pick up" real cases of the disease in question. The higher the test's sensitivity, the greater will be the percentage of cases that are accurately identified as being real cases of illness. Specificity, on the other hand, refers to a test's ability to "rule out" disease in normal people. The higher the specificity, the greater is the likelihood that a negative test result identifies a person who does not have the disease. Few tests in medicine approach 100% sensitivity and specificity; certainly the medical interview will not yield such definitive information, but we want to maximize the usefulness of symptom data as much as possible.

The Sensitivity and Specificity of Symptoms

Here is how the concepts of sensitivity and specificity work when we are dealing with symptoms. A symptom may be extremely sensitive (most people with pneumonia have cough) but not specific at all (dozens of diseases cause cough); it may be relatively specific (nocturnal midepigastric pain relieved by eating in cases of duodenal ulcer) but not that sensitive (most persons with duodenal ulcer do not have that symptom). This relative lack of sensitivity and specificity for individual symptoms is one reason why clinicians often minimize the value of history taking and rush into more supposedly scientific tests. However, an individual symptom is rarely the appropriate unit on which to base decisions; we deal, rather, with symptom complexes, patterns, or stories.

◆ **PRACTICE POINT**

It is important to consider the patient's whole story. A detailed reconstruction of the patient's illness, rather than isolated statements about symptoms—not just one symptom, but many; not just one point in time, but the whole story—will help you to make a better diagnosis.

A complete symptom complex may well be quite sensitive and specific; it may be adequate, in fact, to serve as the basis for diagnosis and therapy. Even when a thorough health history does not contain enough information for a correct diagnosis, the history usually contains *most* of the needed information. Moreover, a thorough history narrows the range of possible problems dramatically and yields a small number of hypotheses to be ruled out, supported, or confirmed by physical examination and further studies. The well-conducted patient interview will usually yield a firm (and large) database on which to design an efficient (and small) diagnostic plan. To achieve this result, however, the clinician must approach the task objectively and precisely.

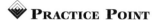 **PRACTICE POINT**
The sensitivity and specificity of a symptom complex are irrelevant in a given situation if the instrument through which the data are obtained—you, the clinician—lacks objectivity and precision.

RELIABILITY

Reliability, or **reproducibility,** is another important characteristic of scientific tests, including medical interviewing. Different observers should be able to obtain the same results. In the medical history, however, reproducibility is tempered by several considerations about human nature and the interactive process.

Different Versions

In caring for a patient in the hospital, three or four observers are likely to obtain three or four different versions of the patient's story. Much of the time, the differences may not be of great importance, but sometimes they will be crucial. Only one of four observers, for example, may note that the patient has had bright red rectal bleeding intermittently for the last 3 months. This fact might be lost in the review of systems (discussed in Chapter 7, Review of Systems, Physical Examination, and Closure) because the patient actually came into the hospital for chest pain and was either too embarrassed to mention the bleeding or perhaps too concerned about his heart to mention a seemingly unrelated problem. It suddenly becomes an important issue when you find the patient has occult blood in his stool or a blood count that indicates anemia. The health care team might have to shift gears from an ischemic heart disease workup to a lower GI bleeding workup.

Of course, just as in the laboratory, data that change from one observer—or one experiment—to the next are suspect. Reproducibility is a characteristic highly valued in testing; this apparent lack of reproducibility in medical history taking makes many clinicians question its value.

There are several reasons why various observers may get varying stories at different times.

Patients Learn to Tell a Good Story

Every patient comes to the hospital or the office with a personal story that includes various symptoms, but most patients have no point of reference indicating which of these are more or less important in explaining their underlying condition. A severe headache may cause more pain than a sudden swelling of the left leg, but the latter could be secondary to lymphatic obstruction by metastatic cancer, whereas the former may have no pathologic significance at all.

The patient learns, in a sense, to "package" the story and make it more efficient or relevant or interesting to the clinician. Therefore, it is likely that later observers will get a more clearly connected and flowing—and certainly different—history than will the first interviewer.

 PRACTICE POINT
Each time a patient relates the clinical story, the patient learns, by virtue of questions asked and interviewer response, what items are of most importance to the interviewer.

Patients Recall New Information

A corollary to this educational process is that patients may learn to emphasize some symptoms that they had not bothered to mention originally. For example, the patient may have forgotten the first episode of syncope or considered an illness that occurred 3 years earlier to be unrelated to the current illness. Repetition and focusing on specific symptoms not only will make the story more coherent but will also refresh the patient's memory or perhaps set the stage for some new insight. Therefore, it is reasonable to assume that later observers may pick up entirely new information that the patient neglected to mention earlier.

Here is how a first interview might proceed with a patient complaining of headaches. Knowing the importance to the diagnosis of differentiating new headaches from chronic ones, the clinician, a student, proceeds:

Clinician **Tell me about your headaches. When did they start?**
Patient   Well, I started getting them about 3 months ago.
          Is that the first time you ever had this headache?
          Well, yes.

So headaches are really new for you?
Well, now that I think about it, I can remember one something like it about 2 years ago. I remember, we were on vacation and I had to stay in the hotel. I thought I had the flu or something.
That's interesting. When did you get the next one?

For the next clinician, the attending physician, who interviews this patient, the story may be revealed as follows:

Clinician   **Tell me when these headaches started.**
Patient   Well, I guess the first time I ever had one was about 2 years ago. But then I only had one every few months or so; they weren't frequent until about 3 months ago, when I started getting them every week.

Although both interviewers asked similar questions, notice how the patient's story is more organized and straightforward on the second account. The first interviewer had to dig harder for the onset 2 years ago and could have missed it entirely.

Patients Have Beliefs about Their Illnesses

Sick people may have already organized their illness in some way that makes sense to them before they see the clinician. They may have tried getting rid of the symptoms on their own and perhaps may have asked for advice from family or friends. They may have read health columns in newspapers, seen a medical commentator on TV discussing a problem similar to theirs, or searched the Internet for information. In addition, patients may have religious or cultural beliefs that frame their under-standing of illness in general and their own symptoms in particular (see Chapter 12, Cultural Competence in the Interview). In these ways, patients develop hypotheses or reasons for their problems and have ideas about what can or should be done about them. Consequently, they are likely to tell their stories in ways consistent with these hypotheses; they will emphasize symptoms that support their theories and minimize or forget symptoms that do not.

 PRACTICE POINT
The primary data—perceived symptoms—are filtered through the patient's beliefs.

In the process of being interviewed by several different people focusing on strict medical hypotheses, a patient's own hypotheses about the data may change. And when the story is filtered through a different set of beliefs, the story's elements—perceptions, symptoms, and attributions— also appear to change.

Patients Change Their Stories

Different histories may be obtained at different times because the patient simply and consciously changes the story. Clinicians often invoke this reason when they dislike the patient or are unable to account for the symptoms. The more the symptoms seem to be unrelated to supposedly objective findings or diagnostic tests, the more likely clinicians are to consider the symptoms exaggerated or even imaginary and, therefore, susceptible to change from one interviewing session to another.

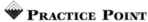 **PRACTICE POINT**

Although some patients, of course, do change their stories, this type of unreliability is a much less frequent explanation for apparent inconsistencies than the other factors that should be considered.

Skill Matters, Too

Interviewing skills play a part as well in the reliability of the data obtained. A skilled clinician who lets the patient tell his or her story and listens carefully is much more likely to obtain an accurate picture than a clinician who asks a list of questions by rote. Interviewing expertise bears a general relationship to the person's experience level (student, postgraduate trainee, practicing clinician), but when one considers an individual interview of an individual patient, this is not always the case. The inexperienced student who has sufficient time to spend with a patient in a nonthreatening atmosphere may learn a lot more than a hurried attending physician.

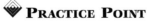 **PRACTICE POINT**

Interviewing skills that maximize objectivity and precision produce accurate data and reduce the rate of false-positive (making a diagnosis that is not there) and false-negative (missing the diagnosis) histories.

SCIENCE AND ART AT WORK: ACTIVE LISTENING

As you develop clinical skill, you will learn techniques to achieve objectivity and precision in gathering data from patients. These techniques make good science and, what is more, allow the patient to "connect" with you in a therapeutic relationship. Thus, the techniques of interviewing that facilitate the scientific collection and analysis of clinical data also serve as preconditions for the art of the therapeutic relationship.

◈ **PRACTICE POINT**

The interdependence of science and art in clinical practice is much like the interdependence in most art forms, such as music or painting, which require understanding theory and the execution of technique as preconditions to producing something of beauty.

Is there a contradiction between a "just get the facts"—scientific—interview and an artful interview? No, they are one and the same. You are unlikely to obtain all the clinically important facts without utilizing active listening skills (see *Active Listening Skills,* page 5). If you try to do so, the "facts" that you obtain may be irrelevant, or worse, untrue. Active listening allows you to achieve objectivity and precision in the interview and is also the first step toward connecting with your patient and establishing a therapeutic relationship.

Establishing a Therapeutic Relationship

A patient's own words can best demonstrate how achieving objectivity and precision goes hand in hand with establishing a therapeutic relationship. The following excerpt is part of an interview in which the patient describes how it feels to be listened to and understood:

Patient   Aw, I'm not usually this able to talk to people like this. I don't really know you ...

Clinician   **That's true. I'm a total stranger.**

And all of a sudden I have gone completely down the line and told you everything I could possibly think of to tell you. I've never been able to do that. I have very few people that I talk to personally or talk to about the way I feel ... um ... I talk to my family but there are only certain things that you can talk to your family about, and I have never had anyone I could talk to. I have always kept everything to myself. And now, all of a sudden, I've just flowed over like a broken toilet.

Was it helpful?

Yes, because I just learned something else about myself. The funny thing is, I have said all these things to you, and most times talking to people, I always think before I talk. I have said everything I have said to you without thinking about it first, and without wondering what you are going to think about what I am saying to you. And I can honestly say that I have never done that with anyone.
Uh huh.
I ... um ... have, maybe, I have a lot of friends but I mean, I even, I even think before I say what I say to them because there's always a chance that someone misinterprets.
Well, I'm glad. Because I like to think it's helpful.
It really is. I feel quite good about the whole thing.

This patient describes being able to say everything "without thinking about it first." He is describing his ability to reveal uncensored data that are vital to the diagnostic process; he was able to do this because he wasn't "wondering what you are going to think about what I am saying to you." This is precisely the aim of competent clinical history taking. Revealing uncensored data was crucial for this patient, who presented with secondary syphilis acquired as a result of unsafe sex. Had he filtered out the story of his sexual activity, about which he was embarrassed and ambivalent, the diagnosis would have been made less quickly or perhaps not at all. He later became ill with AIDS, and the need to communicate openly remained vital to his care.

SAGA OF THE FIFTH WHEEL

It is perhaps inevitable that the beginning interviewer sometimes feels like a spare part, or a "fifth wheel." He or she may have minimal or no responsibility for patient care, and patients may be fatigued and disgruntled at having to interact with a trainee. Besides simple inexperience and the associated anxiety, students have several other realistic concerns about their initial patient interviews. Three major concerns include:

- "I don't know enough about pathophysiology or human behavior to do a good history, let alone to get the diagnosis."
- "The patients are fed up. They have been worked over 10 times already and are generally tired of it all, and sometimes angry, by the time I arrive to examine them."
- "I have no responsibility for the patient and can't help, so I feel like an interloper—a fifth wheel."

Of course, each of these statements has an element of truth, but none of them need be a major constraint in your interviewing and physical diagnosis experience. Let us deal with each concern.

"I Don't Know Enough"

First, "I don't know enough about pathophysiology or human behavior." It is clear that you are not going to characterize patterns of symptoms as efficiently as an experienced clinician, nor will you be able to pick up subtle physical signs. If you are a medical student, you might examine a patient with gastroesophageal reflux before you study the GI tract in your pathophysiology course and complain, "I don't know what symptoms to ask about. I don't know what direction to take." As long as the content of the history (or physical examination) is all that interests you, your lack of knowledge serves as a major barrier. However, the clinical art involves process and method. Your goal is to learn to talk with patients in a way that maximizes both information gathering and therapeutic communication. The diagnosis (although interesting) is largely irrelevant at this point. You want to characterize the symptoms and the person as precisely and objectively as possible and, more importantly, to create an interview encounter in which this can occur. Unfortunately, some studies have suggested that, at least in medicine, the interviewing skills of clinical students actually decline as they progress through their training and learn more about the mechanisms of disease. The point is that the beginner who practices good technique can do well.

"Patients Are Fed Up"

Second, "The patients have often had numerous other examinations and are sick and tired of it all." The anger your patient expresses, or just barely conceals, frequently arises not from the mere fact of repeated examinations, but from the whole situation—being ill, having a backache that no one pays attention to, undergoing uncomfortable diagnostic studies, interacting with doctors who are rude or preoccupied and nurses who seem unsympathetic, and so forth. Know that the anger may be present before you arrive on the scene and may have little to do with you.

How might you deal with this? It is crucial to clarify your role, not just as a student, but as a student simply learning to do an interview and not as part of the health care team. Then, make sure the patient has really consented to your interview and examination with a comment or question, such as "May I talk with you now about the problems that brought you to the hospital?" If he or she does not wish to talk with you and says so, let it go at that. For patients who are tired or in pain, suggest the possibility of your coming back later. If the patient seems angry, acknowledge the anger. This will give you a good opportunity to see how effective "interchangeable" responses can be in obtaining information and developing rapport (see "Levels of Responding" in Chapter 2).

Sick people, like anyone else, may have several conflicting feelings at the same time. A given patient may want to be helpful to a trainee but simultaneously feel angry about the situation, depressed about being ill, or simply exhausted. You can tip the balance in your favor: by being honest and listening carefully, you will avoid exacerbating the patient's anger and may even help to defuse it.

"I Feel Like an Interloper"

Finally, there is the frequent refrain of "There's nothing I can do to help this patient." The issue of responsibility and helpfulness needs another look. Professionalism is not something you put on overnight when you get your degree. You grow into it. As a clinical student, you are demonstrably more a clinician now than you were 2 years ago. Although still a learner, you are interacting with patients in a professional manner. The information you gather is important. Although the disease data you collect may only occasionally be helpful, the personal data you collect will often contribute to the patient's well-being and satisfaction. If the patient has a specific request or complaint, you can discuss it with a unit nurse, resident, or clinical instructor. If the patient has a misunderstanding, you can clarify the problem or find someone else to do so.

Listening Is Therapeutic

The truth is that simply listening to patients in an empathic manner is therapeutic. Listening might not repair the damaged myocardium or lower the blood sugar, but it will make the patient feel better. That is, after all, what the clinical enterprise is all about, although the goal of helping another person feel better often becomes confused, or may seem remote, in a busy office or hospital. The patient experiences a strange environment with a potentially serious or life-threatening illness and is often caught in a system—a health maintenance organization, an office, or a hospital—that is not always flexible or responsive to human needs. If you are willing to take the time to listen, you will be surprised at how therapeutic the encounter is for your patient, even though you feel as though you are "doing nothing."

SUMMARY—Interviewing as a Clinical Skill

In this chapter we state one of the major themes of our approach to medical interviewing: the conversation between clinician and patient is the basis for both the science and the art of medicine, and the active listening that lies at the core of clinical science. We reviewed these skills:

- Objectivity in clinician-patient interactions requires effective listening.
  - Obtaining the primary symptom data enhances objectivity.
  - Jumping to premature interpretations compromises objectivity.
- Precision requires that the information we obtain be sufficiently detailed and unambiguous to use in diagnosis and treatment.
- Sensitivity requires that we use our interviewing skills to maximize our ability to identify "real" cases of illness.
- Specificity requires that we use our interviewing skills to maximize our ability to identify "real" cases of wellness.
- Reliability requires good interviewing technique to enhance reproducibility and to understand why and how patient stories may change and evolve with repeated telling.

Finally, a number of factors lead students who are just beginning to learn clinical interviewing to feel out of place, like fifth wheels. These factors, which may serve as barriers to learning and practicing new skills, include feeling as if you don't know enough, feeling reluctant to interact with patients who are tired and uncomfortable, and feeling awkward because you lack responsibility for the patient. In Chapter 2, we will explore therapeutic core qualities—respect, genuineness, and empathy—that help overcome these barriers.

When active listening leads to symptom and patient data that are objective, precise, sensitive, specific, and reliable, you are on your way to *understanding exactly* what patients are saying when they tell the stories of their illnesses.

Respect, Genuineness, and Empathy

With Simple, Kindly Words

*He longed to soothe her, not with drugs, not with
advice, but with simple, kindly words.*
Anton Chekhov, *"A Doctor's Visit"*

CONNECTING WITH THE PATIENT

It is easy to agree that certain attitudes toward patients, such as respect
and empathy, are praiseworthy. On first hearing this truism, you may
think that these attitudes reflect the clinician's personality and value
structure and are not immediately relevant to the medical interview. You
may not believe that these qualities are skills that can be learned and
used. However, empathy and other qualities should, in fact, be understood as patterns of behavior that can be practiced and learned. These
skills allow us to connect with patients.

Therapeutic Core Qualities

In this chapter, we borrow some concepts from psychologists, particularly
Carl Rogers and his followers, who first identified a number of observable
characteristics of therapists that correlated with good therapeutic outcomes. They called them **therapeutic core qualities,** and the three most
important were respect (or unconditional positive regard), genuineness
(or congruence), and empathy. They found that the content of psy-
chotherapeutic intervention, such as the specific intervention dictated by
a theory, was less important to outcome than was the process of the interaction. Subsequently, other investigators defined specific skills embedded

in that process. They showed that qualities such as empathy, for example, could be broken down into a set of skills in listening to and responding to a patient.

These therapeutic core qualities are important links between the art and science of medicine. They not only improve the interviewer's history-taking ability and the accuracy of the data obtained, but they also lead to better therapeutic relationships in ordinary practice. In Chapter 1, Interviewing as a Clinical Skill, we identified the goal of maximizing objectivity and precision in our communication with patients. In this chapter, we will look at some basic concepts about how to understand and practice these skills.

The following two examples serve to introduce these concepts. In one, the patient is a 50-year-old woman who, on her first visit to the clinic, complains chiefly of abdominal pain that becomes worse when she gets upset.

Clinician	**What happens when you get upset? What do you feel like?**
Patient	Oh, I just feel right nervous, the stomach pains, my arm ... it pains, it seems like the strength is going out of my arm and hands.
	How often do you get upset?
	Quite frequently.
	What's quite frequent?
	Mostly every day it seems like I'm upset. I get something on my mind and that brings on the nauseated feeling.
	So what's the usual sequence? You get upset first and then what happens? You get upset first or does the nausea come on first?
	No. I get upset and then the nausea comes on.
	Tell me about when you started being upset.
	Oh really, right after my mother passed, really, in April, I've been mostly upset.
	What happened when your mother passed away? I understand it must have been a very upsetting event; was she very close to you?
	Yes, I was really close to my mother, and it seems like after she passed, I don't know, something just left out of me, I don't know what it was, you know.

In the second example, a new patient, a 40-year-old man, has come to the office for a checkup. The interviewer is inquiring about his family history and finds that the patient's father, who had divorced his mother, died of a ruptured brain aneurysm.

Clinician **You don't know anything more about that?**

Patient   Well, my understanding is, the context of this is, that my mother was raised in the Catholic Church, and divorce was a terrible scandal in her mind and she tried to forget about it as quickly as she could. It's such a painful subject that there was never any discussion about who he was and so forth. And as a consequence all I've really heard are niblets, and one of the things I understand is that my father was an alcoholic or at least he had a problem with alcohol, but really caused my mother a lot of problems. So, I don't know if that would be a complicating factor in terms of an aneurysm or not.

Not that I know of. How about brothers and sisters?

I have one full natural brother and then four half-brothers.

Medical problems in any of them that you know of?

No.

And you work as?

An editorial writer for the *Journal*.

All we have are transcripts of these tape-recorded visits, so we cannot reconstruct the tone or quality of the language or the nonverbal communication (e.g., head nods, eye contact, gestures). However, the clinician in the first example (who, by the way, is a student) appears to be connecting with the patient, acknowledging both the facts and the patient's feelings ("I understand it's a very upsetting event"). But in the second example, the attending physician does not appear to be on the same wavelength with the patient; the physician's agenda has little regard for the other person. The patient has told the clinician that his father died of a cerebral hemorrhage, but he does not know anything else about it because his parents were divorced. The clinician ignores the divorce, the "painful subject," and the history of alcoholism and abruptly answers the patient's stated question and moves on ("Not that I know of. How about brothers and sisters?"). The second excerpt gives us a feeling that, at least in this segment, the interviewer's history-taking skills lack the qualities of respect, genuineness, and empathy.

- **Respect** is the ability to accept the patient as he or she is.
- **Genuineness** is the ability to be yourself in a relationship despite your professional role.
- **Empathy** is the ability to understand the patient's experiences and feelings accurately; it also includes demonstrating that understanding to the patient.

RESPECT

Respect means to value an individual's traits and beliefs despite your own personal feelings about them and to see patients' feelings and behavior as a valid adaptation to their illness or life circumstances. Some patients have irritating habits: smoking cigarettes, drinking too much, refusing to take medications, or even, at times, being antagonistic to their health care professionals. Other patients have beliefs about illness that try your patience: the man with severe emphysema might explain that his illness has nothing to do with his 100-pack-year smoking history but was caused by a cold he never got rid of in 1966. Another patient frustrates you with devastating migratory pains that refuse to go away, despite a normal examination and negative diagnostic tests. Some patients are unable to keep themselves clean; others do not adhere to your recommendations. Many have value systems different from yours or a healthy skepticism about the benefits of medical technology.

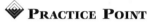 **PRACTICE POINT**
Simply put, respect means being nonjudgmental.

Separating Your Personal Feelings

The skill in having respect is to separate your personal feelings about the patient's behavior or attitudes or beliefs from your primary concern—figuring out what is wrong and helping him or her get well. For example, the patient who believes that his emphysema is unrelated to smoking can still be guided to give a reliable account of his symptoms. Likewise, although the hostile patient makes you feel uncomfortable, you can still try to respect his or her reasons for being angry. Moreover, the emphysema patient's denial and the hostile patient's anger may actually contribute to their ability to tolerate their illnesses; such feelings should be accepted as part of the whole patient, not rejected as threats to "truth" or to the clinician's ego. When patients act in ways that make you anxious or angry, they ordinarily have good reasons—based in their beliefs—for doing so, although their reasons may be difficult for you to understand.

Respect involves valuing the patient as a person and as a historian. The following case example, taken from Platt and McMath (1979), demonstrates lack of respect in several ways.

> *The interviewer failed to knock at the patient's door. He introduced himself in a hasty mumble so that the patient never had his name*

clearly in mind. He mispronounced the patient's name once and never used it again. The clinician conducted the interview while seated in a chair about 7 feet from the patient. There was no physical contact during the interview. On several occasions, the patient expressed her emotional distress. On each occasion, the interviewer ignored the emotional content of her statements.

Clinician   **Exactly where is this pain?**

Patient   It's so hard for me to explain. I'm trying to do as well as I can. [Turning to husband:] Aren't I doing as well as I can?

Well, is the pain up high in your belly, or down low?

I kept getting weaker and weaker. I didn't want to come to the hospital. I was so frightened [weeping].

Did the pain come before the weakness or afterward?

The physical examination was brusque; the examiner never warned his patient when he was going to perform painful maneuvers (for example, firmly stroking the sole of the foot). At the end of the examination, the clinician failed to comment on his findings or plans. He said in parting, "We'll do some tests and see if we can find out just what's the matter with you," and left the room before the patient had an opportunity to question him.

    In this case example, notice how the clinician seems to have his own agenda, ignoring the patient both as a person, by not acknowledging her emotional distress, and as a historian, by not helping to clarify the nature of the pain and weakness. *How to Demonstrate Respect for Patients*, below, presents a number of simple steps you can take to demonstrate respect for your patient.

WHAT TO SAY
How to Demonstrate Respect for Patients

- Introduce yourself clearly: "My name is John Smith; I'm a medical student."
- Do not use the patient's first name during an interview without permission: "May I call you John?"
- Explain your role: "I would like to spend about 30 minutes talking with you about your illness."
- Inquire about and arrange for the patient's comfort before getting started: "Is this a good time for you?"

■ Continue to consider the patient's comfort during the course of your interview and clinical evaluation: "Would you be more comfortable if I lowered the bed?"

■ Warn the patient when you are about to do something unexpected or painful: "I'm going to check your nerve endings by touching you with this pin."

■ Respond to your patient in a way that shows you have heard what he or she has said: "Let me see if I have the story straight."

If the clinician had been demonstrating respect, the previous interview might have gone something like this:

Clinician	Exactly where is the pain?
Patient	It's so hard for me to explain. I'm trying to do as well as I can. [Turning to husband:] Aren't I doing as well as I can?
	I can see it's hard for you to explain and that you're trying hard. Perhaps you can show me where you are feeling the pain right now.
	It's right about here [pointing] but what really frightened me was that I kept getting weaker and weaker and I didn't want to come to the hospital [weeping].
	[Handing patient a box of tissues.] Here, do you need one of these? Was it the weakness that frightened you?

Now the clinician is focusing not only on the symptoms but also on the patient's feelings about the symptoms. In other words, the clinician is communicating respect.

◆ **PRACTICE POINT**
One demonstrates respect by attending to the patient's words and by providing comfort.

GENUINENESS

Genuineness means not pretending to be somebody other than who you are; it means being yourself, both as a person and as a professional. The first time you encounter this concept of genuineness as a problem in the health professions may be in your role as a student. How do you introduce yourself? Should you introduce yourself as a clinical student or as a clinician? Do you allow a patient to address you as "doctor"? How do you respond when patients ask medical questions beyond your expertise or inquire about their own prognosis or care? Or when they say, "You look so young to be a doctor." In all these cases, if you are to be genuine, you must acknowledge what you are: a student. You should introduce yourself as a student and, whenever appropriate, reaffirm to the patient your limited knowledge and limited responsibility (but not limited interest) in the patient's care.

The terms "student doctor" and "student nurse" represent useful concepts. They acknowledge the patient's need to perceive the clinical student in a professional helping role, while also genuinely describing what the student is. These terms also allow students to feel more professional and may facilitate a helping attitude toward the patient.

Interns, residents, physician assistants, nurse practitioners, and practicing physicians all experience situations in which patients ask for opinions or require procedures beyond the practitioner's capabilities. We may be required to call in consultants or refer patients to specialists. This aspect of genuineness is a component of being seen as trustworthy by your patients.

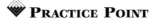 **PRACTICE POINT**

Genuineness requires you to be clear with the patient about what you do or do not know and can or cannot do, and to negotiate a plan for future care based on your capabilities.

Being Yourself

Being genuine also means being yourself in another way: expressing your feelings while staying within the boundaries of a professional relationship. If a patient is in the hospital for a medical or surgical illness but has experienced a recent loss, such as the death of a spouse, it is desirable to respond to this fact with a statement such as, "I am sorry to hear that. How has it been going for you?" However, adding personal details (e.g., you too have lost a spouse or parent) may stress the limits of your comfort in a professional relationship. When patients make sad or comical comments, it is appropriate to respond as a person, with an expression of sympathy or with laughter, as the case may be, and not just as a history taker. Demonstrating your interest in the patient as a person is another way of being genuine.

Professionalism

There are situations, however, when respect and genuineness may seem contradictory. Everyone has bad days, and you may happen to be at a low ebb yourself during your evaluation of the patient. You may have been on call and up all night with a patient in the intensive care unit. You may be having problems in your personal life or be eagerly anticipating a week-end getaway. At other times, you may be outraged about the patient's behavior, such as canceling at the last minute or arriving late for appointments. What is the role of genuineness in these situations? Should you hide your feelings, disguise your bad day, or express your emotions to the patient? Although genuineness means not pretending, it does not mean that you must share all your feelings with the patient. You must distinguish your genuine professional self from the vicissitudes, experiences, or interests of your personal self. The development of a set of core competencies in professionalism is an important part of your training. Although such competencies have traditionally been implied in health care education, they have recently become explicit and required. Thus, for example, medical students and residents must be evaluated on their professionalism in daily practice. This helps ensure that, as you go through training, you gradually develop your professional self into a well-integrated instrument of healing. It is this professional self that serves as the standard for genuineness.

For example, the patient who makes you angry by continually not showing up for appointments can be told that you, as a person, are angry about that, but, as a professional, you try to confine your anger to that aspect of the relationship. For example, you could say, "I know it's hard for you to get here, but when you're late I can't give you the time and the care that you need." At the same time, you try to respect the patient by understanding his or her reasons for being late—chaotic lifestyle, three children younger than age 5, single parenting, the need to take two buses to get to your office, and so forth.

Two Caveats

This discussion leads to two caveats:

- It is rarely helpful to share your personal anger or disgust with the patient in the name of being honest. You may confront the patient with inconsistencies (to you) in his or her story or point out the patient's erratic behavior, if you believe it will help therapeutically; this is not the same as sharing your own negative feelings.

- Sometimes clinicians are tempted to share their experiences and feelings as illustrations for the patient. This may range from such statements as "I have young children, too, and I know what you mean," to detailed personal anecdotes. Here again it is crucial to judge your personal revelations in the light of your professional judgment. Ordinarily, comments of rapport and connection are helpful. The type of car you own, the vagaries of parenting, or your opinions about a football team are not really self-revelations. On the other hand, it is rarely useful in a genuine clinician-patient interaction to describe intimate experiences or specific moral values.

Here is an example of a genuine response by a medical resident who is seeing a woman with asthma, peptic ulcer disease, and numerous psychosocial problems. The patient has just related a personal history of abuse during her childhood, and continues with her story.

Patient   I can write a book. Well, you know, I'm not any more, but I used to be atheist for a while. God made me. I was a little girl, but I think about if you got children, you want the best for your children. If we are God's children, why did I go through what I went through? So that's why I feel the way I do.

Clinician   **I think about that all the time when I see people who are sick. They didn't bring it on themselves. It makes you wonder. No answer to that one.**

Notice how the clinician responds in this scenario without revealing his own religious beliefs.

EMPATHY

Empathy is a type of understanding. It should not be confused with feeling sympathetic or sorry for someone, nor is it the same as the virtue of compassion. Although compassion may well be your motivation for developing empathy with patients, empathy is not compassion. In medical interviewing, being empathic has a well-defined meaning: listening to the patient's total communication—words, feelings, and gestures—and letting the patient know that you really understand what he or she is communicating.

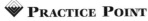 **PRACTICE POINT**

Being empathic is at one and the same time being scientific, because understanding is at the core of objectivity. The skill of

empathy involves maximizing your ability to gather accurate data about the patient's thoughts and feelings.

Demonstrating Your Understanding

There are ways of responding to patients that help you demonstrate to them that you understand. The data that the patient gives you about his or her illness will be associated with feelings and beliefs. When you speak to patients, remember that you are also speaking to a set of beliefs about the world. The elderly gentleman who gives you a detailed description of his abdominal pain may at the same time feel frightened because he fears that the pain means stomach cancer because his father died of stomach cancer. His description will be filtered through his fears and his beliefs; unless you attend to the worry, the patient may not give an accurate account of what he is experiencing. One such patient may magnify the symptom to ensure a complete workup that will not miss cancer; another may minimize the symptom in the hope of being reassured that it is not cancer. If the interviewer acknowledges the fear, it is easier to get an accurate idea about what is really going on.

An empathic response can also be important in helping patients clarify their feelings. At times, the patient will not be in touch with his or her own feelings. By checking within yourself—how you would feel, for instance, on finding blood in your stool—you can formulate a response. Then, by checking back with the patient—by saying, for example, "That can be pretty frightening"—you as the interviewer can find out whether your assessment of what the patient might have felt is valid for that person's experience of illness.

LEVELS OF RESPONDING

It is useful to think of empathy as a feedback loop. You begin by listening carefully to what the patient tells you, both cognitively and affectively. When you think you understand, you respond by telling the patient what you have heard. If you happen to be on the right wavelength, the patient will feel understood and be encouraged to reveal more of his or her thoughts and feelings. If you do not get it right, but have demonstrated your interest by checking back, the patient is likely to feel comfortable in correcting your impression, thus giving you an opportunity to reassess and respond again. This process can be iterative, as in some cases you check back several times to arrive at the most accurate characterization of the experience.

Assessing Your Patient's Feelings

Your assessment of the strength of the feeling that the patient is experiencing will influence what you say to the patient—in other words, your level of response. If the patient believes that you are picking up on everything he or she says and are listening attentively with a nonjudgmental attitude, not only will accurate symptom data emerge, but feelings and beliefs will emerge as well. In formulating a response, it is important first to assess the nature and intensity of an expressed feeling. For example, is the patient upset? If so, is he or she slightly annoyed or furious? Your assessment will include not only what the patient says but also how it is said and how the patient looks when he or she says it.

In clinical interviewing, you must learn a professional way of responding, which is different from the way you might respond in social interactions. In social situations, we often ignore or minimize feelings. For example, when people say, "How are you?" or "How do you feel today?" they do not ordinarily expect you to reveal how lousy you are actually feeling. In the clinical setting, however, you really do want to know the details of the person's mood and feelings. You acknowledge the intensity of any feelings expressed and demonstrate that you understand and accept them. Consider these four categories, or levels, of responding: **ignoring, minimizing, interchangeable,** and **additive.**

Ignoring Response

You either do not hear what the patient has said or act as though you did not hear. You give no response to either the cognitive or emotional content. For example:

Patient   Most days my arthritis is so bad the swelling and pain is just too much.
Clinician   **And have you ever had any operations?**

    and

Clinician   **Do emotional problems at work seem to make it worse?**
Patient   I think it's …
             Do coughing, sneezing, bending, straining at stool, any of those things make it worse?
             I never associated it with those things.

Minimizing Response

You respond to the feelings and symptoms at a lesser level than that associated with the patient's expressed concern. For example:

Patient   I was in agony with the pain and terribly frightened.
Clinician   Well, I'm sure it wasn't that bad.

and

Patient   Most days my arthritis is so bad the swelling and pain is just too much.
Clinician   What you need is something to take your mind off it.

Interchangeable Response

You recognize the feelings and symptoms expressed by the patient and assess them accurately, and you feed back that awareness at the same level of intensity. For example:

Patient   Most days my arthritis is so bad the swelling and pain is just too much. I can't seem to do anything at all any more and nothing seems to help.
Clinician   It sounds as though the pain and disability are really getting to you.

and

Patient   I was in agony with the pain and terribly frightened.
Clinician   Severe pain can be pretty frightening. Was it the pain that scared you or the thought of what might be causing the pain?

The interchangeable response is a good response in clinical history taking. When you give an interchangeable response, you are likely to find that it has a positive effect on the patient's ability to tell an accurate story. This kind of response is essential to being empathic.

◆ PRACTICE POINT
The interchangeable response is a restatement, in your own words, of what the patient is trying to describe and is used to communicate that you understand.

In the following dialogue, the clinician responds to her patient's concerns even though she does not answer all the patient's questions right away.

Patient   But other than that I'm pretty good but it's my breasts I'm worried about. They started bleeding again, doctor. Why? I want you to take a look today. They're all bleeding in the inside. Is it anything to be concerned about?

Clinician **Well, maybe I can look and tell you.**
Okay.
When did that start up again?
It seems like it will come and it will go, but now they're both all red and I noticed a whole lot of blood just drained out, especially this right one, it really hurts down there. This side don't hurt me, but this side hurts me [touches her breasts]. I don't know.
So you want me to take a look at your breasts [interchangeable response]. Is that what's worrying you most today, your breasts? Is there anything else?
No.
Okay, come and let me take a look. [Patient and clinician move to examination table, and she begins checking patient.] Okay, I can see why you're so concerned; it looks pretty raw here. Okay, this is pretty much like it was before.
Yeah, but it really does hurt.
Yeah, I can see that it hurts [interchangeable response]. This one is the worst, huh? Remember how well we were able to clear it up with medication the last time it got this bad?
Wonder what causes that. That's what worries me.
Yes, most women do worry about things that happen to their breasts [interchangeable response]. But this is not serious, although it's very annoying and painful. When bleeding comes from inside the breast, it is serious. But this is from the skin. It's more like a skin allergy. The skin is real sensitive.
Oh, is that what it is? Okay.

How do you achieve an interchangeable response? Two concise ways are through mirrors and paraphrases. A mirror (or reflection) simply feeds back to the patient exactly what is said using the same words, for example:

Patient   I feel really terrible.
Clinician **You feel really terrible?**

A paraphrase conveys the same meaning as the patient's statement but uses different words:

I feel really terrible.
So you're really not feeling well, are you?

Additive Response

In an additive response, you recognize not only what the patient expresses openly but also what he or she feels but does not express. One common activity of clinicians that requires using additive responses is reassurance. Reassurance involves making an educated guess regarding what the patient is likely to be worried about and dealing specifically with those worries. Here is an example of an additive response during a follow-up visit by a young man with headaches.

Clinician   **Well, how are you? Are you still having headaches?**
Patient   Saturday I had a bad one. I wasn't able to sleep for 5 nights; my system is so pumped up I can't sleep. The pills did work. I took one a couple of hours before I went to bed and one just when I went to bed.
You mean the pills I gave you before you went to the hospital?
Yeah. I took them 2 nights and last night was the first night I could sleep without them. I don't like to take a lotta stuff. I was having very strange effects from some of the medication.
Like what?
Well, you know everything else about me, I might as well tell you this. Those green pills made me ... well, I can't describe the feeling—it made me feel ... very strange. They also depressed me, believe it or not, even though you told me that they were antidepressants. I got depressed with them. For 2 days when I was taking them straight and in heavy doses, I found myself breaking into tears in situations ... I don't even cry when I want to [laughs]. It was very, very strange, so I stopped taking them.
Okay. Can you tell me anything more about this strange feeling you had?
Ahhh ... [patient hesitates].
Were you feeling like you were going to lose your mind? [additive response]
Yeah, I felt like I didn't have control over myself. I started to think I would get complications from the illness and how far behind it was making me get in my work because this is a very crucial time in my business. It really opened a lot of stuff for me. I never felt like this before.

The ability to achieve an additive response comes with the experience of listening carefully to patients' stories over time and learning patterns from them. Note that in the previous example, the clinician did not get it quite right. The additive response overshoots the patient's feeling, which was not so much "going to lose your mind" as it was "I didn't have control over myself." One of the benefits of an additive response is in facilitating this kind of correction, thereby improving accuracy.

An additive response also might be used for this patient with arthritis.

Patient Most days my arthritis is so bad the swelling and pain are just too much.

Clinician It sounds as though the pain is so bad that you think that things won't get much better.

If you have not gotten the sense of the statement quite right, the patient may respond:

Patient Well, I do feel pretty bad, but I'm still hopeful.

Here is another example of an additive response, this time in an interview with a 50-year-old woman describing her history of depression.

Patient You know, sometimes I scare myself.
Clinician You mean, you think about killing yourself?
Yeah, I do.

Understanding Exactly Is a Challenge

Despite your best efforts, some situations present unavoidable difficulties in understanding exactly what the patient means. Among these are technical problems, such as language barriers, the patient's state of consciousness (comatose, delirious, psychotic, or demented), and the patient's educational level, culture, or language skills. We review issues related to language and culture in Chapter 12, Cultural Competence in the Interview, and patients with cognitive impairment in Chapter 11, Interviewing the Geriatric Patient. With patients who do not speak your language or who are demented, we ordinarily dismiss the possibility of a useful interview and seek information elsewhere. We may arrange for an interpreter or elicit information from a family member. Other challenges to acquiring accurate symptom data are subtler: language barriers may involve just a few crucial words, or the patient's anger (see Chapter 13, Difficult Patient-Clinician Interactions) may result in an inaccurate response, or responses may be inappropriate or confused. It is useful early in the interview to detect problems that lead to faulty data collection.

USING WORDS PRECISELY

To increase your skill in responding appropriately, you need to pay attention to words, both your own and those of the patient. Professional education can sterilize your vocabulary. You become immersed in the language of medicine, which, although extremely precise in describing some attributes, leaves little room for feelings or emotions.

The Language of Medicine

In medical language, adjectives and adverbs carry little weight, and you are usually discouraged from using them in conversation. This socialization into the factual language of medicine can present real problems when you speak with patients. The world of the sick differs from the world of the well, but the difference does not necessarily include the sick learning the language of medicine. The most obvious problem you encounter with your medical vocabulary is that patients do not understand the words you use. When you say "hematemesis" rather than "vomiting blood" or "paresthesia" rather than "pins-and-needles sensations," your patient probably will not know what you are talking about.

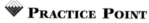 **PRACTICE POINT**

To ensure that you and your patient are speaking the same language, you should "translate" medical terms into words the patient can understand.

Here is an example of a medical faculty member who was trying to ask a patient how much alcohol he drank:

Clinician   **Okay. Do you use ethanol a lot, a little, weekends ... ?**
Patient   Tylenol?
             Daily? Ethanol? Alcohol?
             Drinks? You mean ... alcoholic beverages? ... I usually have a drink every night.
             Okay.

This clinician was thinking "use ethanol" rather than "drink alcohol," and the choice of words created confusion, which in this case was temporary. Fortunately, the patient acknowledged the misunderstanding. Many times patients do not let on that they don't understand. This is a particular problem with yes/no questions and with explanations or instructions in which no response is sought from the patient.

Feeling Words, Qualifiers, and Quantifiers

Another important result of medical language and thought patterns is our often-impoverished ability to describe feelings, qualities, and emotions with accuracy or precision. Empathy requires both accurate understanding and accurate feedback. This skill demands that you identify not only symptoms but also feelings, not only quantity but also quality.

- **Quantity.** Although we are often more comfortable using numbers as quantities, patients frequently use analogies or comparisons to capture the intensity of their symptoms. For example, the patient who describes his pain as being as severe as a kidney stone is giving as precise a description as the patient who says that the pain is 8 on a scale of 1 to 10. Perhaps the former description is even more precise than the latter, because we may not know the patient's "10," but we do know that renal colic is one of the most severe pains a person can have.
- **Quality.** Likewise, we must open up our windows to the world, and learn to use a broad vocabulary of feeling words. Table 2–1, *Descriptive Words for Levels of Feeling*, presents examples of words that describe emotions and their intensity. In giving an inter-

TABLE 2–1

DESCRIPTIVE WORDS FOR LEVELS OF FEELING				
Intensity	*Anger*	*Joy*	*Anxiety or Fear*	*Depression*
Weak	Annoyed	Pleased	Uneasy	Sad
	Upset	Glad	Uncertain	Down
	Irritated	Happy	Apprehensive	Blue
Medium	Angry	Marvelous	Worried	Gloomy
	Testy	Joyful	Troubled	Sorrowful
	Quarrelsome	Delighted	Afraid	Miserable
Strong	Infuriated	Thrilled	Tormented	Distraught
	Spiteful	Jubilant	Frantic	Overwhelmed
	Enraged	Ecstatic	Terrified	Devastated

changeable response, you must "hit" not only the right feeling, but also the right intensity. The patient who says, "I am devastated by this pain" is not likely to believe you really heard him or her if your response is, "So the pain upset you a little?" On the other hand, when the patient mentions that "I feel a little crummy today," the clinician is not sticking to his or her observations if the reply is "Sounds like you're feeling utterly hopeless." Once we accept the idea that medicine is about helping people to feel and function better, it is easy to understand how feelings reveal important data about the patient, which must be described as accurately as possible.

NONVERBAL COMMUNICATION

Nonverbal communication is the process of transmitting information without the use of words. It includes the way a person uses his or her body, such as facial expressions, eye contact, hand and arm gestures, posture, and movements of the legs and feet. Nonverbal communication also includes paralinguistics—verbal qualities such as tone, rhythm, pace, and vibrancy; speech errors; and pauses or silence. It is often through the nonverbal aspects of communication that we apprehend another's feelings. We recognize anger not so much by what a person says as by how it is said. Speech may slow down and get quiet in controlled anger, or the opposite may occur—with shouting and gestures such as pounding on a table. We can often tell when people lie unless they are good liars. They might look away, break eye contact, hesitate, or get "red in the face" (i.e., flush involuntarily). Common medical examples are the pressure of speech in the anxious or hypomanic person, or the flat voice tone of an extremely depressed patient. Patients who are ill often "sound" weak; we may gauge a person's state of health by how he or she sounds ("She's been through a lot of surgery, but she really sounds strong").

Kinesics

Another component of nonverbal communication involves **kinesics**— that is, the use of personal space and how physically close we get to each other while talking to friends, business associates, lovers, or patients. Other factors such as personal grooming, clothing, and odors (e.g., perspiration, alcohol, tobacco) also communicate nonverbal information about the patient. For example, if a patient who is normally careful about personal grooming comes in disheveled and unkempt, you are alerted to the possibility of a problem even before he or she begins to speak.

Matching Verbal and Nonverbal Responses

Even though nonverbal communication may be obvious to you, the patient is likely to be unaware of it. This does not mean that nonverbal messages are invalid; in fact, they may be more accurate than the verbal message, precisely because they are usually unintentional and uncensored. Although it is interesting to note various aspects of nonverbal communication, you may wonder what to do with your observations. Look for consistency: note nonverbal behaviors, and determine whether they are congruent with the patient's verbal message. When congruence exists, the communication is more or less straightforward. However, when there is a discrepancy, an effort must be made to ascertain which one conveys the "real" message.

Here is an example of a patient who came in for a routine follow-up of abdominal pain and reported first that her husband, from whom she was separated, died recently of some sudden and unknown cause (he was 27 years old). David is the child they had together.

Patient	I want to tell you something before we start.
Clinician	**OK.**
	David's dad died. And now, it's like every week it's something new.
	Oh my. [Note the genuine response.] What happened?
	I don't know. He just went to sleep and never woke up.
	My goodness, when did that happen?
	Last Friday, right before the ninth.
	Oh, I am so sorry to hear that. Ah, how is David doing?

The clinician went on to explore how the patient and her son were reacting to this event, but the patient discussed this catastrophe with a bright smile on her face. Although she was separated from her husband, they had remained close because of David, and her cheeriness seemed inappropriate. What did the smile mean here? What kind of problem did this discrepancy suggest? Indeed, the clinician seemed more upset about this news than the patient. It later came out that the patient was having great difficulty, particularly in communicating to her son appropriate ways to mourn and remember his father. Although the clinician did not confront the patient early in the interview, he was alerted to a possible problem and later helped guide her toward a more appropriate response.

Responding to Nonverbal Communication

Often the nonverbal message is more accurate than verbal statements. You may choose in some situations, especially early in the interview, simply to note a discrepancy and use it to help you understand the patient. Or you might use the nonverbal communication to modify your own nonverbal behavior, your conversation, or both. For example, if the patient seems tense, as evidenced by facial flushing or fidgeting, you may modify your voice tone and the way you are sitting in response to the patient's discomfort by speaking in a more soothing way and leaning forward to demonstrate your interest.

Self-awareness

During the patient's interview, you should be aware of your own nonverbal behavior as well as the patient's. For example, if you seem uninterested, never looking at the patient or looking often at your watch, the patient may be unable to provide the details you need. Likewise, if you stand by the door rather than sit by the bed, patients may assume you are in a hurry and, respectful of your time, leave out critical data they decide are unimportant. Attention to your own nonverbal behavior requires a high level of self-awareness and discipline. It is particularly important to be conscious of how you respond to distractions during the interview, such as an emergency across the hall. You need to demonstrate your focus on the patient by maintaining eye contact, an attentive posture, and a seeming lack of awareness that chaos is occurring somewhere else.

 PRACTICE POINT
Remember, at the same time that you are observing the patient's nonverbal behavior, the patient is, perhaps unconsciously, observing your nonverbal behavior as well. As a result, your job is twofold.

Gestures

Although investigators have studied various gestures and suggested specific interpretations, the meaning of gestures must always be judged in context. Interpretation is no problem when a gesture "confirms" the patient's statements or the clinician's hypothesis based on those statements.

◆ PRACTICE POINT

When the patient's gesture or facial expression appears to imply something different than the words, an effort must be made to ascertain which—the gesture or the words—is delivering the real message.

Consider this example, in which a patient is suffering from headaches. The clinician learns that the patient has been under much stress recently.

Clinician	**So, you have a lot of things on your mind.**
Patient	Yes. About them, about some of the members of my family, and, um, mostly it's money worries, mainly money. [Patient puts her hand on the part of her head that has been painful.]
	It's funny, when you say "money worries," you know where you point to?
	Huh?
	You point right where it's hurting.
	Yeah, aha ... that's mostly it, you know.

In this situation, pointing out the relationship between financial stress (verbal) and tension headaches (nonverbal, pointing to head) might well be effective both in demonstrating your empathic understanding and in making explicit a connection the patient may already experience implicitly.

Table 2–2, *Gestures and Possible Interpretations*, presents a list of common gestures and some of their suggested interpretations. Two of these deserve comment. The helplessness or hopelessness gesture is typically biphasic. Both hands are raised briskly to face level, with elbows fixed, palms facing each other; they are rotated slightly outward, fingers spread, and thumb and fingers slightly flexed as though preparing to grasp. This position is held briefly, and then the hands fall limply down to the lap. This gesture suggests that the patient feels helpless about the problem or situation. The first part may represent reaching out for assistance, while the second part (hypotonia and withdrawal) emphasizes the futility of reaching for help.

The respiratory avoidance response includes frequent clearing of the throat when no phlegm or mucus is present. A variation of this is the nose

TABLE 2-2

GESTURES AND POSSIBLE INTERPRETATIONS	
Gesture	*Possible Interpretation*
"Steepling" of hands, that is, joining them with fingers extended and fingertips touching, like a church steeple	Confidence or assurance of what is being said
Slight raising of the hand or index finger, pulling at an earlobe, or raising the index finger to the lips	Desire to interrupt the speaker
Helplessness or hopelessness gesture (see text)	Feeling of hopelessness; request for help is futile
Respiratory avoidance response (see text)	Rejection of or disagreement with what is being said
Raising a finger to the lips	Attempt to suppress a comment
Crossed arms (note the manner in which the arms are crossed and muscular tension, especially in the hands)	Defensive gesture indicating disagreement, a sign of insecurity, or simply a comfortable position
Increased muscle tension, "white knuckle syndrome"	Fear or tension
Crossed legs	Attempt to shut out or protect against what is going on in the interview, or simply a position of comfort
Uncrossed legs, shifting forward in the chair	Receptivity to what is going on in the interview

rub, which involves a light rub of the nose with the dorsal aspect of the index finger. These gestures indicate rejection of or disagreement with statements being made. For example, the clinician asks, "How are things at home?" The patient answers, "Fine," clears his throat, and lightly rubs his nose. He may actually be saying, "Things aren't really going very well at home."

Paralanguage

When you hear a patient's speech, you are hearing pauses, tone, and modulation, also called **paralanguage,** in addition to words. Likewise, the patient hears the pitch and rhythm of your conversation. Table 2-3, *Components of Paralanguage,* lists the elements of paralanguage.

TABLE 2–3

COMPONENTS OF PARALANGUAGE	
Component	Examples
Speech rate	Slow, fast, deliberate
Pauses	Long, short, inappropriate
Pause/speech ratio	Mechanical, halting, flowing speech
Tone or voice quality	Whiny, flat, nasal, bright, breathy
Pitch	High, medium, low
Volume	Loud, soft, wide variations
Articulation	Clear, precise, slurred

SOURCE: Adapted from Cassell EJ. *Talking With Patients. Volume 1, The Theory of Doctor–Patient Communication.* Cambridge, MA, MIT Press, 1985.

Paralinguistic cues can contribute significantly to your understanding of the patient and to the patient's perception of you as a helping person.

Let us deal briefly with just one aspect of paralanguage: pauses. Why does a patient pause a moment before answering your question, or before making her next statement? The functions of pausing include:

- Absolute recall time
- Language formation time
- Censorship of material
- Creating an effect (timing)
- Preparing to lie

People rarely need to pause before recalling a place, age, or date fixed in time. For example, a person readily remembers the age at which a parent died, but might have to think a moment before remembering a living parent's current age. It is easy to answer a yes/no question without pausing, even if giving the incorrect answer: "Do you drink alcohol?" The yes or no response has little meaning. Alternatively, you might ask, "How much alcohol do you usually drink in a day?" or "Tell me about your use of alcohol." These questions demand some thought and integration. Listen carefully. How much of a pause occurs before the answer? How much stumbling or backtracking occurs?

In general, it is helpful to listen to the number, quality, and placement of pauses. Frequent long pauses associated with low amplitude and a "dead" tone suggest clinical depression. Frequent pauses over factual answers throughout the interview suggest dementia or organic brain dysfunction. Pauses over answers in selected areas may indicate sensitive topics, with time required for censorship of material. (We will return to this aspect of medical interviewing in Chapter 13, Difficult Patient-Clinician Interactions.)

SUMMARY—Respect, Genuineness, Empathy

In this chapter we presented three fundamental skills of clinician-patient interactions:

- Respect
- Genuineness
- Empathy

Respect means to be nonjudgmental, and genuineness means being yourself—although a professional self—in the interaction with the patient. Empathy means understanding exactly what the patient is saying and letting the patient know that you understand. To achieve empathy in the clinical encounter you should:

- Strive for interchangeable responses.
- Develop and use a good vocabulary of descriptive words.
- Pay attention to nonverbal communication, especially paralinguistics.

Armed with an understanding of these fundamental skills, you are now ready to begin the interview, as we move on to Chapter 3.

Chief Complaint and Present Illness

Why Should You Come to Consult Me?

*"Never mind," said Holmes, laughing; "it is
my business to know things. Perhaps I have
trained myself to see what others overlook.
If not, why should you come to consult me?"*
Arthur Conan Doyle, *"A Case of Identity" from* The
Adventures of Sherlock Holmes

BEGINNING THE COMPLETE MEDICAL HISTORY

In the next four chapters we will discuss the traditional parts of a
complete medical history: the chief complaint, present illness, other
active problems, past medical history, family history, social history or
patient profile, and review of systems. In each section we introduce,
describe, and illustrate skills or techniques useful for that part of the
interview—skills particularly appropriate to the content or medical objective (e.g., the review of systems requires a different approach than the
history of the present illness). This division of the interview is for
simplicity of illustration only and does not imply that open-ended questions or interchangeable responses, for example, are useful only in the
present illness section. Remember, too, that one does not necessarily
proceed in this order or, for that matter, in one sitting. Sometimes you
learn the family history in the opening moments of the encounter
("My mother had breast cancer, so I thought I'd better come in for a checkup"), or the patient profile may evolve over several encounters with the
patient.

Chapter 3 deals with the interview setting and opening, chief complaint, and present illness. When patients share their stories, they begin
to make sense of their illnesses both cognitively and emotionally; and for

the clinician, gathering the database helps to establish the relationship, as well as the etiology of the symptoms.

INTERVIEW SETTING

In the past, clinicians usually first learned their interviewing skills with hospitalized patients. Although the emphasis is now on ambulatory care, students still frequently begin their experience in the hospital setting. The hospital is an unnatural habitat; as a result, the patient with "dis-ease" may not feel "at-ease." Patients may be similarly uncomfortable, although perhaps less so, in the clinic or emergency room or physician's office. When you see a patient for the first time, his or her blood pressure and pulse are often elevated, the face flushed, the handshake cool and damp, and the gestures clearly nervous. These characteristic signs indicate an autonomic response to the stress of illness, seeking help, meeting a new clinician, and the uncertain outcome. If you appear hurried, indifferent, or unsympathetic, the patient is likely to feel even more uncomfortable; this discomfort creates a barrier to effective communication.

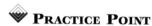 **PRACTICE POINT**
Before beginning your patient's history, make sure that he or she is as comfortable as possible.

OPENING THE INTERVIEW

The opening of the interview sets the atmosphere for the rest of your history and physical examination. Quickly show your respect with a friendly greeting and begin by establishing a sense of privacy for the interview. For example, if there is another patient sharing the hospital room, draw the curtain around the bed. Even though this obviously does not provide a soundproof barrier, it gives the patient a psychological sense of privacy. If the patient can walk comfortably, it may be better to do the interview in a convenient lounge or waiting area, if this would be more private. If the patient has visitors, you might suggest that they wait outside or, if possible, that you will return later to see the patient. Try to seat yourself in a way that will facilitate communication. People have spheres of personal space. Get close enough for a person-to-person interaction, but do not intrude on the patient's intimate space.

Ensuring Patient Comfort

In a small hospital room it may be difficult to place yourself comfortably so that you strike a balance between being halfway across the room and sitting on top of the patient. If necessary, move your chair closer. Try to sit at the same level as the patient; this helps establish good eye contact. Often it is most comfortable to sit at an angle to the patient, rather than facing him or her directly, allowing you to maintain eye contact, but also providing natural opportunities to look away at times. Good eye contact does not mean staring fixedly, which will only make the patient feel more uncomfortable. You can also use your body to demonstrate interest by leaning slightly toward the patient rather than lounging back in your chair.

Consider these guidelines:

- *Introduce yourself and explain your role.* If you are a student, we strongly suggest you introduce yourself as such. Besides being genuine and not using a facade, you will also be helping to define your limited **contract** (what you expect of each other in the interaction) with the patient. When the patient asks your opinion about his or her diagnosis or treatment, asks for pain medication, or requests anything outside your capacity to respond, you can comfortably remind the patient of the boundaries of your contract. You can tell him or her that you will convey the question to the resident or nursing staff, or you may suggest that the patient do so.
- *Don't begin by saying, "I've been sent to take a history and do a physical."* Such a statement is likely to make the patient feel that you have no real interest in him or her and may set the interview off on the wrong track. A better start would be to say, "I'd like to talk to you today to get some information about why you're in the hospital, and then to examine you. Will that be all right?" As part of this introduction, you obtain permission (the contract) to do the history and examination; by so doing, you demonstrate respect for the person.
- *Taking notes is essential.* You will use them for recall and to write up the information you obtain. As you begin, inform the patient of your need to take notes and the reason for it; this will also let the patient know what will happen to the information you obtain. However, don't let note taking control the interview. If you attempt to record the conversation verbatim—with the exception

of the chief complaint—the process of taking so many notes will interfere with conversation flow. Eye contact will be limited, and you are likely to miss the nonverbal communication, thereby interfering with rapport and missing useful data about the person. While you are taking notes, look up frequently; this will demonstrate your interest. You will find with more experience that only an occasional word or phrase needs to be written down to help you remember, synthesize, and later reconstruct the story in writing.

CHIEF COMPLAINT

The **chief complaint** in a standard medical history is the main reason why the patient is seeking medical help. The chief complaint is often elicited by such questions as:

- "How can I help you today?"
- "Can you tell me about your trouble?"
- "What symptoms made you decide to see a doctor or come to the emergency room?"
- "Can you tell me about your problem?"
- "Tell me about the main thing you feel is wrong."
- "What brought you to the hospital?" (Although this question may be subject to concrete answers like, "A taxi.")
- "Tell me why you came today."

◆ PRACTICE POINT
Make sure to record the patient's chief complaint verbatim in his or her own words.

Consider the following example of how one medical resident began an interview with a new patient in an outpatient clinic.

Clinician	**I guess the best place to start is to ask you what brings you here today.**
Patient	Well, I haven't had a physical really for 6 years now, since my daughter was born.
	I am going to be writing some things down on paper here, okay? Is there any particular reason why you chose now to come in?

I figured I kept putting it off and putting it off. I'd make appointments and put them off. There is no particular reason. I just felt as though it was time, I suppose.

Nothing is bothering you at this point?

No, it's just that I am overweight, that's all. I go up and down, up and down.

So that was your major concern, the weight problem?

Yeah.

Can you tell me about that?

The chief complaint, stated verbatim, is "It's just that I am overweight." It took a little digging to clarify that fact; the clinician was appropriately not satisfied with "There is no particular reason."

Sometimes an opening question leads to a clear-cut chief complaint, as in this example:

Clinician **What can I do for you?**

Patient Um, the reason why I'm here is, since the latter part of July up to now, my bowels wouldn't move and I'd have to, in like 4 and 5 days, I'd have to take either milk of magnesia or a bulk laxative, and I just thought it was maybe something that I was eating, and this still continues until now, and it's the reason why I'm here to see you.

In other cases, the same opening question might lead to a much more complex and rambling answer, such as:

Clinician **Now what can I do for you, Mrs. P?**

Patient Well, first of all, I'm here mainly because I've been experiencing that tired, worn-out feeling most of the time. I can go to bed, say 9:00 in the evening, and get up at 8:00 or even later and I still feel very tired. And, I don't know ... I've still been experiencing hot flashes and sometimes now ... I don't experience them as often as I used to, but I still do, especially toward the evening or at night, and it awakens me when I do experience something like that. Maybe that's part of the reason why I felt so tired, I don't know. Anyways, now in the evening when I experience this kind of hot feeling, I just get that craving—I want to eat, you know, or sometimes it works just the opposite where I feel kind of nervous, I get that nervous feeling, and now last week I had headaches just about every day on arising; I had a little runny nose, so maybe, I don't know, maybe I could attribute that to a cold, but I'm just mentioning those things to you. And, sometimes you know my head just feels as though ... it feels stuffed ... when you have a head cold; that's just the way it has felt many times. And I had a hysterectomy, let's see, about 1992 or '93 and since then I just have had no sexual desire or anything. I mean, as far as I'm concerned that doesn't mean a whole lot. I know it upsets my husband a bit.

What is the chief complaint in this scenario? Ostensibly, it is her first statement, "mainly because (of) that tired, worn-out feeling ...," but in context the situation is less clear. What is really bothering her most? Why did she come here today, as opposed to last month or next week? This patient rambles on and on, presenting a challenge to the interviewer that we will discuss near the end of this chapter (see page 66). The clinician permits this lengthy response, and, in so doing, acquires a wealth of useful information about the patient's symptoms and concerns. The clinician will later establish more structure to help the patient clarify her complaints.

Discovering the Primary Reason for Seeking Care

In contrast to the rambling response example, investigators have found that clinicians usually do not allow patients to complete their opening statements. Rather, they interrupt and steer the discussion toward a specific topic, thereby diminishing the chance of getting to the patient's primary reason for seeking care.

The discursive patient is not the only one who presents problems in identifying the chief complaint, however. Often, the actual reason why the person comes to see the clinician lies embedded somewhere else, far from the patient's initial statement (see cartoon). Here is an example of a patient who presents with chest pain that he has had for some time:

Clinician   **I'm glad you came in today. Tell me why you came in.**
Patient   Okay. I been having some problems with my chest; you know it's, it's like pressure and plus I have a knot under my arm, under my armpit.
    Okay. You have pressure.
    Yeah, I have pressure, and I don't know if it's because I smoke a lot of cigarettes, or I don't know what it is.
    Um hum.
    All I know is it's pressure across my chest. It's not what you call a pain or anything—it hurts; it's pressure all across here.
    Um hum.
    And, then, I have this knot under my, under my armpit.
    Okay.

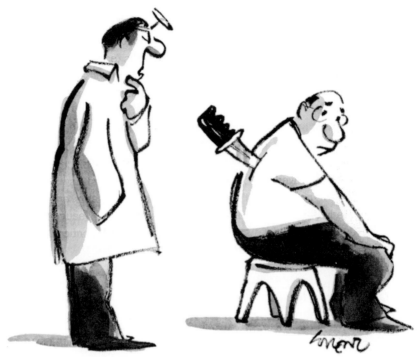

*"It's got to come out, of course, but that
doesn't address the real problem."*

About the size of a half-dollar.

Okay, let's talk about the chest pain first; when would you say it started?

Um, I'd say about a month ago; maybe it might have been longer but I didn't pay it any attention.

Um hum.

You know but I can't jog because if I just start jogging, it bothers me in my chest.

What made you decide to get it checked?

Well, two things actually: I want to get back in shape and I got a note from the Health Department that this test came back positive. See I'm a barber and they test for tuberculosis.

By asking "What made you decide to get it checked?" this clinician not only has the answer to why the patient came in now, but also an important new piece of data—namely, the positive tuberculin test result. We learn that the patient may believe there is a relationship between his symptoms and the positive tuberculin test result. He really came to the clinician because of the test result, perhaps simply to fulfill a legal requirement for his license, and perhaps, in addition, because the test result made him reinterpret his chest problems as being more serious than he had thought they were. In any case, if the workup for tuberculosis is negative, the clinician knows that the patient will need reassurance that tuberculosis isn't responsible for his symptoms.

When you consider why a person might come for medical help at a certain time, it is not enough simply to elicit the symptoms, as they may have been present for some time. Although the answer to a question such as "How can I help you?" frequently contains the core of the patient's problem, sometimes it does not. The *ostensible reason for coming,* as initially stated by the patient in the chief complaint, may not be the same as the *actual reason for coming.* This is most often true with people who:

- Have chronic diseases
- Have vague, chronic, or recurring symptoms
- Say they just want a checkup

Why Now? The Iatrotropic Stimulus

Alvan Feinstein (1967) used the term **iatrotropic stimulus** ("iatrotropic," toward the physician) to indicate precisely why the patient decided to seek care at a particular point in time. Once you can answer the question "Why now?" you have probably uncovered the iatrotropic stimulus or the actual reason for coming. Despite the fact that the person has a clear-cut disease or symptom (congestive heart failure or shortness of breath), it may not satisfactorily explain why the patient is here today, as opposed to yesterday or last week. We list some of these reasons in *Why Patients Seek Care at a Particular Time*, page 53. If you listen carefully, the iatrotropic stimulus will come out during the interview. Sometimes it arrives only at the last moment, when you are about to walk out of the room and the patient says, "Oh, by the way, Doc, I'm sure this has nothing to do with it, but ...." We will touch on the "Oh, by the way," or "hand on the doorknob," phenomenon later, in Chapter 9, Communication in the Office Setting. However, basic respect, empathy, and open-ended questioning (described below) early in the interview go a long way toward minimizing or avoiding this phenomenon. The earlier in the interview you ascertain the patient's reason for coming, the more efficient you will be, wasting less time digging. For example, the patient with the rambling "chief complaint" whom we met earlier in this chapter actually provides all of her concerns within the opening 2 minutes of the interview. The clinician can take notes and come back to each in turn, prioritizing for maximum efficiency. We will return to this technique in Chapter 9, when we discuss primary care interviewing.

WHY PATIENTS SEEK CARE AT A PARTICULAR TIME

Reason for Seeking Care	Timing of Symptoms
Symptoms of the Illness	May increase to the point that they become unbearable and the person simply realizes he or she needs medical help.
Anxiety about the Meaning of the Symptoms	May reach the point where the person seeks medical help, even though he or she may have been sick for quite a while, or may even have had a decrease in symptoms.
Symptom in Chief Complaint May be "Ticket of Admission"	May get the patient to the clinician's office or emergency room; the actual problem may be an entirely different symptom that the patient is at first afraid to mention, or it may be some life stress or crisis.

PRESENT ILLNESS

The **present illness** is a thorough elaboration of the chief complaint and other current symptoms starting from the time the patient last felt well until the present. In the patient interview you generally move from open-ended questions to more specific "Wh" questions (who, what, when, where, why, and how), laundry list questions (menus), or closed-ended questions, as appropriate, to achieve precision in symptom description. We describe each of these techniques in turn.

◆ PRACTICE POINT
The best strategy for the present illness part of the interview is often, first, to let the patient talk, then to use a variety of non-directive and directive questions to clarify and embellish the story.

Open-Ended Questions

Examples of open-ended questions are:

- "Can you tell me more about that?"
- "What else did you notice?"
- "What was the pain like for you?"

Another version of these open-ended questions is to restate them as gentle commands, requesting the patient to elaborate:

- "Tell me more about that."
- "Tell me what else you noticed."
- "Tell me what the pain was like."

Nondirective or open-ended questions are always a good way to start, allowing the patient freedom to talk and the examiner time to sit back and "size up" the patient. They are especially good for eliciting the less structured data of the present illness and the psychosocial aspects of the patient's problem. These questions allow the patient, who, after all, is the one who knows the story, to choose the most important symptoms and to point the way. The most nondirective of all statements are **minimal facilitators**—queries such as:

- "Yes?"
- "Uh huh?"
- "And?"
- "And what else?"

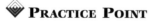 **PRACTICE POINT**

Nonverbal cues, such as nodding your head in agreement or smiling, also may serve as minimal encouragement for the patient to continue talking.

Directive Questions

Wh Questions

Nondirective questioning usually just sketches the picture, without giving precise detail. Patients only rarely volunteer all the needed details spontaneously; a rambling, vague patient may take too much time and still not provide the information you need, whereas a shy, reticent patient may offer little or no information. In a medical interview you move from the general to the more directive, but still open-ended, "**Wh-**" **questions: where, what, when, how, why, who.** These words describe the attributes of the patient's symptoms and specify the story. They are described in *Using" Wh-" Questions,* below.

WHAT TO SAY
Using "Wh-" Questions

Where

Exactly where is it on your body? *or* Show me where it is.

What

What does it feel like? *or* Tell me what it feels like.

When

When did it start? Does it come and go, or does it stay?
When does it occur (episodic, inception and duration, fluctuation, and frequency)?

How

How is it altered by season, by time of day, by sleep, by food, by exertion, and so forth? Describe how your daily activities affect it.

Why

Why do you think it occurs? Why do you think you have this problem?

Who

Who is affected by it? (consequences to patient and other people)

Laundry Lists and Menus

Patient disclosure of relevant clinical information is most strongly correlated with open-ended questions, but directive questions also are usually necessary to develop the patient narrative. **Laundry list questions,** or **menus,** are directive questions that are useful when a patient cannot find words to express a certain characteristic. The following examples include menus from which the patient is asked to select:

- "How would you describe this pain—sharp, dull, burning, or tight?"

- "Would you say the pain lasted a few seconds, a minute, 10 minutes?"

Such questions obviously exclude other descriptive words and should be used only when a nondirective approach ("Can you describe the pain?") and Wh questions ("What is the pain like?") have both failed.

Closed-Ended Questions

Closed-ended questions provide detail; they are good for emergency situations ("What's your name?"; "How old are you?"; "Are you allergic to any drugs?"), for reticent patients, and for structured data, such as the past history and the review of systems. They also are useful as focused questioning when you have already generated hypotheses in the interview and are trying to build a case for one particular diagnosis. Additional examples of closed-ended questions include:

- "Are your parents still living?"
- "Did you actually pass out?"
- "Have you ever been anemic?"
- "Does this pain occur when you take a deep breath?"
- "Do you have double vision?"

◆ PRACTICE POINT

Be aware that a "high control" interview, in which the interviewer asks one directive question after another, will produce false or incomplete evidence, not to mention a discontented patient.

You should not ask yes/no questions in situations in which information may be sensitive, because a lie will close off all access to further information on that topic. For example, it is not useful to say, "Do you drink alcohol?" if you suspect alcohol may be a problem; try, "How much alcohol do you usually drink in a day?"

Types of Questions to Avoid

Finally, there are certain types of questions to avoid:

- *Leading questions,* which encourage certain responses from the patient to fit the interviewer's own hypothesis, such as "You're feeling better now, aren't you?" or "That pain wasn't on the left side of your chest, was it?" This type of query suggests to the patient what you want (or don't want) to hear.

- *"Rapid fire" or multiple questions,* such as "Do you have any trouble sleeping and how about coughing?" Sometimes these slip out, because your mind is working too quickly and dragging your tongue along with it. Slow down; wait.
- *Jargon questions,* which presuppose knowledge of technical language—for example, "Have you ever had an MI?" or "Any COPD exacerbations?" A more understandable way of asking these questions would be:
  - "Have you ever had a heart attack?"
  - "How about your chronic bronchitis (or emphysema)—has it acted up recently?"

Sequencing Interview Questions, below, summarizes the various types of queries used in taking the medical history.

WHAT TO SAY
Sequencing Interview Questions

Start with ↓	Open-ended questions (general): "How can I help you?"
	Open-ended questions (topical): "Tell me more about your sore knee."
	Minimal facilitators: "And?" or "Um, hm …"
Proceed to	Wh questions: "Where exactly do you feel the pain?"
	Laundry lists or menus: "Does it feel sharp, or burning, or like pressure?"
	Closed-ended questions: "What did your mother die of?"
	Yes/no questions: "Do you smoke cigarettes?"
Avoid	Leading questions: "You haven't had any sexually transmitted diseases, have you?"
	Complex/multiple questions: "When did you first notice that sore on your toe? And has a doctor ever told you that you have diabetes?"

Symptom Description

Throughout the history of the present illness, it is important to describe the patient's symptoms as carefully as possible without jumping to conclusions. For example, "I'm having trouble breathing" does not necessarily indicate dyspnea on exertion; it could indicate stuffy nose or the chest sensation of a pregnant patient at term. It is also important to avoid jumping to conclusions about the meanings of words. Many words popularly used to describe symptoms have different meanings to different people. Examples are "diarrhea," "constipation," "tired," "dizzy," "my side," "sick," "weak," "high blood," "low blood," "insomnia," "gas," and "heartburn." The novice has a tendency to establish quantitative aspects of symptoms ("How many times a day?") before establishing the qualitative aspects. The expert interviewer attempts to characterize the quality of the symptom ("Are the stools soft or watery?") before quantifying it. *Pinpointing Symptoms,* below, presents examples of patient statements, followed by either quantitative (prematurely specific) or qualitative follow-up questions.

WHAT TO SAY
Pinpointing Symptoms

Complaint	Qualitative Questions (Ask these first.)	Quantitative Questions (Ask these next.)
I've been having chest pain.	What does it feel like? Where exactly is it located?	How long have you had it? How often does it come?
My side hurts.	Show me where.	How long have you had it?
I have diarrhea.	What do you mean by diarrhea?	How many times a day?
I vomited blood.	What did it look like?	How much?
I can't walk as far as I used to without getting tired.	What do you mean by "tired"?	How far can you walk?

Identifying the Intended Meaning of Words

"Dizziness" presents a prime example of a word that has different meanings to different people. A patient comes in and says, "My main problem is dizziness. It just came on me about a month ago, and it's been getting worse now. I'm so dizzy I can hardly stand up sometimes. What's wrong with me, Doc?" The first problem here is the word "dizziness." At least four symptoms are commonly labeled with this word:

- Vertigo—a definite sense of rotation or environmental motion.
- Presyncope—the sensation that loss of consciousness is about to occur.

- Disequilibrium—the sensation that balance, especially during walking, is impaired.
- Lightheadedness—a vague head sensation that is neither vertigo nor presyncope.

Some people also idiosyncratically label weakness, fatigue, or anxiety as dizziness.

The following exchange is an example of a clinician trying to find out precisely what a patient means by dizziness.

Clinician **Can you describe what you mean with words other than dizzy?**
Patient I feel out of balance. I feel like I might fall down even. I haven't yet, but I get awful woozy when I walk.
Is it mainly when you walk that you have trouble, or do you get this feeling sometimes when you are sitting or resting?
I guess it is mainly when I am up and around.
Can you tell me, then, how you feel bad when you walk? Try not to say dizzy.
Well, I feel I'm unsure of myself. I can't trust my walking.
Does everything around you spin or move, or do you feel like you're spinning?
No, not exactly.
Do you feel like you are going to faint?
I feel like I will fall, not faint.

Notice the mixture of open-ended and directive questions that the clinician uses to characterize as precisely as possible what the patient is experiencing. There is much more to find out about this symptom, but from the exchange so far the patient appears to be describing disequilibrium rather than vertigo, presyncope, or lightheadedness.

Following Up to Clarify the Symptoms

Consider another example; in the following interchange a patient has visited her clinician because of cough. Note how the clinician begins with an open-ended question, but specifies that she wishes to hear about the cough, and then follows up with Wh questions until the symptom is clearly specified.

Clinician **Tell me about the cough that you've been having.**
Patient It's just worse at night. I can't get no sleep.

What happens?
I'm up on three pillows. I'm just miserable, that's all.
You go up on three pillows to try to prevent the cough?
Yes.
How is it miserable?
Well, if I lay flat I can't breathe, and then I start gasping and gasping for breath, and the only way I can stop is when I sit up and watch TV or something.

The patient in this example actually suffered from congestive heart failure with orthopnea: she became short of breath when she lay flat in bed. She experienced tightness in her chest and a sense of "gasping" for breath that she chose to call "cough." Later in the conversation, the clinician learned that she had chest pain and dyspnea on exertion as well as these nocturnal symptoms.

Establishing a Pattern

In this next, longer example, the clinician wants to pin down the exact timing of the onset, duration, periodicity, and pattern of chest pain because he is concerned that this 62-year-old smoker may have coronary artery disease and knows that only precise symptom description will guide the diagnostic process. Each time the patient gives a somewhat vague statement, the clinician follows up with an attempt to clarify.

Patient   … and a little bit too fast, it might just be my imagination though, I don't know.
Clinician   **Uh huh. When did this all start? [Wh question]**
             Well, just since the weather has been hot, like it is, you know.
             Several weeks it's been going on, would you say? [clarification]
             Uh huh, just—now the chest pain is not continuous, like, during the day, I don't have to be doing anything, I can just be sitting.
             And where do you feel it? [Wh question]
             It's in here. And like full, just too full, it's fullness in here.
             And then how long does it last when it comes? [Wh question]
             Not too long.
             Minutes, hours? [clarification, laundry list]
             Not hours, just maybe a half hour, or something—you know, it doesn't last.
             Do you do anything that seems to relieve it? [Wh question]
             No, I don't take anything, just sit and be quiet, or either I'll rest.

Uh huh. [minimal facilitator]
And rest seems to help, when it starts acting up, whenever I could or would be doing around the house, I let it go and just rest.
Does it sometimes come on while you are doing something? [closed-ended question]
Yeah, mostly, if I'm doing something like trying to sweep or clean in the house, or something like that.
How about with walking? [clarification, closed-ended question]
With walking sometimes, and like mostly. I'll go up to the mall every day and that way I am inside walking and they have benches, I'll sit ... when it starts acting up.
And then how long does it take to go away once you sit? [Wh question]
Once I sit, oh, I'll say, half an hour to an hour.
And it will take a half hour or an hour to go away? [clarification]
... Uh huh.
Or do you sit for that long even though it's gone before that? [clarification]
Uh huh. I just sit for that long until it eases.
And it takes a half hour to an hour for it to ease up? [clarification]
Uh huh.

Notice how the clinician in this example tries to establish a pattern of chest pain brought on by exertion and relieved by rest. Perhaps the most critical detail to establish if one suspects coronary artery disease is the length of time it takes for the pain (in this patient, a "fullness" in the chest) to ease with rest. In typical angina, the pain ceases after several minutes or less. This patient's pain is not typical. It is likely that had the response been "less than 5 minutes" to the question "And then how long does it take to go away once you sit?" the clinician would not have requested further clarification.

Clarifying through Summarization and Confrontation

Two techniques that help to clarify what has been established during the patient interview include summarization and confrontation. **Summarization** is a technique by which the clinician feeds back to the patient the main points of what has been said thus far. Frequent summaries help to:

- Ensure that the interviewer has the story straight
- Provide focus
- Serve as transitions from one topic to another
- Keep the interviewer organized

A summary may be as simple as repeating a particularly important statement to confirm it, such as "Okay, as I understand it, the pains you had in 1998 were exactly like the ones you're having now." In other cases, a brief summary helps you get back on track if the patient is wandering and switching topics, for example, "Okay, we'll get to the cough in a minute, but I need to understand your chest pain better. You said it was like a heavy pressure right in the center of your chest, and it lasted about 5 minutes."

Summaries are also extremely useful as transitions from one part of the interview to another. Here is an example of a summary that segues from history of the present illness to the past medical history:

Patient   So that's about how it happened.
Clinician   **Okay, let me see if I have it straight. You felt perfectly well until 2 days ago, when you began to notice an uncomfortable feeling right in the middle here around your belly button, and this has gradually gotten worse, and you are now also having diarrhea. [Patient nods.] OK, I think I understand pretty well what's been going on the last 2 days. How about in the past, have you had any problems with your health in the past?**

Sometimes as you try to summarize, you note discrepancies in the story; and because you want to know exactly what happened, it is usually necessary to point out those discrepancies. When you do this, you are using **confrontation**. This rather dramatic word has connotations of pointing out falsehoods, rationalizations, or neurotic conflicts, and in its everyday usage often implies opposing sides. You need to find out which version is right. For example:

Clinician   **Now let me see if I can understand this. You said before that you were coughing up some bloody stuff with that heavy cough last year. But just now you said, when this cough developed yesterday, it was the first time you ever saw blood come up. Did I misunderstand you?**

In other words, confrontation is a device to clarify the data. You say what you heard, but ask for more detail, perhaps to resolve ambiguities, as in the earlier example of our patient with chest pain.

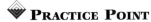 **PRACTICE POINT**

In the medical interview, confrontation is simply an attempt to clarify inconsistent statements; you heard one statement and now it appears that the patient is describing the experience differently, or contradicting an earlier statement.

BEGINNING THE INTERVIEW: THREE EXAMPLES

Here are three transcripts of beginnings of interviews. In each case, we have labeled the clinician's statements or questions with the technique being used. Note the importance, in this part of the interview, of social greetings, nondirective questions, minimal facilitators, clarification, and summarization.

Interview 1

Clinician **Okay, hello again. I'm Dr. Block. Tell me what I can do for you today. [social greeting, nondirective question]**

Patient Well, I have a terrible vaginal itch, and I don't know whether it's the vaginitis or whether it's the urine, urinary tract infection. My regular doctor treated me for vaginitis.

That was Dr. Hill? [clarification, facilitation]

Uh huh. Then I got, um, a urinary tract infection and then the vaginitis came back. But during the whole ordeal, I've never got any relief.

During the treatment for the vaginitis, during the treatment for the urinary tract infection, you still had this terrible itch? [summary, clarification]

Interview 2

Clinician **Good morning. [social greeting]**

Patient [Patient is seated on end of examination table.] Good morning.

Why don't you have a seat back over here, and we can talk a little bit first. Tell me why you came today. [attending to the patient's comfort, nondirective question]

Um, to get my blood pressure checked.

To get your blood pressure checked? What do you know about your blood pressure? [reflective response, nondirective question with topic specified]

Well, I have heard various things over the past couple of years, really, that it has been high, and um …

For several years? [clarification and facilitation]

[Nods] And I went about, oh, it was quite a while ago, maybe 5 or 6 months ago to the health center, um, and the doctor told me it was high, but he could not treat me until I lost approximately 38 pounds, so I haven't been able to take the weight off and I was kind of, well, he did not give me any special diet to follow or you know, what I should cut out of my diet, and I was very discouraged by it, so when I went to the emergency room because I cut my finger, um, the nurse told me that my blood pressure was very high and I should have it checked, and since I don't have a family doctor, she suggested I come here.

Interview 3

Clinician	**It's nice to see you again. What brings you here today? [social greeting, open-ended question]**
Patient	Doctor, I'm not well.

I take it you have not been feeling really well for a while. [summary based on previous knowledge of this patient]

No, well, I haven't been feeling very good for about the last, oh, I'd say about a week, about a week now.

Uh huh. [facilitation]

About a week now, I haven't been feeling good.

What have you noticed? [nondirective question]

Oh, some soreness in here right through here, and some pain in my arm and a, a, a strangulating feeling right in here and a burning in the, in the middle, right here and a burning in my throat, a little bit, and dizzy—I felt real dizzy when I was on the scale out there, you know, and I called you and the nurse, and she helped me and I wasn't real bad and you know, I told her to open a window and she said first, "Do you want me to open a window?" and I said, "Yeah and I want to get near the air."

Does that help? [clarification]

Oh yeah.

CHALLENGES TO ELICITING THE CHIEF COMPLAINT AND PRESENT ILLNESS

The patient's speaking style may present challenges in getting a coherent story. The profoundly depressed patient may not have enough energy to give a detailed, logical story, whereas the anxious and talkative patient may embellish his or her story with unnecessary details. Some patients are so reticent that you find yourself asking a series of narrow, closed-ended questions until the interview comes to a distressing stop. Other patients have so much to say that you feel as though you are losing control in a confusing quagmire. You worry that, when the interview is over, you may know everything but the information you really need to begin to put together a differential diagnosis.

The Reticent Patient

The Problem

The reticent patient says little or nothing. When only a limited amount of information is needed (e.g., a patient with an acute laceration or a sore throat), this may not be a problem. There are other times, however, when lack of detail seriously compromises history taking, such as for the 62-year-old smoker on page 60 with chest pain, in whom a detailed and unambiguous history is essential for making the diagnosis.

The Remedy

The goal here is to guide the reticent patient without asking leading questions; sometimes one way of asking an open-ended question works whereas another way does not. Consider this example:

Clinician   **Can you tell me what the problem is?**
Patient   Uh, that's what I came to see you about, Doc.
            What have your symptoms been?
            Tired, awful tired.

It almost appears as though the interview will come to an end with the first question, but the interviewer simply asks another open-ended question that, this time around, elicits the chief complaint. A "laundry list" or menu is another useful technique. This interview went on:

Clinician   **Can you tell me more about it?**
Patient   No, just tired.
            When you say tired, do you mean a feeling of not being rested or a feeling of weakness in your muscles? Or do you have trouble doing things you used to do because you get short of breath?
            That's it, Doc, just not rested.

The clinician uses a menu to clarify the symptom without leading the patient. Notice the difference between asking the patient to choose from several possibilities and raising the same possibilities in a sequence of yes/no questions. In the latter case, you can never be sure that the patient is not simply saying what he or she thinks you want to hear.

Patients may be reticent because of depression, dementia (simply cannot remember the symptoms), anxiety, denial, a taciturn personality style, or cultural distance from the clinician. Some patients expect to be interrogated like witnesses. These persons may have trouble with an open directive such as "Tell me what happened," and they may respond better to more structure: "Tell me what happened first," and then, "What happened next?" They may need frequent reminders demonstrating your open, relaxed attitude, such as "It is important for me to know exactly how you felt when that happened—tell me as best you can."

The Rambling Patient

The Problem

Some patients embellish their problems with numerous seemingly unrelated details. In other settings such persons might be considered wonderful storytellers, but you have a limited amount of time for the interview and entertainment is not your goal. Sometimes the details seem connected to the story, as with our rambling patient on page 49; at other times it is difficult to see the connection. At times the details are related but unnecessary, as with the patient who has an attack of diarrhea and describes in excruciating detail his or her attempt to find a bathroom.

The Remedy

The goal is to direct the patient back to the task at hand without appearing to be rude or uninterested. One way to do this is to acknowledge your own confusion and feeling of being lost, as well as your need to accomplish the task at hand. Most patients accept this kind of direction well. For example, you might say to the patient with diarrhea:

Clinician   **It certainly sounds as though you had a hard time with that episode; since our time is limited, though, perhaps you can tell me more about the diarrhea itself. Tell me what it was like.**

In this instance the clinician uses a summary statement ("sounds as though you had a hard time") and a reminder of time constraints, followed by a question that directs the interview back to the characterization of the symptoms.

In the case of the rambling patient on page 49, an interviewer's open-ended question ("Now what can I do for you, Mrs. P?") leads to a deluge of disconnected information that would leave most clinicians feeling totally bewildered. Although this patient may have revealed most of her medical history in one fell swoop, it is difficult to sort out. Many clinicians are reluctant to ask open-ended questions because they fear precisely this kind of rambling response. In reality such responses are infrequent. When they do occur, it is best to acknowledge your confusion and try to direct the patient to one topic at a time. One possible reply might be:

Clinician **Okay, I'm getting a bit confused. Let's see if we can take one problem at a time. You mentioned tiredness even though you seem to get a lot of sleep. Other than the hot flashes, is there anything else that seems to wake you up at night?**

Either during or after the interview, you will have a chance to think about why the patient talks this way. Among the causes are anxiety, loneliness, histrionic personality style, thought disorder, or a particular set of beliefs about how symptoms and events are related. Sometimes this kind of response represents the person's conversational style, which is less appropriate in the context of a professional relationship than it is in a social interaction. Sometimes the associations are so bizarre that you must consider psychiatric illness as the cause.

The Vague Patient

The Problem

With the vague patient, the interviewer cannot figure out exactly what the patient is describing. You may wonder whether the symptom itself is vague or whether the patient is simply unable to describe it. Some sensations are difficult to characterize, such as dizziness or poorly localized abdominal pain. When you know the patient, it is easier to judge the source of the problem. The patient who, in the past, has always given a precise history is probably experiencing a vague sensation, whereas a patient who has a vague conversational style may well have a precise symptom that simply requires more work to translate into medically useful words.

The Remedy

One technique for the vague patient is to provide a choice of useful descriptors. For example, you might use a menu such as, "Was the pain sharp, dull, or burning?" or "Was it all over, or in just one place, or did it move from place to place?" Alternatively, you can ask if it resembles a symptom with which both the patient and clinician are familiar, such as (for lower abdominal or pelvic pain in a woman), "Does it feel anything like menstrual cramps?" Another approach is to ask the patient if he or she has ever felt anything like this particular symptom before, and then to ask, "What's different about it this time?" To find the location of a vague symptom, you can ask the patient to point to where it hurts.

In this example of a vague opening, the clinician simply indicates that vague terminology such as "cold" or "flu" ("tell me more about what you mean") is unacceptable, and the patient begins to describe the symptoms in more detail.

Clinician	**What can I do for you?**
Patient	[Clearing throat] I think I've got, um, a cold or flu or something … yesterday I felt terrible, so I feel I just need some kind of a prescription.
	OK. Tell me, you say you have a cold; tell me more about what you mean.
	Um [Clearing throat] fatigue is the most …
	Fatigue?
	Just kind of drained.
	Aha.
	Kind of scratchy throat, not really sore. Ah, a lot of drainage …
	Coughing?
	A little bit, but not getting anything up.
	Just sort of dry?
	Dry coughing, I don't feel as though there's anything collected down there yet. And, that's another thing that worries me, having had a history of asthma, I have a fear of bronchitis.

Sometimes the patient does not respond to simple requests for more precision.

Patient	Well, doctor, well, I got the dizziness, I'm getting more, looks like I'm, looks like I'm getting tired and more tired, I go up the steps and I just, just like dizziness, I, I go like this, I just go dark, I, and I can't see.
Clinician	**What do you mean by dizziness?**

> When I go up the steps and when I get up in the morning, I got that dizziness again, I'm just falling back.
> **What happens to you when you're dizzy?**
> Well, when, when I drink water, if I drink cold water, that's when I get it, then I start having chills, I get real cold, just like I'm shaking.
> **But how do you feel when you're dizzy?**
> I just go back, like this, and then sometimes I, I can't see, I, I have to close my eyes like that and then open my eyes up like that and I still can't just like ...

In this example, we are left wondering whether the patient's description is vague or the symptom is vague. The clinician could have tried asking, "Tell me what you mean, but try not to use the word dizzy." Another possibility would be to provide a menu.

Clinician	**When you say dizziness, is it a feeling that you may pass out or that you may lose your balance?**
Patient	No, not exactly.
	Could you describe it as a spinning sensation as though you or the room is moving, or is it more of a lightheadedness?
	That's it, lightheaded, just lightheaded.

Whether the patient is reticent, rambling, or vague, the clinician's goal is to obtain a story that is clear, internally consistent, logical, and not fictional. Most patients share these goals but may not necessarily share the same criteria for judging the story. Your first approach is to clarify, teach, or demonstrate the kind of story that will be helpful. If this approach does not work, you are probably faced with one or more of these three issues.

- The patient's personality style, perhaps stressed by the illness, interferes with telling an adequate story.
- A strong emotion gets in the way of the patient's telling a clear, logical story.
- The patient's beliefs are sufficiently different from yours that a story that appears incoherent is actually quite logical once you understand the basic premises from which the patient reasons.

We will examine these issues in Chapter 12, Cultural Competence in the Interview, and Chapter 13, Difficult Patient-Clinician Interactions.

SUMMARY—Chief Complaint and Present Illness

In this chapter we discussed, first, how to set the interview stage and get started. Take these steps:

- Establish a sense of privacy for the interview.
- Introduce yourself appropriately and establish a contract.
- Maintain an attentive body position.
- Minimize distractions.
- Take notes but maintain enough eye contact so as not to "lose" the patient.
- Use language the patient can understand.
  The next steps are to:
- Obtain and record the chief complaint in the patient's own words.
- Consider the possibility that the iatrotropic stimulus, or actual reason for coming, is different from the ostensible chief complaint.
- Let the patient complete his or her opening statement.
  With regard to the history of the present illness, we presented the following facilitative techniques:
- Move from the general to the specific, using open-ended questions to introduce each topic.
- Use nonverbal encouragement, such as silence and head nods; and minimal facilitators, such as mirrors, paraphrases, and saying "Uh huh," "And?" or "Yes?"
- Proceed to Wh questions to characterize symptoms.
- Employ menus or direct questions when necessary for specification or efficiency.
- Strive for interchangeable responses to show that you are listening and to encourage disclosure of accurate information about thoughts and feelings.
- Avoid leading questions that reveal the answer you expect or desire, or multiple questions that confuse the patient.
- Give the patient time to answer in his or her own words.
- Clarify and maintain direction for both the patient and yourself by using summaries, clarification, and, when needed, confrontation.
  Among the challenges to obtaining a good narrative are various interactive styles, including those involving patients who are reticent, rambling, or vague. Attention to technique helps overcome these challenges.

CHAPTER 4

Other Active Problems, Past Medical History, and Family History

Transforming Experience into Memory

To hold a true belief about an event in one's past experience is not sufficient for remembering it. There is still a distinctive factor lacking ... Now it sometimes happens that a belief ... transforms itself into a memory.

A. J. Ayer, *The Problem of Knowledge*

CONTINUING WITH THE INTERVIEW

Once you have elicited the chief complaint and present illness, other parts of the history, although tedious at first, are, in a sense, easier because they deal with structured data and specific questions about predetermined topics. The goal is to emphasize the relevant features of past health and medical care experiences without getting too overwhelmed with a mass of detail. Feinstein (1967) has cautioned us to avoid the "Scylla of over-direction" and the "Charybdis of digression." By this he means the ability to keep your inquiry open-ended enough to avoid missing the important events without getting bogged down in endless details about unimportant events.

This chapter and the two that follow—Chapter 5, The Patient Profile, and Chapter 6, The Sexual History—cover parts of the medical interview that fill in the total picture of your patient's health and illness experience. These aspects of the interview provide important details that enhance your evaluation of the person's current illness and your response to it. In this chapter, we discuss the search for other active problems, the past medical history, and the family history. These components provide you with information about the context or setting in which the illness occurs, including the previous state of the patient's health, as well as the presence of risk factors that have implications for both the current diagnosis and the prevention of future ills.

OTHER ACTIVE PROBLEMS

You have just made it through the history of the present illness, working hard to maintain the narrative thread (what happened first, what happened next) without getting sidetracked by distractions, such as a too-early preoccupation with what the diagnosis is. You begin to build the themes of the interview: what the story of the illness is, who the patient is, how the interview is going. You progressively narrow your focus to delineate a single problem or condition that you hope will explain the patient's symptoms and findings. At this point, however, you should step back and ask yourself: What am I missing here? What else could be going on with this patient? In other words, what are the patient's **other active problems** (OAPs)?

Patients often have a number of chronic conditions that may affect their current distress. The notion of a singular "present illness" quite distinct from "past medical history" is not tenable: the patient who comes to the emergency room because of fever and productive cough may at the same time be under treatment for diabetes, hypertension, coronary artery disease, and osteoporosis. In this case, the patient has several medical problems, any of which may contribute to the current syndrome or must be considered in responding to it. Thus, it is crucial to differentiate these problems from the traditional items in past medical history (e.g., appendectomy in 1996, motor vehicle accident in 1999, allergy to ciprofloxacin noted in 2001).

Technique in This Part of the Interview

The search for OAPs may be accomplished by asking nondirective questions at the end of the present illness segment of the interview. A good way to begin might be with a summary statement as to what you have heard so far, followed by a transition to this new topic with an open-ended question. For example:

- "Okay, I think I've gotten the story straight so far. Has anything else been bothering you?"

- "Aside from your chest pain, can you think of other symptoms or problems that you've had recently?"
- "In addition to your diabetes, do you have any other illnesses that have been acting up lately, or that you see a doctor for?"

In this way other problems that relate to, or influence, the present illness may be uncovered early, thereby avoiding last-minute surprises during the review of systems. A patient may be admitted to the hospital with pneumonia but may also suffer from chronic renal failure, diabetes, and hypertension. These chronic illnesses are also current problems that affect the situation at hand because they require ongoing care and may complicate the main problem.

Another good screening question for OAPs, especially in the case of reticent patients, is, "What medications do you take?" ("Insulin shots" may be the response of the patient who forgot to mention she suffers from diabetes.) Regardless of how the patient responds, always broaden your inquiry to include any regularly used drugs, such as oral contraceptives (which the patient may not consider a *medication*), aspirin, cold preparations, pain relievers, herbal remedies, or over-the-counter laxatives. Remember also to ask about vitamins or mineral tablets. Because many people consider these "natural" products and not medications, they may not mention them unless specifically asked.

Prompting with Open-Ended Questions

Here is an example of an interview in which a 62-year-old retired metal worker came to the office for a complete checkup "because I've never really had one." The clinician picks up on OAPs at the end of the present illness segment. Notice the summary statement, followed by a transition with an open-ended question.

Clinician	**Okay, so the main concern you have, aside from wanting a checkup, is this pain in your left side. Are you having any other problems with your health?**
Patient	No, nothing really. As I said, the main thing is to establish a relationship with a family doctor.
	Okay, that's good. Let me find out a little more about you. Do you take any medications?
	Yeah, well, Dr. Gold has had me on that Vasoretic for a few years for my pressure.

Notice how this patient, like many people, requires repeated open-ended prompts to reveal continuing and obviously important details about his health. What is going on here? Certainly, the patient is not trying to hide the fact that he takes medication for hypertension; indeed, high blood pressure may have become so much a part of his life that he doesn't initially label it as a "problem." Most likely, the clinician would have stumbled on this information later in the interview during an extensive past medical history or review of systems, but it is an important feature to know early in a routine checkup. Chronic illnesses such as hypertension make a difference.

ELICITING THE PAST MEDICAL HISTORY

To begin asking your patient about his or her medical history, see *Eliciting the Past Medical History,* below. Patients may respond in general terms such as, "I've always been sickly," or "Well, I used to have stomach problems," or, alternatively, begin to discuss particular symptoms. Adult patients frequently have one or more chronic illnesses, and each of these may have had several exacerbations or have required hospitalizations at different times. They may or may not be relevant to the current illness. You should focus the inquiry on discrete episodes that caused substantial disability or a difference in the patient's usual health status, and attempt to determine the diagnosis that the patient, or his or her clinician, has given to these illnesses.

WHAT TO SAY
Eliciting the Past Medical History

To develop a solid background of your patient's past medical history:
- Begin with a summary statement ("I think I understand what's going on right now.")
- Follow with a transition that introduces the new topic ("So I'd like to find out how your health has been in the past.")
- Follow with an open-ended question, such as:
  - "Have you had any health problems?" or
  - "Tell me about how your health has been in the past."
- Then fill in more detail with open-ended questions that specify certain topics, such as:
  - "Tell me about any serious illnesses you have had in the past, starting from when you were a child."

- ■ Use these other examples:
  - ■ "Tell me about any surgical procedures you have had."
  - ■ "Have you had any emotional or psychiatric problems in the past?"

You should never simply assume that a diagnosis the patient relates is, in fact, the correct medical diagnosis. For example, a patient might tell you that he has had "four or five heart attacks" in the past when, in fact, he has never suffered an acute myocardial infarction; this problem arises because the term "heart attack" means different things to different people. A good question to ask is, "What exactly were your symptoms that made your doctor think that?"

◆ PRACTICE POINT

Never assume that a diagnosis the patient relates is correct. Ask the patient exactly what his symptoms are to make your diagnosis.

There is no point, however, in trying to confirm every item of the past history by pushing the patient on obscure details. Your time and energy and those of the patient are limited. Here is how one clinician, who himself became a patient, expressed his feelings about being asked "ancient history."

Clinician   **It's bad enough that I don't know all my family's medical diseases or what my grandparents, whom I never knew, died of, but I begin to feel positively stupid when at the mature age of 44 I do not know whether as an infant I had measles or chickenpox. I may do a little better with more recent conditions, but the feeling sinks again when it comes to medications I've taken that have given me trouble. "Those little red pills" seems an insufficient answer, and the recording physician's dubious look does not help much . . . . By this point in the interview, when I am asked questions about the specific timing and location of my varying symptoms, I begin to answer with a specificity born more of desperation than accuracy. (Eisenberg and Kleinman, 1980)**

After you acquire general information about the patient's past health, you fill in important categories of past medical history (as shown in *Content of the Past Medical History,* page XX). Old records can and should be obtained when you believe the information will be relevant to caring for the patient.

CONTENT OF THE PAST MEDICAL HISTORY

The categories listed here will lend clues to the patient's current illness. Use them when obtaining the patient's past medical history.

- Serious illnesses, beginning in childhood
- Hospitalizations
- Surgical procedures
- Accidents or injuries
- Gynecologic and obstetrical history (women)
- Allergies
- Current medications
- Immunizations
- Screening procedures (Papanicolaou test, mammogram)

Here are a few pointers on specificity:

- **Dates.** The exact date or year of an illness, if remote, is generally not important. Inquiry that is too precise will lead both to frustration and to falsely precise answers ("specificity born of desperation"). A "hysterectomy in the early 1970s" is usually adequate; it does not matter whether it was 1972 or 1973.
- **Allergies.** You should clarify what your patient means by the term "allergy." A person may tell you he is allergic to flu shots because, after having one, he had several colds that winter, or another may tell you that she is allergic to aspirin because it gives her stomach discomfort. The first case is a personal attribution of a poor outcome, and the second case illustrates an adverse effect rather than a true allergy to aspirin. Be sure to ask specifically about allergies to medications.

Here is an example of a past medical history obtained from a 39-year-old woman at her first office visit for evaluation of headaches. She was found to have elevated blood pressure. Note the ease with which the clinician prepares the patient for each new topic.

Clinician **Okay, let's talk about your past health. Did you have any unusual childhood illnesses, problems at birth or as an infant?**
Patient   Bronchitis.
             Bronchitis. What do you mean by bronchitis?

Well, I'm not sure. That's what my mother told me. I guess I used to get sick a lot when I was a kid.

Were you ever hospitalized? Any serious illnesses or operations?

Well, I've had D&Cs done, and I had my appendix out with part of my ovary.

Part of your ovary came out and ... ?

Well, I have a history of cysts growing on my ovaries. My gynecologist says I'm okay now.

Now, you mentioned you have two children. Any problems with your pregnancies or with childbirth?

With my little girl, yes. I had a lot of water, plus I had a bladder infection.

Did you have high blood pressure with that?

No, but I was sick a lot, nauseated a lot. It was like morning sickness but I had it for 8 months with her.

Doctor put you to bed at all?

No.

Any other hospitalizations, any other medical problems in the past that you had that you can remember?

No, just the D&Cs and the children and that one operation I had.

Do you have any allergies?

I am allergic to goldenrod.

To what?

Goldenrod. Wool. I have hay fever. Anything like flowers—I get around them, I constantly sneeze my head off or get stuffed up. Roses, stuff like that. Right now, I'm having a time because we went up to the lake and we have a lot of goldenrod growing wild.

Do you take anything for it?

This is an example of a fairly typical past history that demonstrates how old news is relevant to present problems. Notice how the interviewer asks exactly what the patient means by bronchitis; although the patient is not sure, she later reports symptoms of allergy. Symptoms of allergy plus a childhood history of bronchitis suggest atopy, with the "bronchitis" perhaps representing episodes of childhood asthma. The patient may now have "outgrown" her asthma but she still has an atopic disposition, as evidenced by the hay fever symptoms. The clinician also uncovers the history of fluid retention during pregnancy. This symptom could indicate preeclampsia, which may be relevant to her current hypertension. Notice how the interviewer asks specifically if the patient had high blood pressure. He also tries to determine if she was treated for hypertension without realizing it by asking, "Doctor put you to bed at all?" Another way to ask would be, "How was that treated?" The question regarding whether the patient takes anything for her hay fever is relevant for at least three reasons:

- To avoid the embarrassment of recommending something the patient has already tried
- To help ascertain symptom severity
- To learn if medications that can raise blood pressure in susceptible persons (such as pseudoephedrine, commonly used in cold and allergy remedies) were used

FAMILY HISTORY

The **family history** is the systematic exploration of the presence or absence of disease in the patient's family that may influence the patient's health or risk of particular diseases. What illnesses and conditions are relevant? They include:

- Hereditary diseases, such as sickle cell anemia or osteogenesis imperfecta
- Familial illnesses, such as coronary artery disease, diabetes mellitus, or breast cancer, in which genetic factors play a significant role
- Family traits, such as short stature
- Illnesses such as bipolar disorder or alcoholism, which may not only be familial, but may also profoundly affect the patient's psychosocial environment
- Current illnesses in the family that may suggest an infectious process or common toxic exposure

What do we actually mean by "family"? To determine the risk of hereditary disease, we generally mean the patient's parents, siblings, and children. The patient's grandparents, cousins, aunts, and uncles are of somewhat lesser importance. The spouse or significant other or partner is a vital member of the patient's family but is of no importance to familial disease. In dealing with contagious disease and toxic exposures, however, we might expand the concept of "family" to include the whole household, perhaps in this instance even including coworkers.

Tailoring the Family History

The family history always enriches our understanding of the patient, whether in making a diagnosis or in managing the illness, but because time and energy are limited, a potentially enormous amount of information must be tailored to the specific situation. How much we want to know depends on the patient, the type of problem, and the ability of the patient to give the information. For example, a family history of breast cancer is obviously of less relevance to a 10-year-old boy with tonsillitis than to a 45-year-old woman with a breast mass. A seriously ill patient may have a very relevant family history but be too sick to give it. This might be the situation, say, in a critically ill patient with an acute myocardial infarction whose father died of a heart attack at age 44; the family history can wait until the patient feels well enough to remember and discuss the details. *Technique in the Routine Family History,* below, presents good ways to begin taking your patient's family history.

WHAT TO SAY

Technique in the Routine Family History

- Start with a transition, such as:
  - "Now, I'd like to know a little about your family."
- Follow with an open-ended question, such as:
  - "Are there any illnesses that seem to run in your family?" or
  - "Has anyone in your family been seriously ill?"
- Then proceed to more specific questions, such as:
  - "How about your parents? Children?" or
  - "Has anyone in your family had heart attacks?"
- Finally, check for emotional content with questions, such as:
  - "Do you have any concerns about problems that you think run in your family?"

In the case of needing to rule out exposure to contagious disease, you must inquire not only about the family but also about other possible sources or contacts. For example:

- "Has anyone else at home or work been sick lately?"
- "Have you come into contact with anyone who has similar symptoms?"

Here is an excerpt of a routine family history that will give you a sense of the flow of this part of the medical interview. Notice how the clinician first provides a transition to the new subject area and then proceeds with a specific question.

Clinician   **Okay. I think I understand the symptoms. Now I'd like to find out a little about your family. How about your parents, are they still living?**
Patient   They're deceased.
             Do you recall what they passed away from?
             My mother had a heart attack 2 months ago.
             How old was she at that time?
             63, I think.
             How about your father?
             About 7 years ago.
             What did he pass away from?
             Lung cancer.
             How old was he?
             Oh, I'd say 57.
             Brothers or sisters?
             Yes, I have nine brothers—I mean I have five brothers and three sisters.
             Do they have medical problems that you are aware of?
             No.
             Is there any history of high blood pressure in the family?
             My mother.
             Your mother, okay. How about diabetes?
             No.

The clinician begins with a general question about problems or illnesses, then follows with some specific yes/no questions about illnesses frequently found in families, such as hypertension and diabetes.

But we observe something else here. Notice that the patient's mother is *recently* deceased. The clinician here faces a choice about how to proceed, given this information. Should she explore the patient's feelings about his mother's death, or continue with the family history? In this instance, the interviewer proceeds with the history, an approach that appears to be useful. Had the patient's mother died at an advanced age after increasing illness or disability, the clinician would expect the patient to feel differently than if she died suddenly at a relatively young age. A potential problem here is that the clinician accepts the stated diagnosis of "heart attack" and learns little more. Was it a sudden event? Were there many previous attacks? Was she sickly for years, perhaps with rheumatic heart disease and a final deadly attack? And what of the resulting effects on this person—the patient—with a sickly mother? The clinician will, later in the interview, return to her recent loss and deal with it more effectively. Everyone has feelings about his or her close relatives, especially parents and children. We must acknowledge, be prepared for, and deal with these feelings in a compassionate way during this part of the interview.

 PRACTICE POINT

Because the family history deals with people for whom the patient has strong feelings, the information is both clinically relevant and emotionally charged.

The Past Shapes the Future

Knowledge about family history shapes the patient's beliefs and worries about health, health risks, and current symptoms. A patient with chest pain may believe that she has a bad heart like her mother, even though she is young and suffering from a totally different condition. A patient approaching the same age at which a parent died may have special concerns about his or her own health. Consider this family history in a 41-year-old woman who came because "it's been a while since I had a good checkup."

Clinician   **Your parents still living?**

Patient   My father is living. My mother died when she was 42.

              How is your father? Is he in good health?

              Uh huh.

              How old is he?

              He was born in 1933.

              So he's 71.

              Yes.

              Any brothers or sisters?

              Two sisters. Both are in good health as far as I know. I don't keep very good contact with them, because I live here and they live out of state.

              Any medical problems? You said there are some medical problems that run in your family. What are they again?

              My mother had a bad heart. Most of it is in my mother's family. Like my grandmother died, she had cancer. She had diabetes, too. When my mother died, she had had a plastic valve put in, then slowly deteriorated. She had sclerosis of the liver and a bad heart. She lived about a year after she had the plastic valve put in.

A woman who dies at age 42 after having a prosthetic valve implanted probably had rheumatic, or possibly congenital, heart disease. Although there is a chance that the daughter may suffer from a similar problem, of more relevance are the daughter's beliefs about the matter. Note that she is age 41 and her mother died at age 42. If she is found to have no signs of heart disease, it will be important to reassure her that her symptoms are totally unrelated to what went on with her mother.

Even the most straightforward questions sometimes lead to double-edged answers:

Clinician	**You said you've been pregnant five times?**
Patient	Yes.
	Do your children live at home with you?
	Yes.
	Five of them?
	Yes.
	How old are they?
	20, 15, 13, 10.
	That's four children.
	Oh, I lost one.
	Did he die of disease?
	No, he died—he had a little growth on his eye and he died in surgery.

The interviewer who uses a mechanical set of family history questions could have simply ignored the fact that she listed only four ages. Although the death of her child seems to have no strictly medical bearing on the case, a parent who has lost a child will certainly have feelings attached to the memory of the event and may also have negative feelings about the medical system, which, she may believe, caused or failed to prevent her child's death.

Keeping It Routine

In some cases, discussion of family history may cause the patient to become anxious. In asking about family diseases, you imply a possible relationship to the patient's current medical problem. It is helpful to emphasize the "routine" nature of the inquiry. Here is an example of a clinician who stumbles on anxiety-provoking information in asking a routine family history question.

Clinician	**Yeah, okay. Very good. Now your mother and father, what did they. … Are they still alive?**
Patient	Um, my mother is alive, my …
	Age?

Notice how the clinician hesitates over the initial question, realizing that the first fact he needs to know is whether the parents are living; then, barely listening to the response, he asks another question. The dialogue continues:

Patient	She is 64.
Clinician	**She have any illnesses you know of?**
	Uh …
	Heart disease, lung disease, anything?
	No, nothing of that sort; she's had a well-known skin cancer and uh, and she seems to have a recurring, it's a problem with her back, but actually it's a nerve that has to be blocked every once in a while.
	Okay. Your father?
	I never really knew that much about my father, but as I understand it he died of a cerebral hemorrhage.
	How old was he?
	Oh, he must have been in his early 40s.
	Was an autopsy done or anything to find out … ?
	There was so little … there was a bad occurrence, bad divorce between our mother and father when I was real young and I never saw him after age 9 months really. So I'm very hazy on the particulars of this.

The clinician here stumbles on two kinds of loaded information: (1) the father died of a cerebral hemorrhage at about the same age the patient is now, and (2) the patient does not know much about it because of a "bad occurrence." The clinician ignores the "bad occurrence" and goes after a possible cause of the hemorrhage, a cerebral aneurysm being relevant here because this condition can be hereditary.

Clinician	**But nobody knew whether it was traumatic; did he get hit or anything?**
Patient	I don't know the details, to tell you the truth. He had, well, I just don't really know enough to talk about it.
	Cerebral hemorrhage at a young age would be an unusual thing. No other causes being known.
	I could find out more, my mother may know more about it.
	If she knew, it would be important to you–if she would know,

for instance, if he had an aneurysm in his brain that burst, which is one of the ways you can have a cerebral hemorrhage at a young age. I think that would be very important, for instance, for your general health information, so perhaps you can find out. Okay? Do you know anything more in terms of other problems?

Note the interviewer's graphic description of "an aneurysm in his brain that burst" and the statement that this "would be very important" while quickly moving on to "other problems." The patient, whom we first met in Chapter 2, Respect, Genuineness, and Empathy, now goes on to talk about the "painful subject" while the clinician completely ignores the affective content.

Patient   Well, my understanding is, the context of this, that my mother was raised in the Catholic church and divorce was a terrible scandal in her mind, and she tried to forget about it as quickly as she could. It's such a painful subject that there was never any discussion about who he was and so forth. And as a consequence, all I've really heard are niblets, and one of the things I understand is that he was an alcoholic, or at least had a problem with alcohol, but really caused my mother a lot of problems. So, I don't know if that would be a complicating factor in terms of aneurysm or not.

Clinician **Not that I know of. How about brothers and sisters?**
I have one full natural brother and then four half-brothers.
Any medical problems in any of them that you know of?
No.

This example demonstrates insensitivity to the patient's feelings and self-disclosure. It also shows that, by pursuing an item of family history, the clinician can increase the patient's anxiety and raise new questions in the patient's mind about his or her own health. A person who tells you that his sister had breast cancer, that his father (who smoked two packs of cigarettes per day for 40 years) developed lung cancer, or that his uncle (an asbestos worker) died from mesothelioma may feel that he is at high risk for developing the same diseases, or some other form of cancer. The more you press for details, the more your patient may believe that there is a connection with his or her present illness. Such a patient may need reassurance that he or she is not at special risk, if the environmental risk factors do not apply.

Another source of anxiety arises from the psychological bias called **availability.** An unusual illness that happens to occur in a family member is highly visible and "available" to the patient. Therefore, it has a greater impact on his or her fears than we, as clinicians, might feel is justified. We look at the disease statistically and understand that it is not familial and that the chance of its occurring twice in a small number of people is extremely remote. However, as a clinical student, resident, or practicing clinician, you will find that availability plagues you all the time, just as it plagues your patients. After you diagnose your first case of glioblastoma multiforme, you are likely to overreact to your next group of patients who complain of headaches. For the same reasons, you must be especially sensitive to the anxieties of the dizzy patient whose sister has multiple sclerosis, or the mother of a child with vomiting and recent varicella whose nephew had Reye's syndrome.

- Make it clear that taking a family history is a routine part of your complete medical interview.
- Listen carefully for any emotional overlay or any connections made by the patient between family illnesses and his or her own.
- Demand no more detail than is required.
- If the patient does become anxious, direct your attention to the anxiety by allowing the patient to express his or her concerns directly. In some cases, you may have to give an additive response (see Chapter 2, Respect, Genuineness, and Empathy) to relate the patient's free-floating anxiety to some unconsciously held causal belief (e.g., the coincidence of the patient's current age and her mother's age at the time she died).

◆ PRACTICE POINT

You can avoid creating anxiety by being clear about why you need the information, being sensitive to the patient's responses, and being informative in your explanations.

SUMMARY — Other Active Problems, Past Medical History, and Family History

In this chapter we discussed the importance of searching for OAPs in addition to the present illness. We learned to:

- Complete the history of present illness and then open up the interview again with a summary statement and transition with nondirective questions to search for OAPs

- Question about current medications or other conditions under treatment, which is a good method of screening for OAPs

The information you gather about the patient's past medical history helps to fill in the context of the present illness. We learned to:

- Introduce the past medical history with a general question or statement, such as "I'd like to know a little more about how your health has been in the past," which indicates the transition to a new topic
- Ask about the details of past illness based on present needs
- Identify what the patient means by "allergy"—making sure to distinguish true allergy from adverse effects

Finally, the information you gather about the patient's family history is helpful for hereditary diseases, family traits, and such polygenetic conditions as heart disease, diabetes, and cancer. Be sensitive to the social and psychological or emotional dimensions of the information you obtain, particularly in the family history.

CHAPTER 5

The Patient Profile

Gaining Richness and Reality

Dialogue ... can exhibit the object from each point
of view, and show it to us in the round, as a sculp-
tor shows us things, gaining in this manner all
the richness and reality of effect that comes from
those side issues that are suddenly suggested by
the central idea in progress, and really illumine
the idea more completely, or from those felicitous
after-thoughts that give a fuller completeness to
the central scheme, and yet convey something
of the delicate charm of chance.

Oscar Wilde, *The Critic as Artist*

UNDERSTANDING THE PATIENT PROFILE

The patient profile, also called the **social history,** is the part of the medical interview in which we attempt to learn about the patient as a person.
Illness is not only disordered pathophysiology; illness happens to a person and involves changes in the person's feelings and abilities. Moreover,
getting sick, seeking care, getting well, and staying well all have social
determinants, sometimes only an influence but sometimes a direct cause,
as with accidents or domestic violence.

◆ PRACTICE POINT
Making therapeutic decisions requires knowledge of the patient as
a person.

The importance of the social history may not be readily apparent in
the acute hospital setting, where diagnostic and therapeutic objectives are

set on an hour-to-hour (if not minute-to-minute) basis. In this artificial setting, knowing how the illness is experienced by the patient or what the patient's lifestyle is like seems much less important than knowing about the disease process. That this view is artificial becomes readily apparent when it is time to discharge the patient, and then the social environment and family support system become critical. You may ask yourself, for example:

- How many stairs will my patient have to climb?
- Who will prepare her food?
- How will he juggle the complicated medication schedule? Can he afford his medications?
- How much will his employment allow changes in lifestyle necessitated by the illness?
- How will this young mother with lumbar disc herniation pick up her baby?
- How will this heavy equipment operator with carpal tunnel syndrome perform his job?

Hospital stays are shorter than they used to be, so patients tend to be sicker when discharged and require more support in the home environment. Moreover, most medical care occurs outside the hospital. Office visits involve chronic and recurrent conditions that interact continuously with the patient's life circumstances.

Traditionally, we place the patient profile in a separate section of the written case history as if the social history were a self-contained aspect of the interview, but this is an arbitrary separation for the sake of organization only. The social history can be critical in helping to make the diagnosis. For example, patients with sexually transmitted diseases and personality disorders are cases where the social history may actually be part of the history of the present illness.

You are continually acquiring social information throughout the interview from "small talk" or "chit-chat," the patient's manner of dress and speech, and demographic information that may appear on the patient's chart. Another important aspect of your interaction is assessing educational level and intelligence, both of which are critical to your ability to communicate successfully; much of this assessment is done automatically as you converse at your patient's level of comprehension and in a manner appropriate to his or her life experience.

How Much Do I Need to Know?

Just as it is a mistake to believe that there is such a thing as a "complete" review of systems, it is also a mistake to believe that there is a "complete" patient profile. You have time constraints. How do you limit the inquiry so as to avoid a lengthy assessment? What is relevant in the limited time you have? What information must be obtained when the patient is first admitted to the hospital or on the first office visit, and what can be developed over the course of a hospital stay or a long-term relationship? Unless the situation is an emergency, your goal is to learn enough, at least, to answer three questions. How do the patient's personal characteristics or lifestyle:

- Contribute to the etiology of this illness?
- Aggravate or limit the severity of illness?
- Interfere or help with getting well?

◆ Practice Point

Begin the patient profile with general questions about the patient's recent life and experience. For example:
- **"Can you tell me a little about yourself? Your family? Your work?"**
- **"How have things been going for you otherwise? At home? At work? In your marriage?"**
- **"Tell me what else has been going on in your life."**

The degree of completeness needed depends on the situation. Some information may emerge in the course of the interview without specific questioning, and often data are not acquired initially, but over time as you get to know the patient and understand what is relevant to his or her care. Keep in mind that the idea is to find out the patient's strengths and weaknesses and the nature of his or her support system, if any. How has this person coped with illness or other stress in the past? How does he or she keep distress within manageable limits?

◆ Practice Point

Remember, more intimate data are easily and reliably obtained when you know the patient better, whether later in your initial history, in the interview, in the hospital, or, perhaps, even years later. Tailor what you need to know to the situation at hand.

Often one of the most useful parts of an entire history is a detailed description of what the patient usually does on an ordinary day and exactly how this is modified by the illness. For example, a person who may be suffering from dementia may describe a typical day that may be more revealing than a mental status examination would be, particularly when the dementia is mild. The description may also be more clinically important, because what really counts is how the patient functions in the environment, not how the patient performs on a mental status test.

EXPLORING THE TYPICAL PATIENT PROFILE

In the following sections we explore the components of a typical patient profile or social history, including:

- Demographics and occupational history
- Nutrition and diet
- Daily activities and exercise
- Alcohol, tobacco, and recreational drug use
- Spirituality and beliefs
- Relationships

The sexual history and alternative lifestyles are discussed in Chapter 6.

Demographics and Occupational History

The patient's age, education, race or ethnic background, religion, and residence are among the most fundamental data in the patient profile. However, we often minimize or forget the occupational history when conducting a medical interview. We may find out that the patient is a lawyer, a plumber, or an information technology specialist, but that is the end of it; for example, "This patient is a 45-year-old farm worker." Period. Nothing further about what kind of farming he does, what chemicals he might be exposed to, or how much of the year he is employed. Yet specific information about employment, school, or retirement is vital to understanding the patient's lifestyle and his or her economic and social support system. Does the patient have financial problems related to unemployment or underemployment? Is the retired person actively involved in hobbies, sports, or volunteer work? Is the patient coping well with being a working wife and mother? How does she unwind from the rigors of a 45-minute daily commute?

Asking about Occupation

Most people spend a significant part of their waking lives in an occupational environment. Moreover, one's employment or profession contributes substantially to one's sense of personal identity. Almost the first question we ask when speaking with a new acquaintance is, "What do you do for a living?" In a certain sense, we *are* what we do. Thus, when you are evaluating a person's illness, or providing a person with preventive health care, it seems reasonable that the answers to "what do you do?" (and "how and where do you do it?") will contribute importantly to your ability to provide appropriate care for the patient. *Essentials of a Quick Occupational Survey,* below, presents one approach for obtaining a brief occupational history, either for screening purposes or, if indicated, as an entrée to more detailed exploration.

WHAT TO SAY
Essentials of a Quick Occupational Survey

- "Do you work outside your home?"
- "What kind of work do you do?"
- "Tell me what that job is like for you."
- "Is that what you've always done? What other jobs have you held in the past?"
- "Do you now—or did you in the past—have exposure to fumes, chemicals, dust, loud noise, or radiation?"
- "Do you think anything at work (or at home) is affecting your symptoms now? How about stress at work?"

Consider the following exchange between a clinician and his new patient being seen for fatigue:

Clinician **And what do you do for a living, Ms. Nelson?**
Patient   I'm a secretary. I've been back to work for about 5 years now.
             You mean after the children?
             Yes, I started back when my youngest went to first grade.
             OK. And how are things at home?

In this case the clinician places Ms. Nelson into the secretarial category and quickly moves on with the interview. Her fatigue may or may not be related to the job—perhaps she has a stressful office environment, which should be explored—but the clinician is unlikely to investigate further the role of chemical exposures in causing her symptoms. However, what might happen if the clinician asks for more detail about Ms. Nelson's employment?

Clinician **And where do you work?**
Patient   At Johnson Environmental, up in Cadiz.
             Johnson? What do they do?
             You know, clean up spills, sewage, that sort of thing. A lot of our work is out East now, you know, in farms and vineyards. We do a lot of that in the summer.
             Do you ever get out in the field?
             Well, in a way. My boss has me working out of our trailer at Stebson Farms for the last 2 months, which is a problem because it's a 45-minute commute and I'm not used to that.

In fact, what the clinician eventually discovers is that there may be more of a problem than the commute itself. The company had a large abatement contract that involved potential exposure to organophosphate pesticides. Ms. Nelson worked in a trailer, which had been placed on-site in a dusty, windy field. As a secretary, she was not required to wear a respirator or protective clothing like the field workers. Her blood cholinesterase levels were found to be significantly low, indicating organophosphate toxicity, which may well have been the cause of her progressively worsening fatigue.

The key details of what the person actually does on the job will reveal more of the patient's occupational history. For example, a patient who works for the phone company may be a manager, a telephone installer, or a maintenance person who works out-of-doors on telephone lines. Similarly, a steelworker may operate heavy equipment, drive a truck, or work in an office. Each specific job exposes the patient to different risks, ranging from chronic stress to chemical exposure to serious accidents.

Nutrition and Diet

Your patients may have strong beliefs about the role of diet in their health and many will have tried popular weight-reduction plans and vitamin supplements. Often you will recommend dietary changes, such as reduction in fats or increase in dietary fiber, for both primary prevention and treatment of disease. Specific food intolerance (e.g., lactose intolerance), food allergies, the condition of the patient's teeth, the ability to shop for and prepare food, income, and ethnic and cultural influences (which may be resistant to change) all affect dietary habits.

◈ PRACTICE POINT

To give appropriate nutritional advice, you will need to understand your patient's eating habits.

An Efficient Nutrition and Dietary Survey, below, provides a guideline for the patient's nutritional history. The question "Tell me about your diet" may be misinterpreted if the patient is not on a weight-reduction diet. Details are important. If the patient has toast for breakfast and a sandwich for lunch, find out what goes on the toast and between the two slices of bread. If your initial screen leaves you wondering if the patient might have an eating disorder (for example, a description of bizarre eating habits), additional directive questions may be helpful in pinpointing the problem. Such questions include:

- Do you think you are fat?
- Do you make yourself sick if you feel you are too full?
- Do you worry about losing control over food?
- Do you feel that food dominates your life?

WHAT TO SAY
An Efficient Nutrition and Dietary Survey

A. Initial screen

■ "Are you happy with your (present) weight? Any recent gain or loss? What did you weigh a year ago?"
■ "Tell me what's been happening with your weight."
■ "Are there any major food groups that you either eat a lot of or don't eat at all?"

B. Then, depending on the answers and the clinical situation: (e.g., is the patient's weight normal? Are there drug-food interactions?)

■ "Tell me more about your eating habits."
■ "How many meals do you eat each day? Do you snack between meals? What about eating in the evening, after dinner, or at bedtime?"

■ "Do you have any trouble taking your medications because some of them need to be taken with food, or on an empty stomach?"

■ Are there any foods that make you sick or that you think you might be allergic to?

C. Then, more specific, depending on the clinical situation

■ "Tell me about your intake of:
  ■ Salt (for patients with congestive heart failure or hypertension)
  ■ Fiber (for patients with chronic constipation, hemorrhoids, or diverticulosis)
  ■ Dairy products (for patients with possible lactose intolerance or patients who need calcium)
  ■ Fat (for patients who are overweight or have hyperlipidemia)
  ■ Caffeine (especially for patients with palpitations, tremors, or anxiety symptoms)"

■ "Tell me what you've eaten over the last 24 hours, beginning with just before you came to the office and working back."

■ "Is this a typical day for you? How is it different?"

Daily Activities and Exercise

How your patient spends a typical day reveals additional factors that contribute to illness or facilitate getting well. For example, the sedentary retired salesman will need an explicit and graded exercise program with frequent monitoring of his progress as he recuperates from a myocardial infarction. People who are constantly on the go, eating on the run, and rarely preparing their own food may need to undertake major and difficult changes to treat obesity and hyperlipidemia.

Describing the patient's type and intensity of physical activity is a major feature in the patient profile. Vague answers such as "I like to play tennis" or "I have a rowing machine at home" are not necessarily indicators of regular aerobic exercise. Perhaps the patient has not had time for tennis for the past several years or the rowing machine has sat unused in the basement. To monitor your patient's health effects, you must inquire specifically about regularity and duration, as well as manner, of exercise. As you do this, you can also assess the potential for various types of trauma that result from sports and exercise programs (e.g., stress fractures in joggers, major knee injuries in skiers).

Alcohol, Tobacco, and Recreational Drug Use

You should ascertain the amount, frequency, and context of the patient's use of alcohol, tobacco, and recreational drugs. For example, when asked, "How much do you smoke?" many smokers reply, "Too much." Notice how there is no quantification in this answer; the reply is colored by the patient's awareness that it is "wrong" to smoke. It may be easier for such patients to talk more neutrally about what age they started to smoke or how many times they have tried to quit.

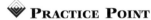 **PRACTICE POINT**

Assessing truthfulness is a common problem when eliciting alcohol, smoking, and drug histories because these are sensitive topics, and most people—both patients and health care professionals—feel that there are "right" and "wrong" answers.

Here is a smoking history obtained from a 40-year-old man presenting with shortness of breath. The interviewer tries to find out exactly how much is "not too much", and also tries to determine whether the patient's current respiratory symptoms caused him to cut down and whether the cumulative smoking history is sufficient to cause such medical problems as chronic bronchitis or perhaps lung cancer.

Clinician	**Okay. How much do you smoke?**
Patient	Oh, not too much.
	How much is not too much?
	Oh, umm, not half a pack a day.
	Is that as much as you've always smoked? Have you ever smoked more than that?
	Uh, when I was barbering, I would smoke more, sometimes a pack. You know, but they would burn out. You know, because when I was doing a customer or something, they'd burn out, so I'd just light up another one.
	Uh hmm. How old were you when you started?
	Thirteen.

A Digression on Truth Telling

Similarly, use of recreational drugs or excessive alcohol intake is seen by most patients as a habit of which the clinician will disapprove. Some will deny the use of these substances, particularly if asked a yes/no question. Here is an example of an interviewer (who can smell alcohol on the patient's breath) trying to elicit the history of alcohol use in a 28-year-old woman presenting for evaluation of hypertension.

Clinician	**You are using some aspirin and Tylenol?**
Patient	Every once in a while. It's not regular, but that's the only drugs I take.
	And are you a pretty steady drinker?
	I have one or two drinks at work, you know. After work I …
	… Okay. Do you have any more than that?
	Sometimes it's more than that but basically …
	Is that something that would be hard for you to give up?
	Well, it's a very social type thing for me, I guess … so … yeah, I'd have to think about it, ha ha.

Often in this situation it is not so much what the patient says, but how she says it. This patient paused and looked away, and began to use phrases such as "you know" and hedges like "basically." She also displayed some nervous laughter. These are often clues that a person is telling less than the truth. You may notice pauses (time to censor material), shifts in position, eye aversion, and hedges in the verbalization, such as "not really" instead of "no." The most revealing question in this example is the indirect one ("Is that something that would be hard for you to give up?"), to which the patient's answer ranges from denial ("Well, it's a very social type thing") to agreement ("I guess so, yeah") to ambivalence ("I'd have to think about it. Another patient with a history of narcotic addiction, when asked about his current drug use, replied, "No, not much. I mean some. Yeah, I'm using." It is rarely useful to tell a patient that you doubt the accuracy of his or her story, especially when you have not already built a relationship. You should make a mental note of the behavior, however, in the hope that in the future you will be able to use the information to help the patient. *Screening Your Patients for Problem Drinking,* below, presents questions widely used to screen patients with suspected alcohol problems.

WHAT TO SAY
Screening Your Patients for Problem Drinking
CAGE Questions

C Have you ever felt you ought to **cut down** on your drinking?

A Have people **annoyed** you by criticizing your drinking?

G Have you ever felt bad or **guilty** about our drinking?

E Have you ever had a drink first thing in the morning (***eye opener***) to steady your nerves or get rid of a hangover?

If all answers are negative, problem drinking is not likely. If one or more are positive, explore further the role of alcohol in the patient's life. Or, ask both:

■ Have you ever had a drinking problem?

■ Was your last drink within the past 24 hours? Or, when was your last drink?

These two questions together have a high predictive value. If the patient answers yes to both, there is a high risk of a drinking problem; those who answer no to both have a low risk of having a drinking problem.

TWEAK Questions

These questions may be optimal to identify women with alcohol abuse or dependence in ethnically diverse populations:

T *Tolerance.* How many drinks does it take before you feel the first effects of alcohol?

W *Worried.* Have close friends or family worried or complained about your drinking in the past year?

E *Eye openers.* Do you sometimes take a drink in the morning when you first get up?

A *Amnesia.* Has a friend or family member told you about things you said or did while you were drinking that you could not remember?

K *Kut down.* Do you sometimes feel the need to cut down on your drinking?

◈ PRACTICE POINT

Recreational drug use and narcotic addiction, particularly when the clinician may potentially be the patient's source of drugs, is a difficult situation that demands careful attention to both the substance and style of the patient's statements.

Spirituality and Beliefs

The existential or spiritual dimension of life includes a person's deepest beliefs and values and includes questions such as: Who am I? Where do I come from? Where am I going? What gives meaning to my life? Spirituality is often expressed as a religion or a relationship with God, but other forms of experience or belief may also constitute spirituality: for example, a passionate love of nature, a sense of oneness with the universe, or a deep moral commitment to helping others in need. Intense involvement with a 12-step program such as Alcoholics Anonymous is for some people also a form of spirituality.

◆ **PRACTICE POINT**

For most patients spiritual values influence their experience of illness, especially their understanding of what the illness means, how they should respond to it, and what the outcome will be. It is important to distinguish between personal spirituality and active practice of a specific religion.

Many patients will express only loose affiliation with a religious tradition, or identify themselves as nonpracticing. Others will express considerable hostility toward "organized" religion in general, or declare themselves atheists. Such antireligious positions do not necessarily mean that the patient lacks deep spiritual values. Alternatively, regular religious service attendance or frequent participation in church activities is not necessarily an indicator of spirituality. Some participate for social or business reasons, or to provide what they believe to be a wholesome atmosphere for their children.

Understanding Religious and Spiritual Perspectives

There are several health-related reasons to learn about your patient's religious and spiritual perspectives:

- *As a potential protective factor for morbidity and mortality.*
  Epidemiological studies consistently demonstrate that people
  who actively practice their religion—any religion—tend to live
  longer and have better health parameters (e.g., less disability,
  less substance abuse, more social support) than nonpractitioners.
- *As an influence on the personal experience of illness and expectations
  for treatment and healing.* This reason may be of particular importance when religious beliefs restrict or prohibit certain forms of
  treatment, such as blood transfusion with Jehovah's Witnesses.
- *As an existential resource for understanding illness and suffering.*
  Although spirituality is potentially an important component of
  any patient's well-being, the more progressive, prolonged, and
  threatening an illness becomes, the more likely it is that the
  patient will turn for strength and support to spiritual values.
- *As a resource for assistance and social support.* Religious groups
  may provide an enormous amount of practical assistance to
  needy and disabled members of their congregations.

As discussed further in Chapter 14, Telling Bad News, spiritual assessment is crucial in the care of dying patients and is often a factor in discussions about living wills or advance directives. *A Stepwise Approach to Spiritual Assessment,* below, presents FICA, a useful acronym for asking about spirituality as part of the complete patient profile. The first three steps (faith, influence, and community) can be accomplished quickly. For example, here is a clinician interviewing a new patient who has come in for an "executive physical":

Clinician	**Now I want to ask a couple of questions about what means most to you. Do you see yourself as a spiritual person?**
Patient	Uh, I don't know … I don't think I've ever been asked that [pauses]. I was raised a Catholic, you know, but haven't practiced, not since the kids were young. … We don't usually go to church. [Another pause] But, you know, I feel that God is everywhere in nature, all around.

WHAT TO SAY
A Stepwise Approach to Spiritual Assessment

F **Faith** Do you consider yourself a spiritual or religious person?
Tell me more about that.
What things do you believe in that give meaning to your life?

I **Influence** Are these beliefs important in your life?
Does this belief influence how you take care of yourself?
How has your belief influenced your behavior during this illness?
What role do these beliefs play in regaining your health?

C **Community** Are you part of a spiritual or religious community?
Is this community a support to you? How?

A **Address** How would you like me, your clinician, to address these issues in your health care?

Adapted from Pulchalski CM, Romer AL. "Taking a spiritual history allows clinicians to understand patients more fully." *J Palliat Med* 2000; 3:129–137.

With a single question, this clinician has learned that the patient comes from a Catholic tradition (see step "F" in *A Stepwise Approach to Spiritual Assessment,* above), but he is not a part of a practicing community (see step "C"). It is unclear how much influence (see step "I") the Catholic tradition has in his life, although he has suggested another deeply felt faith or experience (God-in-nature) that might be of importance to him in coping with illness. It seems unlikely that the clinician will need to go further at this point. However, when patients with serious illness express strong spiritual commitment, it is important for the clinician to ask whether (or how) they wish to have their spirituality addressed (see step "A") in their health care.

Consider this second example, in which a primary care physician is newly evaluating a middle-aged patient with metabolic syndrome (obesity, hypertension, and elevated blood sugar and lipids):

Clinician	**And do you consider yourself a spiritual person?**
Patient	Absolutely not. I'll tell you—my wife was religious. You know, kids in Sunday school, Bible study, the whole bit. What good did it do her? Did God prevent her from getting cancer when she was only 36? Did God save her from suffering? And those condescending bastards from her church that kept coming around and preaching to her.... If you ask me, religion is a disease.

This patient may possibly have other deep commitments of a spiritual nature, but it would be counterproductive to pursue them at this point. The clinician has learned that her patient remains angry about his wife's early death from cancer and that he finds God (or the absence of God) responsible both for her death and his continuing grief. It will be important for the clinician to learn more about his life since his wife's untimely death, both from a clinical (e.g., depression, weight gain), and a social (e.g., job, social network) perspective.

We consider further sociocultural aspects of illness and the impact of the patient's health beliefs and expectations in Chapter 12, Cultural Competence in the Interview, and Chapter 14, Telling Bad News.

Relationships

You have begun to develop an idea of the patient's relationships, including his or her support system, when you know the answers to questions such as:

- Who lives in the household?
- Are there family members nearby who are willing and able to help in times of crisis?
- Has there been recent bereavement? (Widowed persons have higher rates of illness and death, particularly during the first year of widowhood.)

- What kind of help does the young mother have with her new baby?
- Who will care for the elderly, demented woman when her husband (who normally cares for her) has his hernia surgery?

As you answer these questions, you also develop a sense of the patient's relationship with his or her spouse or significant other. You may not need to ask direct questions about it. Because patients may regard this information as intimate and possibly unrelated to their illness, it is often best to ask questions in a somewhat indirect and open-ended manner, which permits patients to reveal as much or as little as they wish. You may begin, for example, with questions relating the patient's illness to the current state of the relationship: "How has your being on chemotherapy affected your husband?" Such questions allow the patient to say anything from "Okay" to "Well, we've had our rough spots but things are pretty good right now" to "To tell you the truth, I wanted to leave him, but I'm too sick now." Once the patient has indicated an interest in discussing the relationship, more specific questions are useful, such as:

- "What are some of the good and bad aspects about your present relationship?"
- "What would you change?"

In addition to the impact of illness on relationships and of relationships on illness, certain diagnoses or clues to diagnoses reside in the story of the patient's relationships. For example, the criteria for diagnosing certain personality disorders lie in the patient's history of difficult relationships with family, friends, and employers.

Domestic Violence

Domestic violence, also known as *intimate partner violence*, was long considered a strictly "private" matter by both health professionals and law enforcement. Now it is recognized as a serious public health problem, sufficiently prevalent to justify screening in the medical setting. *Detecting Domestic Violence: The "SAFE" Questions*, page 102, outlines an approach to screening for domestic violence that begins with less threatening and somewhat general questions, and progresses to more specific queries that focus on the patient's safety. Note how each question allows the patient to answer from his or her own point of view, avoiding judgmental wording and remaining open ended.

WHAT TO SAY
Detecting Domestic Violence: The "SAFE" Questions
Stress/Safety

- What stress do you experience in your relationships?
- Do you feel safe in your relationships?
- Should I be concerned for your safety?

Afraid/Abused

- Are there situations in your relationships where you have felt afraid?
- Has your partner ever threatened or abused you or your children?
- Have you been physically hurt or threatened by your partner?
- Has your partner forced you to have sexual intercourse?

Friends/Family

- If you have been hurt, are your friends or family aware of it?
- Do you think you could tell them if you have been hurt?
- Would they be able to give you support?

Emergency Plan

- Do you have a safe place to go and the resources you need in an emergency situation?
- If you are in danger now, would you like help in locating a shelter?
- Would you like to talk with a social worker (a counselor, or me) to develop an emergency plan?

◆ PRACTICE POINT
Detecting relationships that are physically or emotionally abusive is an important function of the patient profile.

Here is an example of a 52-year-old professional, a victim of domestic violence, with a history of breast cancer and recent treatment for clinical depression. She is seeing her clinician for a routine office visit.

Patient   The other thing I wanted to talk about is going back on Zoloft because it works for me but I'm not sure I need it.

Clinician   Tell me more.

Well … my husband and I may be separating, so things are stressful. In the morning I feel pretty low and I don't want to get out of bed, but then once I get to work I feel okay and then I feel okay for the rest of the day.

Any sleep problems?

No.

Any problems with your energy, concentration, being irritable?

No, no, I'm okay that way.

[Knowing the past history of an abusive relationship] You know, with this going on at home, how are you feeling about your safety?

[slowly] Okay, right now.

Do you know what to do if you don't feel safe?

Yes, I have to leave. I have friends I can go to, and I have the number of the women's shelter.

Notice how the clinician asks in an open-ended and nonjudgmental way about the patient's safety and ensures that she has a plan. The clinician should also perform a quick screen for depression.

THE PATIENT PROFILE IN PRACTICE

Here is an example that demonstrates the importance of the patient profile, or social history, in the diagnosis and management of medical problems. A 61-year-old woman with diabetes and hypertension urgently scheduled a visit to her family clinician complaining of chest pain, headache, and increasing concern about her blood pressure. The clinician, confused about which problem was really the chief complaint, because the symptoms were chronic and the blood pressure under control, asked the patient to clarify her concerns:

Clinician **Uh, what, what would you say is worrying you the most right now?**

Patient Well, mostly, is how, getting those bills paid. See, I'm on, I'm on assistance.

Oh, I see. Tell me more about this worry. Did something new happen?

Mostly it's a gas bill and then, um, see I own a house. I have the taxes, keeping up with them, and, ah, just finances generally.

Did you recently get your gas bill?

Yes, I did.

When did that come?

Yes, ah, it came the other day.

The clinician had in mind a menu consisting of the three ostensible problems—chest pain, headache, and blood pressure—and was actually trying to ask the patient to choose among them in order to direct her focus to the patient's main area of concern. Instead, she asked the question in a more open-ended manner and used the word "worry" to describe what she was looking for. This technique provoked an entirely unexpected response. In this instance, the social problem was *the* problem. Notice how the clinician then looked for positive or confirmatory evidence that it was the patient's inability to pay the gas bill that was really bothering her. This doesn't mean that her chest pain, headaches, and high blood pressure weren't "real," but it was helpful in answering the "why now" question—that is, why the patient sought care at this particular time for symptoms that had not changed.

SUMMARY—The Patient Profile

We close this chapter with key elements of the patient profile and some typical questions you might ask to begin to explore them. These questions are simply examples of how one might choose to screen for these elements on an initial visit with the patient. Keep in mind the basic technique of going from general to more specific questions, and less intimate to more intimate topics as you develop your relationship with the patient.

KEY ELEMENTS OF THE PATIENT PROFILE

Topics	*Typical Screening Questions*
Demographics and Occupation	
Age, gender, race, ethnic group, religion, marital status, education, occupation	• Now that I know something about your symptoms, tell me a little about yourself. All I know is that you're 53 years old and married.
	• What kind of work do you do? What exactly does that job involve?
Lifestyle	
Nutrition and diet	• Tell me a bit about yourself.
Daily activities and exercise	• What is an average day like for you?
Cigarette, alcohol, and recreational drug use	• What's your diet like? Tell me what you eat on an average day.
	• Do you have time for regular exercise?
	• Do you smoke cigarettes?

Topics	Typical Screening Questions
Relationships	
Family and household composition	• Now tell me about your family. You've been married how long? Do you have any children?
Support system	
Marital and other significant relationships	• Any stresses or problems with your family?
Sexual history	• Any problems in your marriage?
Spirituality	• How is your sexual relationship?
	• Do you consider yourself a spiritual or religious person? Tell me more about that.
Health Beliefs and Expectations	
Personal health beliefs (see Chapter 12)	• What are you hoping to get out of this visit today?
Culturally determined health practices (see Chapter 12)	• Do you have any concerns about taking medication?
Use of complementary and alternative medicine (see Chapter 15)	• Do you take care of your health (or health problems) in other ways, or use other, nonmedical kinds of treatment?
Provision for surrogate decision making (see Chapter 14)	• Do you have an advance directive or living will?

CHAPTER 6

The Sexual History

Sex Is Something I Don't Understand Too Hot

Sex is something I really don't understand
too hot ... I keep making up these rules for
myself, and then I break them right away.
J.D. Salinger, *The Catcher in the Rye*

UNDERSTANDING THE SEXUAL HISTORY

Sexual functioning is an essential part of life experience and is also an important factor in caring for patients. Every day, clinicians deal with issues related to sexual functioning, from conception and contraception, infertility, sexually transmitted diseases, and erectile dysfunction, to rape or incest and abuse. Sexual contact may be the source of the patient's illness, as with HIV, hepatitis B, and human papillomavirus; and knowledge of the patient's sexual orientation and behavior drives your diagnostic hypotheses and guides your plans to screen and educate the patient. In addition, depression, anxiety, and anger may be related to the patient's underlying sexual problems; conversely, many physical diseases or medications can lead to sexual dysfunction.

Despite its importance and place as part of the "routine" patient profile, most of us find sexuality a difficult topic to address in our conversations with patients. We live in a culture that is, on the one hand, characterized by lack of information and secrecy about sex and, on the other, by sexually explicit entertainment and advertising, not to mention easy access to pornography over the Internet. We may find questions about sexual orientation and behavior difficult to ask, and patients may find them difficult to answer. A young person may readily accept your question about sexual preference, whereas an older adult may think you are being inappropriate. Likewise, patients of different cultures

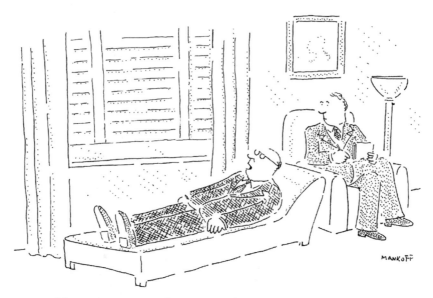

"Frankly, I've repressed my sexuality for so long I've actually
forgotten what my orientation is."

may have radically different views about the propriety of discussing
sexual issues.

Here's how one patient describes the reaction of her physician to
discussing a sexual problem:

Patient   There's something I need to talk to you about; it's from last time and I
            thought I could set it aside but I can't. ... This is really hard. Okay, when
            I started to talk about my sexual relationships you sat back and went
            like this [patient demonstrates folding arms across chest] and it made
            me feel like I had done the wrong thing by bringing it up. And then
            when I called you, I felt that you really rushed me off the phone and I
            figured you were mad at me because of what I had said about my sex
            life. Because I used to jump into bed with every guy and I feel so
            ashamed. Now I think, what's the point?

Next, consider this not uncommon example of how an outpatient,
whose chief complaint relates to a sexual problem, dances around the
issue, digresses, and finally gets to the point with open-ended prompting:

**Clinician   Hi, good morning. Long time no see, it's good to see you. Why
            did you decide to get a physical now?**

Patient	Well, it's just that, well [patient seems anxious] you know, I'm getting older and I kinda figured it's been a while.

Yeah, it has, it's been almost 5 years since I last saw you and did a physical on you.

Well, I've been in more recently than that and saw someone else. Actually I wanted to mention that to you because you see I have this way of clearing my throat [patient demonstrates a kind of half cough] and I do it constantly and your associate put me on Claritin for it and I thought that was a lazy approach, without actually figuring out what's causing it. I mean, shouldn't I have been tested for allergies or something?

Well, I'll make that a part of our evaluation today. Let me get an idea, first, what else is on your list?

Well, this is embarrassing to talk about. But my sexual performance, I'm concerned about my sexual performance.

Tell me more. How long has it been going on?

Well, it started about 18 months ago [patient having difficulty going on] …

And is it that you're having trouble maintaining an erection?

Well it's the strength and the duration. Maybe I'm just getting old, it's an age thing. I didn't tell my wife I was going to talk to you about this.

Techniques for Facilitating the Sexual History

What are some techniques to make the sexual history part of the interview easier? First, if the patient answers a general question about sexuality in the negative, no more need be said; you have, however, indicated that sexual concerns are legitimate fare for discussion, for either you or the patient to initiate. You may continue with other aspects of the history, at the same time building rapport, and return later to the sexual history, if necessary.

◆ PRACTICE POINT

Remember, there is no requirement to get a "complete" sexual history from every patient. Sometimes a few screening questions may suffice, such as "Are you having any sexual problems?" "Are you concerned about your risk of any sexually transmitted diseases?" These questions may be asked during the review of systems.

Second, once you know more about whether the patient is married or living with someone, it is easier to ask about sexual preference and activity. When in doubt about the patient's sexual preference, you should use the term "partner" rather than gender-specific terms such as "boyfriend" or "wife." If you ask only about opposite-sex partners, the patient may infer that you anticipate only heterosexual activity, and a homosexual patient may avoid relating his or her actual sexual preference. (On the other hand, the married 75-year-old male patient may well be offended by use of the term "partner.")

 PRACTICE POINT

Finding out more information about your patient as a person facilitates asking more specific questions about sexuality.

Third, delaying the sexual history until later in the interview allows you to become familiar with the patient's language, therefore making it easier to use words that he or she can understand. As with other intimate bodily functions (voiding and defecating), patients may describe their sexual functioning with words conditioned by their age, education, and cultural background. Other descriptions may be idiosyncratic and obscure. Never assume that your patient knows what such words as "relationship," "birth control," or "safe sex" mean.

 PRACTICE POINT

Open-ended questions permit the patient to use his or her own words; in your follow-up questions, you then can use the patient's own words, thereby ensuring a common basis for understanding.

INITIAL SCREENING

Beginning the Sexual History, below, presents some useful ways to initiate the patient's sexual history. If your patient indicates problem areas, then proceed with more detailed questioning.

WHAT TO SAY
Beginning the Sexual History

To begin the patient's sexual history, use introductory statements and transparency, which can ease the transition to a potentially difficult topic. Here are several examples:

- "I always include questions about sexual problems in my routine history because they're so common. Have you had any problems?"

- "I know sexual concerns can be difficult to discuss, especially with a total stranger, but it sounds as if you have some concerns. Tell me more."
- "It's important that I ask about your sexual partners and about when you first started having intercourse so I can help you avoid certain illnesses. Is that okay?"
- "Are you having any sexual problems?"
- "Do you have any questions or concerns about sexuality or sexual functioning?"
- "Many people who are ill experience a change in their sexual function. Have you noticed any change?"
- "Has your interest in sex changed recently? Since you've been ill?"
- "A lot of men have sexual problems when they take blood pressure medicine. Have you noticed any problems?"
- "It sounds as though your marriage has been a good one. How about your sexual relationship?"
- "Many girls (or boys) your age have questions about sex and birth control. How about you?"
- "Many people these days worry about AIDS. Do you have any concerns about being at risk for AIDS?"

◈ PRACTICE POINT

As with the patient profile, proceed from less intimate to more intimate and from open-ended to closed-ended questions. Another useful technique in this part of the interview is revealing why you are asking certain questions, what we call transparency.

The sexual history should be more extensive, for example, when a patient requests birth control, fears a sexually transmitted disease, or has a sexual problem, such as erectile dysfunction or change in libido, as a presenting complaint. Consider this example of a 41-year-old male whose chief complaint is "no desire":

Clinician	Hi, I haven't seen you for a while. How can I help you? (open-ended question)
Patient	Well, doc, I just have no interest in sex at all. I thought maybe I needed to work out so I started going to the gym. I thought maybe it was that and I started a dietary supplement, I've been taking GNC men's formula. I'm playing racquetball. And then I started reading stuff and read something about testosterone levels so that's why I'm here.

Okay. How long has this been going on? (facilitation, open-ended question)

Well it started maybe a year, year-and-a-half ago. My wife's afraid it's her but our relationship is better than it's ever been. We're going to church together now, we have these two great kids, our jobs are good; we're so lucky.

Uh huh. (facilitation)

We are pretty tired, I'm really tired. I get home from work and all I want to do is eat supper and get into bed.

When you do have sex, do you have any problems? (topic specified but question open-ended)

Well, that part is fine, at least it was until about a month ago and that's when I made this appointment because I couldn't keep my erection. But that was the first time that happened.

Have you noticed anything else? You know, sometimes when a person loses their desire, it's part of some physical or emotional problem. Have you felt sick in any way? Weight loss? Headaches? (transparency, open-ended to more closed-ended questions)

No, nothing like that. Overall, I feel good.

Any feelings of depression, or loss of interest in other things? Any trouble or change in enjoying things you've always enjoyed?

No, that's what's funny about this.

Using Open-Ended Questions, Facilitation, and Transparency

The key to getting the patient's sexual history started is to observe good basic interviewing technique as the clinician does in this example. Start with open-ended questions and facilitation so it is unnecessary to ask very specific questions. This clinician also displays transparency, disclosing the reasoning behind certain questions to make the patient more comfortable with what otherwise might seem as obscure or intrusive.

If this patient had been more reticent, the clinician may have had to ask specific questions about change in libido, such as "Are you as interested in sex as you used to be?" or about problems maintaining an erection. Choose words that the patient can understand. If you are not sure you are being understood, ask "Do you understand what I am asking?" As much as possible, you should employ questions that permit patients to answer from their own point of view and in their own words (e.g., "Do you feel satisfied?" as opposed to "Do you have an orgasm?").

EXPANDING ON THE SEXUAL HISTORY

When you need to know more, for example about the patient's risk factors, or if you suspect a sexually transmitted disease, it is necessary to find out about sexual orientation, number and regularity of sexual partners, and whether they are same- or opposite-sex, and to ask your patient if his or her partner(s) have had any sexually transmitted disease symptoms. For example, a woman's age at first intercourse is a risk factor for human papillomavirus and cervical cancer. Prepare the groundwork for questions by using transparency so you will not be startled by the 40-year-old female who tells you that her first episode of intercourse was at age 8, when she was abused by her father. Incest or a history of child abuse, a sexually transmitted disease, and multiple partners are difficult topics about which many patients are reluctant to speak. Patients may want to be open and cooperative, but at the same time may not want to acknowledge that a partner has gone outside the relationship or that they were victims of incest. They may feel anger and guilt or may perceive the clinician as judgmental.

Consider this example of a 54-year-old married financial consultant who presented to his doctor (of many years) with a rash on his palms and soles:

Patient   So what do you think this is?
Clinician **Well, most likely it's a virus of some sort. But because it's on your palms and soles the list of possibilities is rather short, but it includes syphilis.**
           Syphilis?! Isn't the only way you can get that by sexual contact?
           That's correct. And I'm not jumping to any conclusions here, but you need to know it's on the list. [Pause] Let me get the requisition for some lab work for you and I'll be back. [The clinician decides not to ask a direct question and, instead, gives the patient some time to absorb this information by stepping out for a moment.]
           [When clinician returns] I feel terrible, I have to deal with the consequences, but I did have unprotected intercourse with someone not my wife. Can we figure out what this is as fast as possible?

Maintaining Objectivity

You should express your questions in the same neutral way that you talk about other illnesses or infections, such as "Are you concerned that you might have gotten this from someone?" or "Is there any chance that you have been exposed to someone with a similar infection?" Sometimes it helps to introduce a difficult question with a statement, such as "I think you may have an infection that is acquired only during sexual intercourse, but I don't want to make any assumptions about your sexual relationships. Is it possible that you've been with someone who has the same infection?" If the patient says, "That's impossible," accept that statement as representing the patient's belief. You can still add, "If you do think of anybody who might have this, it would be good if you could tell them to get checked." Do not argue with the patient. If the diagnosis is uncertain, say so and outline the plan for making the diagnosis clear. In the case of reportable sexually transmitted diseases, the clinician might say, "By law, I am required to report this illness, and someone from the health department may contact you about who else you know that might have it."

Here is an example of a common sexual problem that arises frequently in patients. The clinician's task is to determine if the problem is the result of the illness itself, adverse effects of medication, difficulties in the personal relationship, or some combination of factors.

Clinician	**Are you living at home now? Living with your boyfriend?**
Patient	He's like 16 years older than me and we've been together for about 15 years, but see there's a, a little bit of a problem when we have to, 'cause see since I've been on those steroids, you know it messes with your sex life, too. I don't have any.
	You don't have any desire?
	No, and uh, that creates a problem. I just have no desire. It was like if he put his hands on me, I might get real evil, you know, like "get your hands off of me," you know.
	I see. How are things between you and him otherwise? Are things strained in general?
	I wish he would get out of my life.

Notice how the clinician discovers that the likely cause of the patient's sexual difficulty is not what she initially seems to think, namely that it has something to do with her chronic steroid therapy, but rather that the relationship itself is not working. *When You Need to Know More,* page 114, presents some useful ways to elicit information when you require more information than what your patient is revealing.

WHAT TO SAY
When You Need to Know More

- Start with open-ended questions, proceeding to more focused questions.
- Use introductory statements to create transparency:
  - "I always include sexuality in my routine history. Tell me first about your relationships in the past. How about recently?"
  - "What else do I need to know about you to provide you with good health care?"
  - "I want to understand more about this problem. Does anything seem to trigger your lack of desire (interest) or make it harder for you to maintain an erection?"
  - "Tell me more about how you keep from getting pregnant."
  - "Tell me more about how you keep from getting sexually transmitted disease."
  - "Certain sexually transmitted diseases are more common or affect different parts of the body, depending on a person's sexual practices. Tell me more about what you do. Do you have or perform anal or oral sex?"
  - "In the past, have you been sexual (or had relationships) with men, women, or both? How about now?"
  - "How do you see yourself (with regard to sexual orientation)? Gay? Straight? Bisexual? Or something else?" Or "Are you more attracted to men or women?"
  - "I need to know more about your sexual relationships in order to understand your risk for certain disorders. How old were you when you started having sex? How many men or women have you had sex with? Do you know if your partner(s) have had sex with anyone else?"

Moreover, many patients may also want to know what is "normal" in sexual matters and discern whether they fit some hypothetical standard. They may even ask your opinion. Some questions that patients may propose are clearly inappropriate, such as "What would you do? Would you have an abortion?" or "Did you have sex before you got married?" In these cases, it is best to answer in a polite and straightforward manner, such as "Well, we're not here to discuss what I think. I'm more interested in finding out about how you feel." By responding this way, you will help the patient explore his or her own feelings and symptoms as opposed to your own, which are not the focus of the interview.

 PRACTICE POINT

During the sexual history, do not confuse being genuine (see Chapter 2) with giving personal details of your own life.

SEXUAL ORIENTATION IN THE INTERVIEW

Your patient's sexual orientation affects not only his or her risk factors for specific illnesses but also may influence medical care in various ways. For example, many same-sex couples in committed relationships want to have or adopt children or want the right to make medical decisions for their partners should the other individual be unable to do so. As their clinician, you need to know whom to consult if life-and-death matters arise, but you also need to know what your legal constraints may be. (We will deal with these issues in greater detail in Chapter 16, Ethics and the Law.) Same-sex couples may also experience increased tension related to attitudes of their extended families, abandonment by traditional religious groups, or work-related discrimination despite laws that supposedly protect them. These issues may lead to unique stressors in these relationships, which may contribute to clinical depression, sexual dysfunction, or poor control of other medical disorders, such as hypertension or diabetes. At the very least, your gay or lesbian patient may face prejudice-based challenges in maintaining an adequate support system.

The following example presents a patient in whom a variety of lifestyle factors contributed to his illnesses, which include obesity, headaches, and secondary syphilis. It is a touching reminder that sexuality, spirituality, and health can be all muddled together.

Patient   The thing that is interesting to me is I am busy and I am constantly on my feet and I must put in at least 4 miles each day, but it doesn't affect my weight because of the types of things I eat. I don't eat heavily, it's just the things I eat.

Clinician   How do you mean?

When I have not eaten for a whole day, I go to some deli and grab a creampuff and go to bed. That gives me sugar, and sugar helps me. Sugar really helps me keep elevated. I have a terrible—well, I have to drink orange drink. I don't eat breakfast, as a matter of fact, I only eat one meal a day, but it's a junk meal. And I'm very hooked on, I have to have a sugar-type drink in the morning to get elevated. Could use one now!

Now that you know all these things, is there any way you can change something? Like when you go to New York, can you find some time for yourself, even if it's sitting down for 10 minutes, instead of 10 seconds?

I lived there for 2 years, and when I started the business, I didn't realize at the time that the business was going to grow as quickly as it did, and I found out I was going to New York more and staying in hotels. Hotel living is disgusting. This is the part where it gets into the personal part of it. My lifestyle changed quite a bit; a lot of things changed for me. I have always felt that I had very strong religious convictions and things like that. When I moved to New York, my lifestyle totally changed. I went to parties where everybody was having sex with everybody else and you really didn't even get to know the person. You may never see them again and that type of thing. Well, all these things happened to me in this period. And I have to be honest with you, they frightened me, but I enjoyed them. I knew they were wrong, but there was a part of me that enjoyed them. So I was getting very confused. I felt that it was time for me to come back.

You felt that this was a way of coming back home?

Exactly. What happened to me recently was that because of me going back to the way I wanted to be and things not working out the way I thought they should, so I figured why should I make sacrifices and be this person. You know, and not getting the results I want from it. I'll go back to being the other person. And I went back to being the other person and I got [laughing loudly] a social disease! Now you know my life story. That's it in a nutshell.

Skillful Questioning

Note in this patient interview how the clinician skillfully uses open-ended questions ("How do you mean?") and interchangeable responses ("You felt this was a way of coming back home?"). The patient speaks in code, "being this person" (the straight one) as opposed to the "other person" (the gay one) who gets punished with a "social disease" (syphilis). This patient (whom we met briefly in Chapter 1) acquired syphilis, probably at a party at which he had multiple sexual partners. He was finding his obesity difficult to control and was experiencing constant fatigue and stress-related headaches. The rash caused by his secondary syphilis became public evidence of what he saw as religious transgression (i.e., his religion taught that homosexuality is a sin). He was dreadfully afraid that he had been exposed to HIV during his semi-anonymous gay sex. His anxiety and guilt made it difficult for him to work as hard as he felt he needed to in order to keep his business going. This patient did, indeed, acquire HIV and subsequently developed AIDS and died about 2 years later.

SUMMARY — The Sexual History

The sexual history is a vital part of the patient's profile or social history and contributes both an understanding of who the patient is as a person as well as critical information to determine the etiology of symptoms and risk for specific disorders. It is a difficult part of the interview, for both the clinician and patient, but these difficulties can be overcome by attention to technique, including:

- Using simple screening questions to determine how much you need to know
- Delaying this part of the interview until you know something about the patient as a person
- Ensuring that you and your patient are using words that have the same meaning
- Proceeding from less intimate to more intimate questions
- Sequencing your questions from open-ended to closed-ended, depending on the degree of detail you need
- Using introductory and transparent statements to help the patient understand why you are asking what might otherwise be interpreted as intrusive questions

Once through this difficult part of the interview, you are ready to complete the patient's assessment with the review of systems and physical examination, which we will explore in the next chapter.

CHAPTER 7

Review of Systems, Physical Examination, and Closure

No Air of Finished Knowledge

*A physician of this kind never gives a servant any
account of his complaint, nor asks him for any;
he gives him some empirical injunction with an
air of finished knowledge in the brusque fashion
of a dictator, and then is off in hot haste to the
next ailing servant.*

Plato, *The Laws*

REVIEW OF SYSTEMS IN CONTEXT

The **review of systems** (ROS) demonstrates your responsibility for the
total patient and may uncover significant symptoms or problems not otherwise elicited. Clinicians who feel uncertain about how to conduct an
interview, or about their ability to integrate data, often take refuge in a
long, detailed ROS. They ask in great detail about every possible symptom, as if it were actually possible to get all the information simply by
asking an exhaustive set of closed-ended questions. Others look upon the
ROS as a formality with little value—in other words, a burden—but they
ask an endless series of questions regardless.

What, then, are the objectives and goals of the ROS? The first is
to uncover any additional active medical problems not yet discussed,
and the second is to identify additional symptoms that may be related
to the symptoms for which the patient is seeking help, or may influence them. The interviewer may ask questions to address these ends at
any time.

◈ **PRACTICE POINT**
The ROS as a specific segment may be "emptied" when the relevant information is obtained elsewhere in the interview.

In a classic study, Platt and McMath (1979) observed more than 300 clinical interviews conducted by medical residents and delineated five syndromes of "clinical hypocompetence." They called one of the syndromes "flawed database" and illustrated it with this case. The clinical interview took 44 minutes to complete. Time allocation was as follows:

- Introduction = 1 minute
- Definition of chief complaint (cardinal symptom) and development of present illness = 15 minutes
- Major past medical events, health hazards (smoking, alcohol, medications), and family illnesses = 8 minutes
- Review of systems = 20 minutes

In this case, the interview was poorly structured and inefficient in generating data. A large portion was devoted to the ROS; this is generally unnecessary when one uses earlier parts of the interview to develop an understanding of the patient's life, personal habits and interests, and other active medical problems, as well as to skillfully explore the current illness. A more functional allocation of time might be:

Introduction = 1 minute
Understanding the patient's life, personal habits and interests =
    5 minutes
Definition of the chief complaint and present illness = 15 minutes
Definition of other active medical problems = 5 minutes
Major past medical history and family history = 8 minutes
Review of systems = 3 minutes

As you gain experience, much of the ROS may be conducted while you perform the physical examination. For instance, as you examine the patient's ears, you might ask if he or she has had any problems with hearing, ear infections, and so forth; as you examine the eyes, you might ask if he or she wears reading glasses. This method of conducting the ROS, however, requires a high level of competence. You may also run the risk that the patient may think you are asking your question (e.g., "Are you having any headaches?") because you have uncovered a problem during the physical examination. This may create anxiety and distort the patient's response. Thus, it is important to preface your examination, or at least your questions, with a comment that you will be asking routine questions for the sake of completeness rather than questions specifically related to the patient's illness or your physical findings.

Using an ROS Questionnaire

Some clinicians approach the ROS with standardized questionnaires that the patient fills out before the interview. Using questionnaires, however, does not replace the ROS section of the interview but merely changes its character. Instead of asking directly about symptoms, the clinician reviews the questionnaire and asks for more details regarding positive responses. The clinician must also determine whether the patient has understood the written words well enough to answer the questions accurately. A questionnaire is perfectly acceptable, but it is useful for the novice clinician to conduct a complete ROS without the benefit of such tools. Then, after you have developed a comfortable style, you might create a personalized questionnaire for future use.

 PRACTICE POINT

You must also check out pertinent negatives, that is, symptoms a patient has *not* reported that would support one of your diagnostic hypotheses. If a patient presents with cough, for instance, a pertinent negative might be lack of shortness of breath.

TECHNIQUES TO SUPPORT THE ROS

Several techniques are useful in learning about and conducting a productive ROS:

- Avoid asking detailed questions about every symptom related to each organ system. For example, you should ask, "Are you having any trouble with your vision?" rather than "Is your vision decreasing?" or "Do you see double?" In other words, ask the patient about general difficulties with each system, then focus on details of existing symptoms, and finally be sure to check out pertinent negatives.

◆ PRACTICE POINT

Expand the net of your questions by first emphasizing the symptoms related to the patient's chief complaint and then continuing with general, as opposed to specific, yes/no questions.

- Use ambiguous terms, such as indigestion, bowel trouble, or fatigue, during the initial screening. If the patient responds with a positive answer, the symptom can then be defined more precisely.
- Conduct the ROS section of the history at the end of the interview so that you have time to "size up" the patient and ascertain how to assess his or her responses (e.g., denial or obsession with the trivial).
- Abbreviate or eliminate the ROS in emergency situations; it can also be completed at a later date if the patient is too tired or too sick to respond to a tedious inquiry.
- Anyone, even someone in perfect health, is likely to have some positive responses on a complete ROS. With each positive response, obtain enough detail to indicate whether the symptom is significant or trivial.

◆ PRACTICE POINT

Significance **relates to severity and duration, meaning the more severe and chronic the symptom, the more likely it is to be important.**

See *Question Style for the ROS,* below, which presents questions that demonstrate these techniques for obtaining the ROS.

WHAT TO SAY
Question Style for the ROS

These are examples of questions useful in initiating and conducting a productive ROS. To begin:

- "I'd like next to ask some general questions about your health to make sure I haven't missed anything."
- "I'd like you to think especially about things that may have bothered you recently (or in the past year since your last checkup). Okay?"
  To continue:

■ "Have you had any headaches or problems with your head and neck?"

■ "How about with your vision and your eyes?"

■ "What about your ears, nose, or throat? Any allergy or hay fever symptoms?"

■ "Any problems with your skin? Lumps or bumps or moles that concern you?"

Sample ROS

The following sample transcript is neither comprehensive nor ideal, but simply a reasonable example conducted by a medical house officer. As you read through this interview (in which there are some good and some not-so-good features), think about how you might have phrased these questions, whether you feel important information is missing, and if you believe any questions are excessively detailed.

Clinician	**I'm going to ask you a bunch of questions I ask everybody. They are very general questions, and some of them have short answers. Do you find that you get fevers often?**
Patient	No.
	How about chills? Have you had any chills recently?
	Yes, but I just took that as being, you know, my hormones for my hysterectomy. That's what I took it as being.
	Okay. Do you get night sweats?
	Yes.
	Do you soak through all your bed clothing?
	No.
	How much do you weigh now?
	202.
	How much did you weigh a year ago?
	About 180–190.
	What is the most you have ever weighed?
	This.
	You certainly aren't losing weight right now. Is that right?
	Right.
	Do you get headaches?
	Sometimes. Maybe I'd say once a month. Maybe once every other month.
	Do you have problems with your vision?
	No.

Do you ever have double vision?
No.
Ever see spots in front of your eyes?
No.
How about blurry vision?
No.
Have you ever passed out?
No.
Blacked out?
No.
Do you often feel lightheaded?
No.
Do you hear ringing in your ears?
No.
Do you get a pain in your throat?
No.
Sore throats often?
No.
Does your neck hurt?
No.
Have you noticed any lumps or bumps anywhere in your body?
No.
Do your joints ache?
Yes.
Which ones?
Here.
Okay, you are pointing to your left knee and your back. How about other joints in your body?
No.
Do your muscles ache?
I just thought that it was my muscles in my leg.
Okay, fine. Do you get short of breath when you exercise?
I haven't exercised.
How about just walking around town?
No.
Can you climb stairs without becoming short of breath?
Yes.
Do you get pain in your chest?
No.
Have you ever gotten pain in your chest while you were exercising?

No.

Have you ever felt your heart fluttering or racing very quickly?

I don't think so.

Do your ankles swell on you?

No.

Are you able to lie flat in bed without becoming short of breath?

Yes.

Do you ever wake up in the middle of the night short of breath?

No.

Do you have to cough often?

No.

Ever cough up blood?

No.

Have you noticed any change in bowel habits, your bowel functions?

Yes.

How have they changed?

I don't pass my bowels as often as I did before I had surgery.

How often do you pass your bowels now?

Maybe twice a week.

Is the stool shaped as it was before or is it different? Is it thicker or thinner?

Thicker. Yeah, because a lot of times I have to chew some Feenamints to make it go myself.

Do you have diarrhea intermixed with this at all?

No.

Have you noticed any tarry black stools?

No.

How about blood in your stools or on your stools?

No.

Have you had any belly pain?

Yeah.

Where does your belly hurt you?

Right where I had my incision. Sometimes like only when I laugh.

It hurts you along the incision?

Uh-huh.

How about somewhere else in your belly?

Right here.

Okay, you are pointing to your right groin area.

It's just like—mostly like when I see something real funny and just like when I laugh. There is not any pain, it's just there. I just get a pain when I start laughing.

Have you noticed if you are very thirsty often? Do you find yourself drinking a lot of fluids?

Sometimes.

Do you think that you get cold more easily than some of your friends? Do you find that you put on heavy clothing when other people are not wearing jackets and things?

No.

Does the heat bother you more than you think it bothers other people?

No.

What is your energy level like?

So-so. It's moderate.

Do you become fatigued easily?

Sometimes.

How's your appetite?

Great.

What are the good and not-so-good features of this ROS? Among its good features are its completeness—almost every body system is covered—and the way in which it is introduced. Also, the interviewer asks one question at a time and gives the patient sufficient opportunity to respond. However, there are also some problems. For example, the clinician introduces medical jargon with such terms as "night sweats" and "change in bowel habits"; although many patients understand these terms, keep in mind that some do not. The more striking problem—and one common to the ROS—is the variation between lack of detail for some symptoms and overly elaborate detail for others. For example, the patient's complaints of headache, joint pain, and thirst are not further characterized; the clinician seems to have dismissed these symptoms as unimportant without additional inquiry. On the other hand, there appear to be too many specific questions about vision and cough and various types of shortness of breath; one question, such as "Do you have any trouble breathing?" would suffice.

The goal when conducting the ROS is to achieve balance. Because the interviewer is asking questions presumably unrelated to the main problem, the ROS serves as a screening device. The questions are not hypothesis-driven, and the probability that a positive response indicates significant pathology is low.

◆ **PRACTICE POINT**

A positive answer to a screening question in the ROS generally conveys less useful information about the patient's clinical condition than do the patient's spontaneous statements (e.g., in the history of present illness) reporting the given symptom or symptom complex.

RESPONDING TO THE POSITIVE ROS

Some patients give a literal interpretation to the questions in the ROS, answering "yes" to almost every question. When this happens, the task seems to be interminably tedious, and the interviewer fears that the history will never end. Sometimes, in addition to being positive, the answers about relatively trivial matters are also given in great detail. For example, although you may want to know if the patient wears glasses, you may have little interest in the fine details of how the patient's refractive error has changed in the past 5 years or what the patient feels about his or her optometrist.

The Problem

A difficult ROS might begin this way:

Clinician   **Now I'd like to ask you a series of questions just to make sure we haven't missed anything important, okay?**
Patient   Fine.

         I'll start with your head, and we'll work our way down. Do you get headaches?
         Oh, I'm used to terrific headaches all through my life, and one doctor said it was high blood pressure, though I didn't know it at the time.

Already, this situation seems to be off to a bad start because we do not expect or desire a severe, chronic problem to surface first in the ROS. So, instead of zipping through the questions, the interviewer is forced to stop and ask for more details about the headaches. When this happens, usually one of two scenarios is occurring: either the clinician has failed to inquire in an empathic way about other active problems and significant past medical history, or the patient has simply overinterpreted the question.

The Remedy

The best way to deal with this situation is to prevent it by asking about other active problems and significant past medical history soon after the questions concerning the present illness. Not only does this maneuver uncover such problems early in the interview, but it also facilitates making connections between these problems and the present illness. If this technique fails or if you forget to use it, you might try one of a number of other approaches:

- Bring the patient back to the present with a reminder that the focus is on currently distressing symptoms.
- Make the questions general, such as "Have you ever had any stomach or bowel trouble?" and ask for further details only when the response to the initial screening is positive.
- Encourage filtering out of unnecessary details by reminding the patient of time limitations, or by asking him or her to pick out the most important symptoms.
- Undertake much of the ROS while performing the physical examination.

Responding to the Positive ROS, below, provides some examples of how to achieve focus and brevity during this part of the interview.

WHAT TO SAY
Responding to the Positive ROS

■ Focus on current distressing symptoms: "You've checked almost every symptom on the list here. Aside from what we've already talked about, what's bothering you the most right now?"

■ Help the patient filter out unnecessary details: "I am especially interested in any additional problems you've noticed in the past few months."

■ Keep questions general by specifying the topic but avoiding focused yes/no questions: "Any stomach or bowel trouble lately?"

■ Continue the ROS during the physical examination: "Since our time is limited, let me ask you about all these concerns while I do your exam. Would that be okay?"

TRANSITIONING TO THE PHYSICAL EXAMINATION

Medical interviewing, unlike other forms of clinician-patient interaction, usually also involves a physical examination. The history and physical examination are different parts of the same process; if we focus on data gathering, it is difficult to pinpoint exactly where the history ends and the physical examination begins, or vice versa. For example, from the first moment the patient walks into your office or you walk into the hospital room, you begin to make observations about the physical condition of the patient. You observe skin color, affect, behavior, clothing, and mental status. The entire mental status examination, although part of the interview in that it involves no touching, is more properly considered part of the systematic physical examination (see Chapter 11, Interviewing the Geriatric Patient).

◈ PRACTICE POINT
As you perform the physical examination, continue to interact with your patient, striving to obtain not only physical information but also personal and symptom information.

It is difficult, at first, to go from talking to touching your patient. Early in your clinical training, it is especially difficult to unglue yourself from your chair and actually approach the patient. In the hospital, paying attention to the patient's comfort, such as offering a drink of water or changing the window blinds, may be appropriate. Ordinarily, when in the clinic or in your office, you will be interviewing a patient who is fully clothed. Although having a patient disrobe and put on an examination gown prior to the interview is often conducive to good office functioning, it is rarely conducive to patient comfort. It undermines respect for the person. Thus, the patient should be fully clothed, and you will need to ask him or her to get undressed when you are ready to start the physical examination. *Making the Transition to the Physical Examination,* below, presents a procedure for being direct and clear about what is going to happen and why.

WHAT TO SAY
Making the Transition to the Physical Examination

- First, give the patient an opportunity for the last word. For example, "I think that's about it for now. Is there anything else we haven't covered or that you'd like to tell me before I examine you?"
- Second, tell the patient clearly what the game plan is. For example, "Next I'm going to do your physical examination, and then after that, we can sit down and talk about your problems and what tests you might need."

- Third, be very specific about what clothing the patient should remove, where to sit or lie, and in what position. For example, "I am going to step out of the room for a moment now. Please get undressed down to your underpants and put this gown on with the opening in the back. And then sit on the end of the table up here."
- Finally, let the patient know your focus is still on him or her: "I'll review your file while you're getting undressed and then I'll be back."

Here is how one clinician begins an examination of a new patient. Take note of the explicit directions as well as the ROS-type questions asked at the beginning of the examination.

Clinician **Do you have any questions before we do your exam?**
Patient No.

Okay. Why don't you climb up here, and just sit there, just step around, and come around there. Okay. I am going to cover you and you can just sit there. I'm going to check your thyroid and your lungs and your heart, and examine your breasts. Have you had any thyroid trouble?

No.

At this point, it is best for you to leave the examination room, or pull a curtain across the room if one is available, while your patient gets undressed. In the hospital, of course, this is usually not a problem, but even there patients may want to use the bathroom or remove a dressing gown or robe before the examination begins. In office practice, when you are doing only part of a physical examination, it may be appropriate for the patient to remove only his or her shirt or unbutton several buttons. For specific parts of the examination, you might ask the patient to disrobe that area or, alternatively, say, "I'm going to untie (or unbutton or remove) ...." Or you might ask a female patient who has large breasts to assist in the examination by moving her breast for you to listen to her heart.

◆ PRACTICE POINT

By asking your patient to participate in the physical examination, you will avoid making him or her feel like a victim, but rather an active participant.

CONVERSATION DURING THE PHYSICAL EXAMINATION

Although maintaining a conversation during the physical examination allows you to continue to gather data, it may serve other essential functions as well. Here is how one patient describes his feelings about the physical examination.

Patient   Whether it be horizontal, or in some awkward placement on one's back or stomach, with legs splayed or cramped, or even in front of a desk, the patient is placed in a series of passive, dependent, and often humiliating positions. These are positions where embarrassment and anger are at war with the desire to take in what the doctor is saying. In this battle, learning is clearly the loser.

◆ **PRACTICE POINT**

Use your communication skills to put the patient at ease, encouraging the patient to feel like an active participant in his or her own care, and diminishing the perception of a difference in power between the clinician and the patient, which becomes more marked during the physical examination.

Conversation will demonstrate to the patient that you remember the complaint about abdominal pain while you are performing the abdominal examination. In other situations, "small talk" can be used to distract the patient so his or her muscles will relax, making the abdominal or pelvic examination easier for the patient and more accurate as well. As a beginner you may find it difficult to converse while you also are concentrating on the sequence and techniques of the examination. However, it is not difficult to make such statements as:

- "I'm going to look into your ears now."
- "I'm feeling for your thyroid gland. Can you swallow now? I know it's difficult to swallow like that when someone asks you. Good."
- "I'm going to do a rectal exam now to check your prostate gland. It will make you feel like you are going to have a bowel movement, but don't worry, you won't."

◆ **PRACTICE POINT**

During the physical examination, continue to talk with the patient to reassure him or her, and to explain what you are doing.

Using Transparency

The preceding statements are excellent examples of transparency, describing what you are doing and why in order to open up what may otherwise be a "black box" for the patient. It is also easy for you, and reassuring for the patient, to indicate that parts of your examination are normal. It is usually not particularly helpful to comment on every little detail, but if you know the patient is concerned about a particular system, it is helpful to note your findings about that system right away. For the patient who presents with chest pain, a comment that the heart and lungs sound normal can be quite reassuring (the patient need not be bothered at this point with the information that the heart may sound normal even when there is heart disease).

Here is an example of a clinician-and-patient conversation during the physical examination, which involved listening to the lungs and heart and palpating the breasts and abdomen. Notice the clinician's inclusion of a few ROS-type questions, education about breast self-examination, and attention to the patient's comfort (e.g., "Tell me if I hit any sore places") as parts of the body are examined.

Clinician	**Okay, I am just going to loosen this [unties gown in back]. How long have you been smoking?**
Patient	About 3 years.
	And you want to quit?
	Well, yeah, I've been thinking about it.
	Take a deep breath. Okay, out, good, and again. ... Good. Now I am going to ask you to slip your arms all the way out and I am going to listen to your heart. ... Okay. Sounds good. Now I'm going to check your breasts. I want you to put your hands up like this [demonstrates] and I'm just going to look at them first to see if there are any bumps.
	Uh mm.
	Okay, have you ever tried examining your breasts?
	No, not really.
	We recommend that everyone do it once a month; the best time is right after your period has stopped. Do your breasts get sore before your period?
	Yes.
	Okay, well, that is why it is best to wait until after your period starts, when usually the lumpiness goes away and they're not tender to touch. ... I am going to ask you to just hold this up ...

and I want you to put your arms up over your head. What you do when you are checking is to do exactly what I'm doing. ... Go all around the outside of your breasts like this ... up here is breast tissue and also up here ... so you are going to go in kind of a circle like this ... then spiral in until you get every part including under the nipple. Okay? Now I'd like you to lie down and we'll check your breasts again. ... We always check them in two positions. ... And I am going to check your heart. ... Do you have any indigestion or trouble with your bowels? Now tell me if I hit any sore places.

For the female patient, the pelvic examination is a particularly personal and anxiety-producing experience. To alleviate your patient's discomfort, explain clearly what you are about to do and what the patient is likely to feel. Ask the patient if she has had a pelvic examination before. Whether she has or not, it is very reassuring to say, "I'm going to pretend that this is your first pelvic examination and explain everything that I'm doing." The less experience the patient has had, either with pelvic examinations or with you, the more reassurance she will need. You should first touch the patient's inner thigh and then firmly but gently conduct the examination. You should describe the anatomy to the patient as you are doing the examination, another opportunity for transparency. As you become more experienced, you will be able to help her relax her muscles through your calm tone of voice, your gentle palpation, and your instructions about deep, slow breathing.

Here is how one clinician introduced a patient (who had requested a diaphragm for birth control) to her first pelvic examination. Each step is described with a relaxing, almost hypnotic, tone of voice; gestures are slow and deliberate (no sudden moves); and the clinician continuously looks at the patient's face to gauge her reactions.

Clinician **The next thing I am going to do is a pelvic exam. These are all the things I normally use, but I may not use all of them on you. Okay. These are the slides on which the Pap test is done, and these are the little brushes that I use to do the Pap test. See how soft they are? And this also, which I will roll around the cervix just like that [demonstrating], see, it is not sharp. ... We usually do a culture for infection at the same time.**

Patient A culture?

Yes, and that is to check for infection. This instrument is cold, and that is really the worst thing about it. It is called a specu-

lum and this is inserted very gently into the vagina and then opened very gently like that [demonstrating] so that I can see your cervix and see that it is normal. Okay? [Patient nods.] What I will ask you to do is to put your feet into these things, which are called stirrups, these metal things, that's good, and now I want you to pull yourself all the way down to the end of the table like that, and practically feel yourself like your bottom is coming off the end of the table. Okay? That's fine. I am going to put this pillow under your head right there, okay, and I am going to shine a light on you so that I can see what I am doing and as I do things I will tell you what I am doing. Okay? Are you more or less comfortable?

I guess so.

All right, it is not very comfortable, that is true. Okay. Now what I am going to do is to look at the outside of you first. If you can just kind of relax, that's good. Now what I am doing is checking the labia, or lips. Good. Now you are going to feel my finger at the edge of the vagina, feeling where your cervix is. Do you know what your cervix is?

No.

Okay, that is the opening to your womb or uterus. Okay, I am just kind of locating it first, and that is just my finger again. Okay, now you're going to feel the cold metal which I tried to warm up a little bit, but usually it's still cold. Is that okay?

Mm hmm.

Now I insert it just until I can see your cervix so that I can do the Pap test. Okay, now I can see your cervix very clearly now. ...

Is that where I put the diaphragm?

Exactly, that is exactly where to put the diaphragm. Okay, now I am just using that soft brush to do the Pap test, okay?

Mm hmm.

And now I'm going to use one of those scrapers and sometimes you feel that scraping feeling, but usually what you feel is the pressure of the speculum being in place there. ... Now I am just spraying those glass slides that I just took and that preserves them so they can be checked later. And now I am taking the speculum out. Are you still with me?

Yeah.

Now I am going to just check back inside your vagina, okay, and where my fingers are is where you put the diaphragm.

Now I am going to ask you that when you go home you practice feeling where your cervix is. I am touching it right now. On you, it is a little bit off to your left side, okay, and it feels like the tip of your nose when you touch it. Okay. When I put one hand over here, between the two hands I can feel where your uterus is. ... And I am touching it right now and it feels normal. Now I am checking on each side for your ovaries. ...

Can you feel all that?

Yes, I can feel all that, especially in someone like you, because you are very relaxed and I can feel everything. Okay, the next thing I am going to do is check your rectum, and that will make you feel as though you have to have a bowel movement, right, that is just my finger in your rectum. That's kind of an uncomfortable feeling. It feels completely normal.

Notice in this situation how the clinician keeps talking, but frequently checks back with the patient, and is educating the patient all the while about her body and about the normality of the findings. Indeed, the proof that the technique is effective is in the patient's pleasure and wonderment (e.g., "Can you feel all that?") at the ability of a pelvic examination to tell so much and her ability to completely relax her muscles.

◆ PRACTICE POINT
Your continued conversation with the patient during the physical examination provides clarification and reassurance, and it increases your efficiency.

Your ability to gather new information will gradually develop as you become more comfortable with the procedures of the physical examination, so that concentration on the actual techniques can sink into the background and you can focus more thoroughly on your immediate observations. Until you are experienced, do not try to complete the entire ROS during the physical examination. However, if you are looking at the eyes, for example, and this reminds you of an eye question you forgot to ask, go ahead and ask it. The physical examination is also a good time for "chit chat" with the patient, enabling you to find out more about his or her life and lifestyle.

Finally, the physical examination itself has not only a diagnostic but also a therapeutic role. Simply touching the patient—the "laying on of hands"—may cause him or her to feel better and be reassured. Tactile communication opens up a channel of interpersonal response that can be vital in healing.

◆ PRACTICE POINT
Pay special attention to the painful areas of the patient's body, which demonstrates that you have listened, understood, and are concerned about the patient's suffering.

ENDING THE INTERVIEW

When you have completed the physical examination, you will revisit the interview to terminate it. The goal of a good closure is no different from the goal during the entire interview, and it will be easier to achieve if the patient understands from the outset the purpose of the interaction. The purpose will vary, depending on whether you are a medical student, resident, physician assistant, nurse practitioner, or attending physician with a long-term role in the patient's management. Overall, the patient should expect to feel understood and not abused in any way. In history taking, this means that you have gotten the story straight and shown appropriate concern for his or her comfort, privacy, and modesty. The techniques of being accurate, empathic, respectful, and genuine apply to the closing of the interview just as they do to all the other parts.

◆ PRACTICE POINT
It is always a good idea to give the patient the opportunity to have the last word.

To allow the patient the opportunity to have the last word, use such statements as:

- "Anything else?"
- "Do you feel there is anything about what you have told me that I have not understood?"
- "Is there anything else you'd like to tell me or ask me?"

If you are a student, this may be the end of your contact with the patient. When you close the encounter, you should do all of the following:

- Provide a summary of what the patient has told you
- Be sure to let the patient have the last word or ask any additional questions
- Give a pleasant thank-you and goodbye

If the patient asks a question you cannot answer about a particular disease or medical care, you should respond by saying, "I am not able to answer that, but it is a good question to ask your physician." This is a truthful response whether you are unable to answer because you do not know, or because, even though you do know the answer, the question should be answered by the patient's physician.

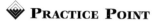 **PRACTICE POINT**
When you are responsible for the patient's care, the typical closure implies a continuing contract between you and the patient; it acknowledges responsibility (both the clinician's and the patient's) for solving problems and providing care.

In this general context, ending a patient encounter, whether an initial evaluation or a short office visit, should include these actions on the part of the clinician:

- **Sharing the differential diagnosis or hypotheses.** What you share depends on the patient—how sick he or she is, how knowledgeable he or she is, and whether or not he or she has other sources of information. What you share also depends on the illness; some findings are pertinent to the illness, and others are incidental or trivial.

PRACTICE POINT
In ending the patient encounter, avoid discussing topics or material that is interesting to you but irrelevant to the patient.

- **Devising a problem list with priorities.** This is painstaking and difficult at first but becomes easier with experience. It is important to realize that your priorities often differ from those of the patient. Patients may be interested first in feeling better, second in their overall prognosis, and third in the specific diagnosis. Clinicians share these concerns but often (especially while in training) are more interested in making the diagnosis than in treating the symptoms. Treating the symptom is often not the same as treating the disease. Many trivial illnesses (e.g., simple upper respiratory tract infections) do not in themselves require specific medications but have symptoms that patients want treated. On the other hand, many significant illnesses (e.g., hypertension) have no symptoms but, from the clinician's point of view, demand specific treatment.

- **Educating and negotiating.** You should provide information so that the patient can make informed decisions about the illness and treatment. Then answer questions and engage in negotiation to determine the optimal course of action that is consistent with the patient's beliefs and values (see Chapter 18 for a discussion about patient education and negotiation).

- **Agreeing on a plan of action and clarifying responsibilities.** Determine what will happen next and who will do what. The clinician may agree to order and interpret diagnostic tests, talk with consultants, write prescriptions, provide information, or perform procedures. The patient may agree to take medication, modify diet, keep the follow-up appointment, or report further symptoms.

◈ PRACTICE POINT

Ideally, medical care is a partnership in which you negotiate an agreement or contract with the patient, but the character of that contract depends on the acuity and severity of the patient's illness (e.g., emergency care versus chronic antihypertensive therapy), and on the patient's willingness to accept responsibility.

To conclude this chapter, here is an example of the closing moments of an interview with a 72-year-old woman with severe degenerative joint disease of the hips who is contemplating hip replacement surgery. She suffers also from a variety of other disorders, including diabetes, which is poorly controlled, and hypertension.

Patient	Well, I'm not sure I want to have that surgery. I'm scared 'cause I'm too old.
Clinician	**Tell me what's too old about 72.**
	Like I hear on TV …
	Like what?
	Like last week, I heard that having hip replacement surgery causes more deaths than automobiles.
	Let me tell you how we can figure this out. You do have risks with surgery and you do have more risk with the diabetes. The diabetes affects your whole body, how it heals, how your heart and blood vessels work and deal with the stresses of surgery.

Well, I listen to a lot of doctors, but I listen to you more because you know me so well and you stuck by me.

By your x-ray, you are ready for this surgery. But there are two things that help you make this decision. The first is pain and ...
... and my pain is not that bad ...

... and the other thing is disability, how much trouble you have getting around. So pain and disability. Pain and disability. If you're not there yet, you don't need the surgery.
But it does bother me, I limp and use my cane. But it's not day and night. And I don't want to have it if I don't need to.

The way we'll know is if the pain is too much or you can't get around. What we would do is try to minimize the risk to you, especially by getting your diabetes in control before the surgery. You will have to help with that.
I know I will. Will you talk with Dr Jones (the orthopedic surgeon)?
I'll be happy to.
When I take my medicine, I really see the difference.

So I'm writing your prescriptions for the diabetes and blood pressure medicines. Did we get through everything? I still need to talk to you about your lab results and they're not here yet, so you have to call me on Friday during my call-in time. Is that okay?
Yeah, okay. You know I have more confidence in people I know.

So, here are your prescriptions; I'll get your lab results and we'll talk about that when you call me. I'll call Dr. Jones and see if he needs to see you again, and I'll see you back, how 'bout six weeks? It's your job to take your medication and get your diabetes in control. Sound okay? Anything else?
One more question. I still have my Medicare, but now I have that medical assistance. Do you think they'll accept my insurance?

In this example, notice how the clinician shares the findings and clarifies the plan of action—using clear descriptions and repetition—including what he will do and what he expects the patient to do. Note, too, how the patient brings up a last-minute concern about her insurance coverage. It is not at all unusual for important questions to surface in the closing moments of the interview when the patient feels comfortable and can see that he or she is being listened to. It is vital, therefore, that you demonstrate your open-ended attitude even as you close the encounter, as this clinician did with the final, "Anything else?"

SUMMARY — ROS, Physical Examination, and Closure

The objectives and goals of the ROS are to:

- Identify active problems not yet discussed
- Associate additional symptoms with the current illness

The ROS may occur late in the interview, or parts of it may occur during the physical examination, when you chat with the patient in order to:

- Obtain more ROS-type information
- Learn more about the patient as a person
- Make the patient more comfortable

After the examination, close the clinical encounter by:

- Summarizing what you heard and what you found
- Devising a problem list and negotiating priorities
- Outlining a plan of action and responsibilities
- Continuing to educate the patient
- Giving the patient the opportunity to have the last word

CHAPTER 8

The Clinical Narrative

I Shall Enumerate Them to You

At least I have a grip of the essential facts of the case. I shall enumerate them to you, for nothing clears up a case so much as stating it to another person.
Sherlock Holmes to Dr. Watson in "Silver Blaze"

CREATING THE NARRATIVE

After you interview and examine your patient, you walk away, possibly with pages of cryptic notes in your hand. The most important single part of your patient's workup is complete, but before progressing further, you need to put the story on paper, or "do the write-up." From the morass of symptoms and experiences, you have to create a narrative and then choose what to include in the written clinical record. How do you abstract what you need? And how do you structure the story to make it most useful?

Because this text is limited to the skills of clinical interviewing, in this chapter we focus on how to conceptualize, format, and write the clinical history. However, the patient record is, in fact, a unique literary genre with its own objectives and standards of practice. In this genre, a patient history does not normally stand by itself. Its proper context also includes physical and laboratory data, an assessment or formulation (e.g., clinical hypotheses), and a plan for diagnosis and therapy, not to mention subsequent entries such as flow charts and progress notes. Consequently, to give a more complete picture of the clinical record, we also present some guidelines for the other elements of your write-up, as well as privacy guidelines and suggestions for formal case presentation and other forms of oral communication about patients among health care professionals.

TURNING THE HISTORY INTO THE WRITE-UP: THE CLINICAL NARRATIVE

Just the Facts?

Recording the history is not a question of "just the facts, ma'am." It is the end product, if you will, of a long process of selection, interpretation, and editing. The written history is created through at least four sequential processes of screening and interpretation.

- The first process involves the **patient's conscious experience** or raw data—that is, the actual facts as they happened and what it was like for the patient to feel the throbbing headache or experience the room spinning.
- The next process is the patient's **conceptualization of the experience**—that is, how the patient organized the facts to construct a story that lends meaning and coherence to the experience. This conceptualization draws on the patient's values and beliefs, and it results in an internal narrative.
- A third process leads to the **clinical tale,** the story you generate by means of the clinical interview. Because you speak a medical language and live in a medical culture, you may reconstruct the patient's story with different characters (e.g., groupings of symptoms) and a different plot development than are present in the patient's original narrative.
- The final process is your selection of items from this story to include in the **write-up.** To do this, you apply certain canons of literary form. There are rules and guidelines appropriate to the write-up just as there are rules and guidelines appropriate to the short story or the nonfiction essay.

When we call the final product the "clinical history," it is easy to forget the selective and interpretive processes that went into producing it. You are not simply a transcriber: you cannot repeat everything the patient says. In this respect, diagnosis and problem solving in the clinician-patient interaction is, metaphorically, similar to interpreting a text. What seems at first glance to be "just the facts" is actually an interpretation of the facts. You try to understand the meaning of the patient's story much as a literary critic tries to understand a text. The quality of your interpretation depends on your skill and experience, as well as on the text's underlying readability. No single interpretation of a book or of a patient's illness is final; continuous reevaluation is necessary. In clinical practice, as in

literary criticism, a "true" interpretation turns out to be one that is vali-
dated through open discourse among peers and consultants.

Recording Personal Information

Because we tend to believe that what is written in the chart is *prima facie*
true, the patient's medical record can become a powerful source of misinformation. Errors, such as mistakes in observation or clinical judgment,
tend to be perpetuated because so much emphasis is placed on the
written word.

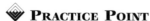 **PRACTICE POINT**
**Keep in mind that, when recording personal data about your
patient, a wrong diagnosis or a judgmental remark, once written,
is difficult to eradicate.**

What should you record? Here are some guidelines:

- Be cautious about recording the patient's attitude, lifestyle, expectations, and health belief system. Although these factors are useful
  to know, it is not always important to record them. Unless a
  patient's personality characteristics are out of the ordinary range,
  privacy and efficiency dictate silence. If you need to communicate
  a patient's style or idiosyncratic beliefs to others because they may
  play a significant role in patient care, then the information should
  be written in a descriptive, nonjudgmental way.
- Avoid recording certain types of personal information, such as
  explicit description of sexual habits, problematic relationships, or
  criminal convictions. Imagining the chart being read by the
  patient or patient's family is a useful criterion for what is appropriate to write.
- Include the patient's own words whenever possible, and not just
  in the chief complaint. For example, recording that the patient
  describes the headache as "a deep pain like someone is twisting
  a screwdriver inside my brain" tells a lot about the patient and is
  less judgmental than writing "patient describes the headache in a
  bizarre fashion," or "patient is histrionic."
- Minimize distortion by avoiding language that "pathologizes." In
  clinical practice we often use words that turn people, experiences,
  or feelings into "pathologies," rather than using the plain language
  of human experience. For instance, we like to use "depressed"

rather than "sad," and rarely do we describe patients as "discouraged" or "courageous." To make the record more expressive of personal narrative, avoid such words as *apathy, anxiety, denial, depression,* and *manipulative.* Try instead to use words such as *determined, discouraged, hopeful, optimistic, brave, fearful, sad,* or *hopeless.* Likewise, beware of saying that the patient *refuses,* or *has failed,* the measures you prescribe.

- Use behavioral or functional descriptions to convey personal information. By describing how the patient spends his or her day, what his or her hobbies are, or what he or she does on weekends, you can sketch important features of the person without getting too personal. Such statements fit well into the medical record and are not judgmental.

FUNCTIONS OF THE CLINICAL RECORD

Memory Aid

Originally the medical record served only as a stimulus to jog a clinician's memory. Most clinicians kept brief notes on index cards or patient log books. The "text" was not written on the card but kept in the clinician's mind. Although today we use more extensive records, we should remember many details about our patients' lives and experiences that we have not written down.

Communication

The medical record serves to communicate with other health professionals. In the modern hospital or clinic setting, health care is a multidisciplinary team activity; typically, 50 or more professionals may have legitimate access to an inpatient chart at one time. Most of them will want to communicate their observations and recommendations to other members of the team. This communicative function necessitates conventions regarding what information to chart and how to chart it.

Quality Assessment and Research

A senior clinician evaluates his or her trainees, at least in part, on the basis of the patient record they write. Hospital quality assurance and utilization review committees monitor performance of physicians and other health professionals by reviewing their chart entries. The clinical record also serves as a data source for case control studies and other clinical research protocols approved by local Institutional Review Boards.

Administrative and Legal Matters

Health care insurers audit medical records to verify diagnoses and to establish that claimed services were actually provided. Quality control and cost-containment strategies involve ascertaining "quality" at least in part on the basis of recorded data. Finally, the clinical record is legally discoverable and can be used as evidence in court.

FORMAT OF THE CLINICAL RECORD

Table 8–1 presents the elements usually included in a clinical write-up. Although there is broad consensus on these major features, agreement

TABLE 8–1

ELEMENTS OF CLINICAL CASE DESCRIPTION

The format of the clinical record should include subjective, objective, and integrative elements. Use this outline when preparing your patient's case.

Subjective

History
- Identifying Data.
- Chief Complaint: Use the patient's own words.
- Present Illness History: Organize the story.
- Other Active Problems: Outline what else is going on.
- Past Medical History: Note hospitalizations, surgery, allergies, and important illnesses.
- Family History: Use a genogram or table.
- Patient Profile: Write with care.
- Review of Systems: Record significant positives and negatives.

Objective

Physical examination
Results of diagnostic tests

Integrative

Assessment: The Problem List
Plan

about subdivisions and details vary from hospital to hospital, clinic to clinic, and practice to practice. Some institutions use highly structured forms for most of the record; some use paperless computerized files; and others still rely on old-fashioned handwritten notes. The following discussion is a generic one into which most institution-specific formats should fit.

IDENTIFYING DATA AND CHIEF COMPLAINT

The write-up begins with a succinct statement that identifies the patient and tells why he or she is seeking medical care. Often the chief complaint, stated in the patient's own words (for which you should use quotation marks), is the most effective descriptive statement to use. For example:

- Mr. Steven Maringo is a 47-year-old construction worker who came in because "I've had a sore throat for a month and it won't go away."
- Ms. Alice York is a 41-year-old chemist at Alcoa, with a history of "ulcers," who came in now because "I've had a burning pain under my ribs all week."
- Beth Salisbury is a 10-year-old fourth grader who came in because "my ear hurts since yesterday."
- Mr. Fred Jones is a 32-year-old computer programmer referred by Dr. A. Zinger for evaluation of a persistent "washed-out feeling" and lower extremity weakness.

When a patient has been referred, as in the last example, it is important to record that fact. Some patients may not have a chief complaint as such because the purpose of their visit is a routine checkup or a physical examination for a driver's license. Whatever the reason, record it in the patient's own words.

Other particularly relevant data may also be included in the introductory statement. For example, "Mr. Fred Jones is a 32-year-old, unmarried, Korean-American computer programmer who works at Ibex Industries." However, one should not try to pack this sentence with too many identifying features. Is the fact that Jones is unmarried or Korean-American relevant to his "washed out feeling"? Maybe, but many other features might be relevant as well. Although it is best to strive for simplicity here, many facilities have their own conventions about how to begin the write-up. Some, for example, might insist that you identify all patients by race and occupation, in addition to age and sex, no matter what their medical problems are.

Present Illness

The Present Illness section should reflect your interpretation and organization of the patient's story. Although the diagnoses may be in doubt, you should have a good grasp of the patient's problem(s) to organize the written narrative accordingly. The description should be succinct, with emphasis on:

- Time course
- Symptom characteristics
- Functional deficits

◈ PRACTICE POINT

Use the patient's own words and voice when possible, but remember that *you* are the author of the clinical narrative. Just because the patient rambles or has several different complaints doesn't mean that your written report should ramble on as well. Make sure that your organization and choice of material should reflect *your* thinking about how the symptoms fit together, not the patient's.

For example, consider the transcription of an opening statement presented in Chapter 3, Chief Complaint and Present Illness. The written Present Illness section might begin like this:

> *Mrs. P has been feeling "tired" and "worn out" even when she gets as much as 11 hours' sleep. Her sleep is interrupted by "hot flashes," although these are becoming less frequent.*

You may choose to put the patient's concerns about nervousness and loss of libido under the Other Active Problems (OAP) section (to follow), or include them in the present illness, if he or she considers them aspects of the same problem (a depressive disorder, for example).

You will frequently encounter patients who have had multiple hospital admissions and specialty consultations, and who have records inches thick. In these cases, it is tempting to construct the present history from old chart data, with little input from the patient. For example:

> *Mrs. Ely was first found to have carcinoma of the breast in May 1998, after which she underwent a left simple mastectomy, followed by a course of local irradiation. In June 2001 she was noted to have bone mets in T4 and L1 ... [list series of medical interventions]*

> *... and today [insert date] is admitted for consideration of further chemotherapy.*

Obviously, this is not a history of an illness; it is a chronicle of medical events. Does Mrs. Ely currently have symptoms? Why is chemotherapy being considered at this time, rather than last year or next month? In addition, the patient's voice is lacking in this history.

◆ PRACTICE POINT
Medical records can often shed light on the patient's current problem, but it is never appropriate to construct a narrative based on old records and call it the present illness.

Other Active Problems

It is useful to consider Other Active Problems (OAPs) in a separate section, although sometimes they may be integrated into the Present Illness section. Patients often have complex and chronic medical problems. A given episode of illness may well be an exacerbation of a chronic problem, or it may interact with another ongoing disease. Because of this, it is important to separate continuing problems (i.e., other active problems) from the Past Medical History and provide details about their current status. In the preceding example, if Mrs. Ely had been admitted for pneumonia, her history of breast cancer would be relevant, and it should be recorded in detail in OAPs.

Past Medical History

The Past Medical History section begins the more standardized, or routine, part of the write-up. By definition, it includes only those problems not currently active or seemingly relevant to the current problems. The format, as described in Chapter 4, Other Active Problems, Past Medical History, and Family History, should include:

- Significant illness or patterns of illness from childhood to the present, including hospitalizations
- Surgical procedures
- Accidents and injuries
- Pregnancies, deliveries, and complications
- Allergies, especially to foods and medications, including a description of the allergic response

- Current medications, including over-the-counter drugs, with dosages and schedule (these may also be listed under Other Active Problems)
- Health maintenance data, including immunizations and screening tests

Family History

The Family History is best presented in a genogram, which shows relationships in a diagrammatic form (see Figure 8–1). Squares represent

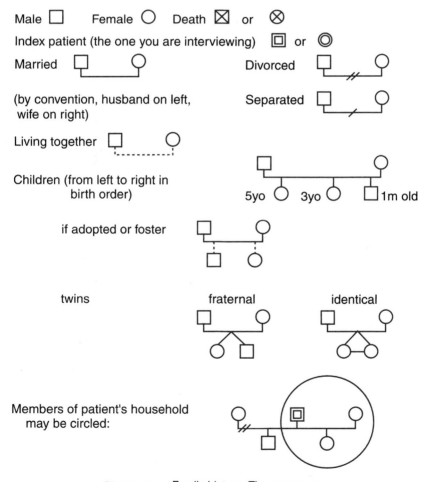

Figure 8–1 Family history: The genogram.

males; circles, females. A diagonal line or "x" through a name indicates that the person has died. Diseases may be indicated above or below the symbols. Alternatively, the family history can be presented in tabular form. This method is more efficient if the patient does not have much medical information about his or her family. Relationships can be indicated by abbreviations such as MGM for maternal grandmother and PGF for paternal grandfather. Such a family history might look like this:

- MGM (d. age 60s), unknown cause
- MGF (d. age 70), heart attack
- PGF (92), arthritis, forgetful

Patient Profile

The object of the **Patient Profile** is to give a picture of the patient as a functioning person and to record health-related behavior.

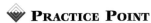 **PRACTICE POINT**

As a harried clinician, you should avoid the tendency to make the patient invisible by, for example, recording only that he or she smokes cigarettes or drinks alcohol. On the other hand, you should also avoid becoming too discursive or personal.

Approach writing the Patient Profile with a standard outline in mind, even though, in a given case, you need not necessarily write something for each item.

- Brief biography (e.g., place of birth, education, military service, and years in this locality)
- Current marital, family, and home situation
- Occupation and occupational history, including toxic exposures and stresses
- Lifestyle (e.g., religious affiliation, spirituality, personal interests, hobbies, travel, and exercise)
- Diet and nutrition
- Personal habits (e.g., use of tobacco, alcohol, and "recreational" drugs)
- A typical day's activities (this may be placed under Present Illness when a change in functional status is an important descriptor of the illness)

- Relevant feelings and beliefs (e.g., work satisfaction, perceived stresses, understanding of the illness, and attitudes toward health care)

Review of Systems

Data obtained in the review of systems (ROS) may be incorporated into the Present Illness narrative, if relevant to the current problem(s); placed in a structured system-by-system ROS section; or simply left unwritten. Beginners should include a fairly comprehensive ROS to develop the discipline of considering each system in turn. More experienced clinicians will usually write a few positive findings and pertinent negative findings. They will then indicate that the rest of the ROS was "unremarkable" or "negative."

PHYSICAL EXAMINATION

Although there are many local variations, the overall format for the physical examination is standard. Begin with a statement about the patient's general appearance and continue with vital signs (respiration rate, blood pressure, pulse or heart rate, and temperature) and the results of the examination of the skin, head, eyes, ears, nose, throat, neck, lymphatic system, chest, back, breasts, heart, abdomen, rectum, genitourinary system, extremities, musculoskeletal system, nervous system, and, finally, mental status. Although you generally collect mental status data by talking rather than touching, they are recorded as part of the physical examination.

Laboratory Tests

Results of diagnostic studies may be included as part of the initial write-up if they are routine or are available shortly after your initial interaction with the patient. In such cases, the results constitute part of the initial database. There is no standard method of recording laboratory or x-ray findings, although it is clearer and more efficient to use appropriate flow sheets. Nonetheless, it can be useful to provide a snapshot of basic studies (e.g., complete blood count and differential, urinalysis, serum chemistries, chest x-ray, and electrocardiogram) in the initial write-up. Each institution has its own policies or standard practices regarding routine laboratory tests, especially for patients admitted to the hospital.

However, in this age of evidence-based medicine, the emphasis is on selecting diagnostic studies, based on initial clinical hypotheses, rather than on standardized or routine panels of laboratory tests.

Problem-Oriented Assessment and Plan

To organize your assessment and plan effectively, use the principles derived from the problem-oriented medical record (POMR) system. There are numerous variations of the POMR system, but these basic elements contribute to patient-centered care:

- **Database.** Each record (or electronic file) includes a database that consists of the written clinical history, physical examination, and basic laboratory data.
- **Problem list.** Each record includes a list that enumerates the patient's identified health problems, including currently active problems and those that have resolved. This list should be updated regularly. The problems may include expressed concerns of the patient, as well as observations and interpretations made by the clinician. Thus, a problem might be any of the following: a symptom or diagnosis; a physical sign or laboratory finding; or a personal, social, existential, financial, or functional difficulty.

◈ Practice Point
As further information about the patient develops over time, the initial problems may be clarified, condensed, divided, or resolved, and others may be added to the record.

- **Structured entries.** Usually a structured format is used for each problem initially and in subsequent hospital or office notes:
  - **S**ubjective, including symptoms and personal data
  - **O**bjective, dealing with physical signs and laboratory results.
  - **A**ssessment, expressing the clinician's analysis of the problem
  - **P**lan, stating the measures to be taken
- The acronym **SOAP note** acknowledges these four structural elements in each entry and requires that person-oriented (subjective) data be incorporated regularly into clinical notes.
- **Flow charts.** The record may include preprinted flow charts and other devices to jog the clinician's memory, organize and display complex data, and enhance patient care.

Professionalism and Confidentiality

Professional oaths from virtually every tradition and culture impose a duty on clinicians to maintain confidentiality, that is, to keep information about their patients to themselves. In Chapter 16, Ethics and the Law, we discuss confidentiality in more detail, as well as important exceptions to the rule of confidentiality. However, at this point it is important to understand that members of the patient's health care team may share information among themselves to the extent that it is necessary for providing patient care. Thus, nurses, physicians, social workers, physical therapists, care coordinators, and medical specialists may freely discuss relevant aspects of the patient's story with one another. They may also read and make entries into the clinical record. As noted earlier, it is surprising how many personnel have legitimate access to a patient's record, especially in the hospital setting. More importantly, however, the vast majority of individuals, even in the busy hospital or clinic, do *not* have legitimate access to a specific patient's record.

Recognizing the importance of confidentiality and the need to protect privacy, the U.S. Congress passed the Health Insurance Portability and Accountability Act (HIPAA) of 1996, which sets up stringent privacy standards for personal health information. For example, every clinical site must have a set of procedures to protect the privacy of patients' oral communication, as well as their medical records. As a health professions trainee, you will need to complete a training session to learn HIPAA privacy requirements before you are allowed to see your first patient.

Here are a few points to remember in the context of your patient write-up and presentation:

- Do not share your patient's story with friends or family. It should be shared only with your clinical preceptor and other team members.
- Do not discuss your patient, even with another health care team member, in public places, such as the cafeteria, classroom, hall, or elevator.
- Do not leave your write-ups in places where others have access to them. This includes computer disks or drives that do not require passwords and logoff from multiple-user computer screens.
- In your write-up, always avoid demeaning comments about the patient. Likewise, use descriptive language, rather than interpretive or judgmental language, in writing about personal characteristics.

PRESENTING THE PATIENT

The oral case presentation is the day-to-day currency of clinical practice. Trainees and clinicians communicate rapidly and effectively by sharing well-organized vignettes that "capture" the patient and his or her clinical problem. As a student you may first encounter case presentation on rounds in the hospital, where the resident gives a succinct summary of the case, ending with a differential diagnosis and plan of action. Less experienced trainees are generally expected to give longer, more thorough case presentations, often lasting for several minutes. As you become more familiar with case presentation, you will notice that some presenters seem assured and energetic, so that you feel that you can actually *visualize* and *understand* the patient they describe. Other presenters come across as tentative and disorganized; images of their patients remain elusive. Not infrequently, disorganized presenters will attribute this problem to their patients. "The story isn't clear," they'll say, "because the patient is a poor historian."

Oral case presentation is a clinical skill in its own right. In the next section we briefly outline the major features of case presentation and present some guidelines.

Guidelines for Effective Case Presentation

Know Your Patient

Clearly, if you have taken a good history, performed a physical examination, thought the case through and completed your workup, you should be able to meet this threshold criterion. We can't emphasize enough how important it is to have a thorough grasp of the patient's story before condensing for oral presentation. If you have questions about the story, go back to the patient. If you have questions about how items fit together, discuss them with one of your colleagues or supervisors.

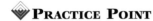 **PRACTICE POINT**

To present a patient effectively, you have to understand the story and have an idea of how the clinical evidence fits together.

Know Your Listener

What is the purpose of your presentation? It makes a big difference whether you are presenting your patient on work rounds, on teaching rounds, or to a specialty consultant, such as a cardiologist or a social worker. Bear in mind your listener's expertise and interest.

Understand the Power and Limitations of the Spoken Word

Readers can linger as long as they wish over a text, but listeners have to comprehend what you are saying as you say it. Clarity and organization are high priorities. The other side of the coin is your opportunity to engage listeners and direct their attention by telling a good story.

Sell the Story

To capture the power of the word, your style of presentation is crucial. You need to "sell" your patient and the narrative you've constructed. You should seize the opportunity to bring the clinical data together in an effective and convincing way. At the end of your presentation, your listeners should have a vivid picture rather than a series of disconnected data points.

Format of the Case Presentation

1. Opening Statement. Begin with an opening statement much like the opening of your write-up. This statement should provide a quick look at the patient as a person while, if possible, introducing the chief complaint in the patient's own words. You should not try to fully characterize patients and put them into pigeonholes, but rather to give a glimpse of a living, breathing person. For example:

- "Mr. B is a 69-year-old retired salesman with diabetes, hypertension, coronary artery disease, and high cholesterol who developed severe chest pain while he was driving his car to the mall this morning."
- "Mrs. R is a 47-year-old school teacher from Bayshore who presents with 3 days of increasing chest pain and productive cough."

2. The Illness Narrative. Present the history of the present illness and other active problems in a concise way. Remember that you are telling a story, not reciting a medical textbook or describing a random occurrence. You are also "selling" the story. Don't be afraid to be enthusiastic.

The more structured sections of the history—past medical history, ROS, family history—can usually be handled by presenting only positives and relevant negatives. It is perfectly appropriate for an oral presentation to contain a statement such as:

- "Past medical history includes gallbladder surgery in 1969 and chronic open-angle glaucoma diagnosed sometime in the 1980s. As far as the patient knows, there is no pertinent family history. The review of systems was essentially negative."

3. Patient Profile. You would be surprised at how a patient can "come alive" by presenting a few human details. Yes, you do want to indicate whether the patient smokes, drinks, or uses recreational drugs. But it is easy enough to say, in addition, that he is a married steamfitter who lives with his wife and has two grown children; or she is an attorney who lives alone and plays semiprofessional baseball. These items give your patient a human face while adding only a few seconds to your presentation.

4. Physical Examination and Laboratory Data. Your presentation will also include a targeted statement of physical findings and relevant laboratory data.

COMMUNICATION AMONG PROFESSIONALS

The complexity and size of the health care team has increased enormously from the time when the patient, the doctor, a nurse, and possibly a single consultant were the only players. Good health care now involves a multidisciplinary team effort. We often use the term *collaborative care* to describe the contemporary model. In collaborative care, one clinician, sometimes called the primary care provider, or PCP, serves as a coordinator and integrator of the patient's total care. Other specialists collaborate both with the patient (in providing specific services) and with the primary clinician (in making their contribution to the whole picture). The problem is that collaborative care is often *not* collaborative because clinicians fail to communicate promptly, appropriately, or completely.

Requesting Consultation

As professionals we are expected to communicate effectively with colleagues, consultants, and team members. Here are some pointers to keep in mind:

- Be specific about your reason for consultation. Remember that technical consultants (such as radiologists) need to know the nature of the problem and something about the patient as well. Thus, you should provide a short patient vignette when requesting a procedure. For example, rather than simply scrawling "mammogram" on a requisition form, you might write, "Ms. B is a 49-year-old woman with fibrocystic breast disease who is very anxious about a tender new mass she discovered last month in the inferior lateral quadrant of her left breast."
- Make the request in an appropriate manner and indicate level of urgency. In some cases you will simply send or fax a request to the consultant's office; in urgent cases you will speak directly with the consultant.
- Be sure the consultant can easily contact you to obtain additional information or answer questions.
- Ensure that the patient (or the patient's family) is aware of the consultation, understands its purpose, and has consented.
- Provide follow-up as a courtesy to your consultant.

Providing Consultation

- Clarify what the questions of interest are and focus your evaluation on answering those questions.
- Respond to the request promptly and flexibly. In addition to a written note, it is often appropriate to call the referring clinician with your observations and impressions.
- If you continue to follow the patient, keep the referring clinician informed about progress or developments.

SUMMARY—The Clinical Narrative

In this chapter we presented guidelines for translating your interview experience into a case write-up as well as an oral case presentation. The write-up and other parts of the medical record serve as memory aids, methods of communication, data for quality assessment and research, and administrative or legal documents. A typical format for the case description is outlined in Table 8–1, *Elements of Clinical Case Description,* page 144.

We also discussed a number of additional points about clinical narratives and medical records:

- The present illness is a narrative of the patient's experience; it should read like a story.
- The problem-based medical record system includes several useful concepts that enhance patient care:
  - An initial database
  - Flow sheets
  - A problem list
  - Respect for subjective data
  - A broad human perspective, rather than a narrow disease perspective
- When recording personal information, be careful to respect the patient's privacy as much as possible.
- Use language that describes but does not pathologize.

Finally, we discussed the oral case presentation that serves as the basis for day-to-day communication among health professionals about patient care. Formal presentations should be concise, well organized, and designed to convey a clear picture of the patient's story, your findings, and a summary of your thinking about the case. Consultation and other forms of communication among professionals should be focused on improving patient care through efficiency and coordination.

PART TWO

BASIC SKILLS IN PRACTICE

CHAPTER 9

Communication in the Office Setting

The Real Satisfaction

*It's the humdrum, day-in, day-out, everyday work
that is the real satisfaction of the practice of medicine; the million and a half patients a man has
seen on his daily visits over a forty-year period
of weekdays and Sundays that make up his life.*
William Carlos Williams, *The Autobiography*

UNDERSTANDING THE INTERVIEW
IN THE OFFICE SETTING

Because of its longitudinal nature, ambulatory care practice presents
many opportunities to use interviewing skills to enhance patient care and
develop effective relationships. However, interviewing in the office setting also presents particular challenges. Outpatient practice can be complex and unpredictable. In a typical day, one patient may come in with a
simple acute problem such as a sore throat; another, for follow-up of a
chronic disorder like arthritis or hypothyroidism; a third may arrive with
unexplained symptoms like malaise or fatigue; and a fourth for palliative
care of a terminal illness. Often, a patient we believe has come in for a
follow-up visit surprises us with a new complaint or asks, "What was my
last cholesterol level, and why haven't I had it checked lately?" Normally,
the clinician does not have an hour or more to spend with each patient,
nor do patients expect to spend their day sitting in a clinician's office;
thus, efficiency and thoroughness may seem to be at odds.

   Although hospitalized patients today are sicker and have shorter stays
than in the past, interviewing them is, in some ways, straightforward.
Frequently only one principal problem has caused the hospitalization
(chest pain, for example, or rectal bleeding), even though chronic disor-

ders (such as diabetes or hypertension) will influence the patient's care. Thus, what we call a linear approach to the patient's history makes sense: a complete exploration of the chief complaint and history of the present illness, followed in order by other active problems, past medical history, and so forth. We can start at A and proceed to Z. However, it is not unusual for the ambulatory patient to present acute, chronic, and preventive issues during a single 15-minute visit. This requires a more complex, nonlinear approach.

The first section of this chapter introduces various ways of gaining efficiency and focus in order to improve communication in the clinical office setting. Subsequent sections consider special issues: problems of communication in office practice, including those associated with managed care; the interview as a tool in preventive medicine; and the crucial role that confidentiality and truthfulness play in everyday clinician-patient interactions. These skills convert sources of frustration into opportunities for better patient care—"the real satisfaction."

GAINING EFFICIENCY AND FOCUS

In ambulatory care, the patient's needs dictate the character and completeness of your clinical history at any given time. One history might be a database on a healthy person seeking guidance about cardiac risk factors; another patient may have an acute illness that demands immediate attention; and others are returning for follow-up of chronic conditions that are influenced by medical, emotional, and social factors. Additionally, chronically ill patients may present with acute, perhaps unrelated, problems. *How to Achieve Efficiency and Focus in the Office Setting*, below, presents a short list of skills for achieving efficiency and focus. In the following sections, we address each of these issues in turn and illustrate how good interviewing skills allow the clinician to be both thorough and efficient.

WHAT TO SAY
How to Achieve Efficiency and Focus in the Office Setting

Solicit the patient's agenda.

- "Tell me more about why you scheduled this visit."
- "What would you like for us to accomplish today?"

Negotiate priorities.

- "You have a lot of concerns. Would it be okay if we deal with the worst one first?"
- "I agree that we have to deal with your sore throat, but I'm also worried about your weight gain."

Orient the patient to the flow of the encounter.

- "Let me find out first what your symptoms are; then I'll examine you. That way I can figure out what's wrong. Is that okay?"

Maximize patient understanding.

- "Now when you say you're worried about your mercury level because you eat a lot of fish, what do you mean? Tell me what you've heard about what mercury does to you."

Soliciting the Patient's Agenda

At times a desire for efficiency tempts us to abandon an open-ended interviewing style in favor of more focused questioning. We think that if we ask just the right questions or follow an algorithm, we will save time. If the patient has chest pain, we will stick to chest pain questions; if he has an upset stomach, we will concentrate only on gastrointestinal (GI) questions, and so forth. Another temptation is to interrupt the patient before she finishes the opening statement, or perhaps even the chief complaint. It might be difficult to imagine a medical history without a chief complaint, but consider the following examples:

Example 1

Clinician **Hello. You're here because of back pain?**
Patient Yes, I have lower back pain. And …
How long have you had it?

Example 2

Clinician **Hi, how have you been? Let's see, I had you come back today to see how your depression is doing.**
Patient That part's okay. But …
How many pills are you up to now?

Example 3

Clinician	**How's it going?**
Patient	Not too well, lot of discomfort here [puts his hand on back] down the arch and here under the arm and, ah, here, and this here …
	How about the pacemaker clinic, were you there this morning?

Notice that the clinician, not the patient, has stated the chief complaint in each of these examples. The clinician has closed the inquiry to other problems or symptoms by indicating what topics may be discussed. In the third example, the clinician completely ignores the patient's obvious back discomfort because he thinks of him as a patient with cardiac problems. A landmark study of practicing physicians found that the average time a patient was allowed to speak before being interrupted was only 23 seconds. Patients who are initially cut off are likely to be dissatisfied and try again and again to return to *their* concern, or they may simply give up and not have their problems addressed. How often does the patient with heart problems fail to have his arthritis evaluated because aching joints are not on the clinician's agenda?

Paradoxically, *you save time by remaining quiet and allowing patients to have their say.* Open-ended questions and listening to the entire response allow you to generate hypotheses quickly: you can sit back and think while the patient is talking. Although questions such as "How's your diabetes?" or "How's your chest pain?" may sometimes be useful, they should be delayed until later in the interview.

Here are examples of better ways to initiate the encounter:

Example 1

Clinician	**Hi, Mrs. Jones, I'm Dr. Walker. Nice to meet you.**
Patient	Same here.
	What brings you here today?
	I'm having a problem with my back. It's still bothering me. And for the past 10 years, I've had a chronic problem with phlebitis in the legs, and I have some problem with my feet swelling at times and therefore circulation in both legs. But right now I'm having a devastating problem with my lower back. It's been going on ever since about the 20th of October. And I would like to see if I could get into a diet program.
	A diet program?
	Uh huh.
	First, why don't you tell me about your back.

Example 2

Clinician	**What brings you here today?**
Patient	Well, for several weeks now I've had these lumps on my head; they're really itchy. My neck hurts, too. I think it's from when I had that accident, you know, it keeps acting up. Since I am here, I might as well have it checked.
	Okay. Have you had any other medical problems recently?

Example 3

Clinician	**Tell me why you came today.**
Patient	Well, I haven't had physicals on a regular basis. I'm feeling like I'm getting to a point where I ought to do that.
	So, you need a good physical?
	Right.
	You sure it's not a specific problem you noticed?
	Not really.
	Okay. But if you think of something while we're talking, don't hesitate to mention it. How has your health been?

These examples depict clinicians who begin with open-ended questions that permit the patient to state a chief complaint and elaborate on other concerns, so that the full range of patient concerns is "on the table." In the third example, the clinician notices the patient's apparent hedge ("Not really," as opposed to "No, not at all") and reassures him that he is welcome to bring up symptoms as the interview progresses. In the second transcript, the clinician listens to the patient's full response, and then encourages additional disclosure: "Have you had any other medical problems recently?" Studies have shown that patients who are permitted to state all their concerns use only a few seconds more on average than patients whose clinicians interrupt or redirect them. However, those who *are* interrupted more often bring up additional concerns later in the interview, thus prolonging the interaction. Undisclosed agendas lead to missed diagnoses, not to mention angry patients (who feel that they did not get what they came for) and frustrated clinicians (who get telephone calls the same day from patients who have just left the office and now have "new" complaints).

◆ PRACTICE POINT

The extra seconds you invest in listening to the patient's opening statement may be the most critical time of the interview, ensuring

that the patient's "hidden" agenda does not remain hidden. Do not interrupt! Remember, listening saves time.

Negotiate Priorities

What if the patient offers more complaints than you can handle in the time allotted? When the patient presents several concerns, you must establish priorities and set an agenda. What has to be attended to today? What can wait until next week or next month? What problem is of most concern to the patient? To the clinician? Here is an example of a woman scheduled for a routine follow-up visit. She had developed a new symptom and some nonmedical concerns. The first-year family practice resident summarized the situation as follows (*we have annotated the text to indicate the different types of problems*):

> L.B. is a 50-year-old divorced woman whom I am seeing in follow-up for newly diagnosed diabetes mellitus and hypertension [*chronic diseases*]. She has been on metformin and her concerns for this visit are that about 1 week ago she experienced a dramatic change in her visual acuity [*acute problem*]. She states that even with her glasses she is still unable to read as she had before. She can't see; her vision is blurry. She denies headaches or eye pain. She denies any other neurological deficit. No numbness or tingling, no swelling of her extremities. Ms. B's other concern is that the Department of Labor states that if she has been ill, she is unable to collect unemployment benefits [*economic and social concern*]. She requests a note stating that she is medically cleared to continue seeking work and, therefore, eligible for unemployment benefits. Her other problem is that she can't sleep because of anxiety, both about her job and also because of her former husband, who keeps threatening her [*emotional and social concern*].

Given this complexity, you frequently cannot attend to all the issues in one visit. Fortunately, you do not have to. It is the clinician's responsibility to take the lead in negotiating (see Chapter 18, Education and Negotiation) priorities.

◆ PRACTICE POINT

The complete patient database evolves, develops, changes, and extends over the course of your ongoing relationship with the patient; you do not need to obtain it all in one visit.

Consider this example of a 72-year-old woman who came for a routine follow-up visit.

Clinician	**Hi, It's nice to see you. What are we doing today, your routine blood pressure check or are there other things?**
Patient	No, I'm fine, just my blood pressure check. And then there are some things I want to ask you about.
	While I'm rechecking your pressure, why don't you tell me what's on your mind so we have enough time to cover everything?
	Well, my sister wants to know why I haven't had that screening test for ovarian cancer, and she's on blood pressure medicine too but her blood pressure is kept much lower than mine and she said I'd better tell you about this, I had in my chest, not a pain but it went into my jaw and my shoulder and I felt a burning in my throat. I stopped taking my Zantac.
	Okay, I hear you have several concerns. Tell me more about your chest pain first, as this concerns me.

Note how, after the patient's opening statement, the clinician encourages the patient to "lay the cards on the table" by specifying all of today's concerns, which she does. This initial phase establishes the range of problems and their breadth, but not their depth. It may be likened to the overture of a musical score in which each theme is briefly introduced but then set aside to be developed more fully later. In music, certain conventions and the composer's artistry determine the order in which the themes or melodies may be developed. In clinical interviewing, the clinician and the patient then negotiate how to proceed. When one problem is not clearly more urgent than another, the patient may be the one to decide how to use the limited time. But when there is an urgent problem that the patient does not recognize, or if the patient is not capable of making decisions, the clinician must play a more direct role in setting the agenda. In this example, the patient's chest pain clearly takes priority. The clinician must develop this theme first in order to ensure the patient's safety and an appropriate response to what could be new-onset symptoms of coronary artery disease.

Non-urgent Health Problems

When a patient has several non-urgent problems, a summary statement followed by a question and an explanation of your strategy may help:

Clinician	**You've mentioned three concerns—your weight, this pain in your foot, and the premenstrual symptoms. Since our time is limited, which one would you like to focus on today [or first]?"**
	or
Clinician	**I can see that you're really bothered by this itching in your feet [*summary statement and interchangeable response*]. But I noticed that your weight is up about 10 pounds and you seem a little short of breath. Since our time is limited, is it okay if we check out your heart and lungs first?**

New Health Problems

It is easy to overlook new problems when a patient is scheduled for what looks like a routine follow-up visit and you start the interview off with, "How's the diabetes doing?" as opposed to, "How have things been going lately?" The latter is totally unrestricted and may even invite nonmedical responses like, "My health is great, but my job is driving me crazy." "How has your health been?" or "How have your medical problems been doing?" are intermediate queries restricted to whatever concerns the patient perceives as health related. "What can I do for you today?" is a good beginning; it is open-ended, yet indicates the desire to focus on "today."

Chronic Health Problems

Here is an example of how you might begin an interim history for a patient with a number of chronic health problems.

Clinician	**Tell me why you came in today.**
Patient	Just my regular visit. Dr. Smith said I had to come back for a checkup.
	A checkup?
	Yeah, he said I needed to have my blood sugar rechecked after he changed the medication.
	Okay, fine. We can certainly take care of that. Anything else I should know about or that we should discuss before we get to that? Are you having any other problems?
	Well, since my last visit I've noticed some trouble with my breathing.

Notice how the interviewer sets the stage for establishing priorities by making sure nothing else is going on. The blood sugar may not be an immediate concern if the patient has developed shortness of breath, possibly suggesting congestive heart failure. This search for other active problems (OAP) (see Chapter 4, Other Active Problems, Past Medical History, and Family History) is an essential part of every initial or follow-up outpatient interview in order to clarify what needs to be addressed today. Unlike the initial interview of a hospitalized patient, where the discussion of OAPs tends to occur after the complete development of the history of the present illness, the discussion of OAPs occurs early in the ambulatory setting, particularly for those with chronic disease.

◈ Practice Point

The search for OAPs is essential in setting the agenda to make efficient use of your time with the patient and to prevent the "hand-on-the-doorknob" phenomenon (see Chapter 3, Chief Complaint and Present Illness, and below).

Hidden Health Problems

We illustrate this section with a 60-year-old woman who scheduled an appointment because she had been having chest pain. Notice the clinician's confusion as the patient states her chief complaint, which is not the chest pain for which the clinician thought the visit had been arranged.

Clinician	**How are you feeling today?**
Patient	Oh, not too good. I still have that goofy headache.
	You still have the headache?
	And it's, I would say, one side, just sick. It's on the right side, and it starts here and it goes to the top of my head.
	Have you ever had a headache like this before?
	Oh, I've had headaches ever since 1965. I would take attacks and my blood pressure was very high and the doctor gave me medication.
	I see. Is there anything different about this headache that you have right now compared to your other headaches that you've had?
	Compared to the other headaches, this one is not quite as bad. But I've had it several days and it started about Sunday, and I'm worried about my blood pressure. Then I started having those chest pains.
	And you've been having chest pains? Tell me about them [search for OAPs].
	Well, they're right here. [Patient points to right pectoral area and then reaches around to her back.] It's right up in here and down around in there. Sharp. Like I went to pick up something off the dresser and it just grabbed me.
	Okay. And you're also worried about your pressure? [OAP]

> When I went to the store, I took it on the machine. It was a hundred and ninety something.
>
> **Okay. What would you say is the thing that's worrying you the most right now?**

Notice that the clinician has established both the range of problems (at least three) and their urgency (none seems particularly urgent—the headaches are old and no worse, the chest pain is probably musculoskeletal, and the blood pressure taken in the office is 140/90). Given the limited time available, the clinician now turns the agenda over to the patient, who will dictate which concern to deal with during this encounter. (By the way, this is the patient we met in Chapter 5, The Patient Profile, who actually answered the last question by saying her main worry was "how to get those bills paid." So the agenda in this case was, indeed, completely hidden until the patient was permitted to decide how best to use the visit.)

Orient the Patient to the Flow of the Encounter

Part of figuring out what you are going to address at a particular visit—and ensuring that the patient is satisfied—is to orient patients to the flow of the encounter. How an office functions or what to expect at a particular visit is something of a "black box" for patients. Most have no idea about how much time has been scheduled for them, and they often do not differentiate between routine follow-up care, visits for acute problems, and visits for comprehensive assessments, such as annual physicals, preoperative evaluations, or routine gynecologic care. The clinician may choose between appearing rushed and dismissive (of problems deemed trivial) or explaining limitations in time (e.g., "There are other patients waiting," or "Can we keep to the schedule so that other patients are taken care of in a timely fashion?") and the original purpose of the visit. Here are some examples:

Example 1

Clinician **I can see you have a lot of concerns that you want me to take care of today. Perhaps we should have scheduled you for more than just a 15-minute visit. But since that is the time we have, we can use it best by checking the most important problem. Then I will get you on my schedule ASAP for a longer visit so we can do a really thorough evaluation. Does that sound okay?**

Example 2

Clinician   Gee, I guess I thought you were coming in for a repeat Pap test to follow up the one that was abnormal. But I can see you have other concerns. If we have time after your Pap, we can get started on these other problems. But then I will have to have you schedule another visit so we don't miss anything. Are you all right with that?

Example 3

Clinician   I would really like the opportunity to listen carefully to your concerns. These are the kind of problems that deserve more time and attention than I can give today.

Notice how the clinician uses positive as opposed to negative statements, such as "We don't have time," to describe the constraints of the schedule and helps the patient feel valued with the statement "Your problems deserve," rather than giving the patient the feeling of being dismissed by, for example, ignoring the unexpected complaints, looking at the clock, or performing other actions that would show lack of interest or respect. All of these statements focus on the patient, and they are also examples of *transparency*. There is a tremendous difference between looking at your watch, which will leave the patient with the thought that "he was in a hurry," and stating that, unfortunately, you have another patient waiting, which allows the patient to process the situation as "he had to work in an emergency so I'll get a thorough assessment at another visit."

Maximize Patient Understanding

Another way of improving efficiency and focus is to help the patient better understand the issues and, in essence, to become a more informed participant in the office visit. Nowadays, by the time patients approach a clinician about a health problem, they frequently have gathered a great deal of information about their disease (whether self-diagnosed or not) from newspaper or magazine articles, television, self-help health books, and especially the Internet. Depending on their general health beliefs, they may have also sought specific information elsewhere—from a natural health food store, for example, or from a massage therapist. Unfortunately, although the information they have gathered may sometimes be accurate and may therefore enhance the efficiency of the encounter, it may just as well be fragmentary, misleading, contradictory, or otherwise confusing (see Chapter 12, Cultural Competence in the Interview). If so, it may actually *detract* from efficiency and focus because of "hidden knowledge"; in other words, the clinician's attempts to prioritize or explain compete with the patient's alternative priorities or explanations, of which he or she may be unaware. Moreover, treatment may often be compromised because the patient simply does not understand the nature and severity of the illness, the nature of the medication, the specific directions for taking it, or the expected outcome of treatment.

We explore these issues again in Chapter 18, Education and Negotiation, in the context of clinician-patient negotiation. Skillful attention to good educational technique in the interview will likely lead to better outcomes, as well as empowering the patient to make more informed decisions. However, in this chapter we want to emphasize that attention to educational technique will also enhance the efficiency and focus of office visits by improving the patient's ability to participate. Here is an example of the final part of a diagnostic interview in which, among other problems, the clinician appears to pay little attention to conveying understandable information.

Clinician	**Okay, Mr. H., you've been having these problems for some time and I think they warrant further investigation. I'm not quite sure right now: some of your symptoms seem to be upper GI but some seem to be colonic as well. It could be an ulcer problem, or it could be inflammatory bowel disease. I think the first thing to do is to schedule a colonoscopy and then we'll go on from there. I can arrange for the colonoscopy early next week. The nurse can give you an exact time, and meanwhile we'll consider getting you scheduled for an upper endoscopy.**
Patient	Is that test you mentioned, is that the one where you insert a tube in my rectum? I had one of those a few years ago. I could hardly stand it.
	Well, it's not the most comfortable thing, but it is important, and we give you some sedatives. It's the only way you can get to the whole colon, look at it, see the problem. It's not as bad as you think.
	The main problem I'm having is this bloated feeling, and the indigestion. I didn't think it was so serious. I thought it was probably my stomach. Isn't there some medicine?
	As you said, it's been bothering you for quite some time, so I think we ought to get to the bottom of it. You can never be too careful. The problem with the GI tract is that, a lot of times,

symptoms blend together and it's hard to know what you're dealing with unless you look.

Do you think it might be something serious, I mean like an ulcer or something?

Well, it could be an ulcer, but it's not typical. I think we'll just have to do the workup and see. In the meantime, I'm going to give you an antispasmodic drug to take; you can take it with every meal and at bedtime. And I'll also give you one that suppresses acid. Two prescriptions. We'll see what happens.

Let us focus first on the clinician's initial statement. How could he have presented the information in a way that would have decreased the patient's uncertainty and improved his understanding? First, the clinician could have used words and phrases the patient was more likely to understand. He should not have used the terms *inflammatory bowel disease, colonoscopy,* and *upper endoscopy* unless he intended to explain them, or at least he should have determined whether the patient knew what they meant. Medical jargon can easily creep into conversations with patients, but it need not. You should be able to describe in plain language what you believe is going on in the patient's body.

Second, the clinician could have been specific about the problems being considered, the steps in the diagnostic plan, and the benefits and risks of his approach. Instead, he spoke in general terms: "further investigation" and "go on from there." What does this mean? Although he had not yet made a precise diagnosis, he could have been more explicit about options and, more importantly for the patient's peace of mind, the likely outcome: "Will I get better?" "Is my condition serious?" "Is it likely that I'll need surgery?" Eric Cassell coined the term "vague reference" to characterize this technique of tangential communication with patients, which often leads to increased, rather than decreased, anxiety about the problem because it encourages the patient to imagine the worst. Increased anxiety prolongs visits.

Third, this clinician could have stated the most important information concisely at the beginning. Patients are more likely to remember the initial chunk of information than they are to remember data presented later. You should hook the patient's memory by giving a succinct statement that puts the problem in a frame of reference and leads to "Here's how we'll deal with it." The clinician might then employ another technique, repetition, to bring home the salient points later.

Finally, at the end of the segment, the clinician could have asked how much the patient understood, listened, and then given some feedback.

This feedback process substantially increases patient satisfaction as well as accurate recall of information. The clinician could also have encouraged questions. These techniques for maximizing patient education also help avoid the "hand-on-the-doorknob" phenomenon (see Chapter 3, Chief Complaint and Present Illness).

Taking the example as a whole, we see that the clinician's approach creates new questions in the patient's mind while leaving the old one ("Is it something serious?") unanswered. The next visit, or an intervening telephone call, may well need to start from scratch as far as prioritizing and keeping on target. However, let us look at how the same clinician, on a better day, shares his findings and suggests a plan.

Clinician	**Well, Mr. H., you've had a difficult time with this problem, but I believe we'll be able to get to the bottom of it and find out what's wrong. We will have to do some additional tests, though, before we can say for sure. Your main symptoms, the cramps you get and the loose bowels, are most likely caused by a problem in your colon, one that we call irritable bowel syndrome. That means that there's a spasm in the muscles of your large bowel and that gives you the cramps and so on. But your other symptoms, that bloated feeling in the stomach and pain up there, they also suggest an acid problem, like ulcer or gastritis.**
Patient	Are any of those serious?
	They're all medical problems that can be treated or cured. There's nothing to suggest that you have something really serious like cancer, for example. It could be an ulcer, but I think it's more likely that irritable bowel syndrome can explain all of your symptoms.
	I really want to get to the bottom of this; I just can't take it any more. I just can't get my work done feeling like I do now.
	It sounds as though these attacks have really gotten to you.
	I'd say I'm almost paralyzed.
	Okay, I understand. What I'd like to do is to schedule some tests today. The first one is a colonoscopy; that's a procedure in which I insert a flexible tube into your rectum. I can look through it and check the lining of your whole large bowel, like for irritation or diverticuli—they are little pockets or outpouchings in the bowel that sometimes cause pain and other symptoms in persons your age. You'll come to our outpatient suite at the hospital for that. You'll have to prepare for the test by

cleaning out your bowel, taking some laxatives and a Fleets enema over the night before we do it. Before you leave today, check with Sarah. You and she can work out a convenient time to schedule the colonoscopy and then she'll give you a brochure that explains everything; it's like a question-and-answer format.

But do you think it might be something serious, like an ulcer or something?

Is there anything specific you're thinking about? Possibly it could be an ulcer ...

Well, ulcers can kill you, can't they?

It sounds like you heard something bad about ulcers.

My uncle bled to death from one. First they said it was an ulcer, then it didn't heal, he couldn't eat anything. Finally they found out it was cancer.

And you're worried that this could be cancer, even if the tests show something else?

I don't know. Like I say, I can't take it any more. My nerves are part of it, maybe.

Let's take this a step at a time. First, your symptoms and my examination do not show any suggestion of cancer; we have no reason to suspect it. As I said, it really sounds like either irritable bowel or an acid problem. That's the most likely. I'm suggesting the colonoscopy just to make sure we don't miss something, such as the diverticuli, like I said. Let me explain that a little more.

This time the clinician has used several techniques that will enhance patient understanding and cooperation. (See *Enhance Efficiency Through Patient Understanding,* below). He also actively elicited the patient's beliefs with the statement, "It sounds like you heard something bad" and considered them in his explanation. This patient is likely to approach subsequent visits as a more satisfied and focused patient.

WHAT TO SAY
Enhance Efficiency Through Patient Understanding

- Use plain English, rather than medical jargon.
  - "Let's check your cholesterol." (not "Let's do a lipid panel.")

- Use concrete and specific language; avoid vague reference.
  - "We will monitor your symptoms for one week; then we will know if this medication is working." (Not "We'll see what's what.")
- State the important message first, then use repetition to reinforce it.
  - "This is not cancer; it is a growth, or tumor, but it is not cancer." (Not "You have a tumor that needs to come out.")
- Ask the patient to restate the message.
  - "Do you mind telling me what I just said so I can be sure you understand?"
- Give corrective feedback.
  - "That's not exactly what I meant. This IS something we need to take care of, but it is not serious."
- Provide opportunities for questions.
  - "I want to be sure you understand. Do you have any questions?"

CHALLENGES TO COMMUNICATION IN OFFICE PRACTICE

In U.S. clinical practice insurers often "manage" the services available to a given patient by offering comprehensive systems of care that range from preventive services and primary care through subspecialty and tertiary care. Managed care programs require each person to identify a participating primary care provider who coordinates the patient's total health care, ideally with an emphasis on prevention, including programs for health promotion and behavioral medicine (e.g., smoking cessation).

One troublesome feature of managed care arises not so much from the concept as from its current implementation. Because health insurance in the United States is overwhelmingly employer based, people often must change their insurance when they change jobs or when their employer signs a contract with a different insurer. These changes often require patients to change their primary care provider. A second troublesome feature arises from making the primary care provider integral to the system. Because many patients are accustomed to dealing with several different specialists, they may perceive the requirement to obtain referrals from a primary care provider as burdensome. Moreover, when generalists attempt to provide care that is more rational by limiting the fragmentation of services, thereby acting as the patient's advocate, some patients believe them to be acting as "gatekeepers" to prevent access to a desired service. These conflicts in beliefs and expectations, what we call coerced change and dueling agendas, may fuel dissatisfaction among both patients and clinicians.

Although some clinicians and patients believe that these problems originated with managed care, they are, in fact, general features of clinician-patient interactions and not limited to certain settings. Hence, we consider them as additional challenges in office practice.

Coerced Change

Consider this opening exchange between a patient and her new clinician, whom she identified from a list of participating providers in her new health insurance program.

Clinician What can I do for you, Ms. B?

Patient   Well, they told me I had to come in and see you. What happened is, my health insurance changed and now I can't see my regular doctor anymore. I've been going to him for about 10 years now. He knows my whole history, everything.

This clinician has a serious handicap: the patient seems upset that she can't see her "regular" doctor and has come only because "they" told her to. The patient's opening statement is not about her symptoms, but about her frustration and possible anger. One temptation here is for the clinician to ignore or minimize the patient's concerns and try to proceed immediately with the chief complaint. For example, he might say, "Okay, but tell me what your medical problem is," or "That's too bad, but we can get copies of the records. ... Now what is your problem today?" The latter statement acknowledges the situation, but fails to consider the patient's feelings. It implies that the clinical record captures everything that's important in a clinician-patient relationship, that clinicians are interchangeable. A second temptation might be to respond to the patient's negative tone with a challenge or hostile clarification. For example, "Well, actually you could continue see your doctor, but you'd just have to pay part of the bill." Or, worse yet, "Look, that's your problem, but if you want me to be your doctor, I have to take your medical history."

Alternatively, how might this clinician respond in a more effective way? Consider the following two responses:

Response 1

Clinician [After a few seconds' pause.] It sounds as if you had a good relationship with your doctor.

Response 2

Clinician **It must be really frustrating when that happens. You probably just picked my name out of the book and you don't know what to expect.**

In both cases the clinician gives an empathic, interchangeable response (see "Interchangeable Responses" in Chapter 2). The first response demonstrates an understanding of the cognitive content (previous relationship); the second focuses on the affective content (current frustration). Either is appropriate in this situation, but the second response goes a bit further because it addresses an additional area of concern: the patient's uncertainty of what to expect from a new clinician. It gives the patient permission to verbalize her fears. For example, this conversation might continue:

Patient   Well, yes, I just had to go through my new insurance carrier's list, so I tried you because it's pretty convenient to get to your office. My regular doctor was Dr. Samuels, just up the road in Port Jefferson. He's been treating me for years for my diabetes and arthritis.

Clinician **Oh, I know Dr. Samuels. He's a very good internist. I understand why you hate to be forced to leave him. Well, I'll try to do a good job for you, too. And with your permission we can send for a copy of your records at Dr. Samuels's office.**

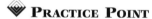 **PRACTICE POINT**

In situations of coerced change, you should apply the general rule of engaging active listening skills at the beginning of the patient interview in order to remove barriers to effective communication as soon as you identify them.

Dueling Agendas

At times your understanding of your role in caring for a patient is totally at odds with the patient's expectations. Consider this example:

Clinician **How can I help you, Mr. C.?**

Patient   They told me I had to see my PCP [primary care provider] to get these referrals. [Brings out a list.] I have an appointment next Tuesday with Dr. Nephron, who treats me for blood pressure, so I need that one today. And then my regular follow-ups with my allergist, my diabetes specialist—by the way, my sugar's high—and my cardiologist are due. So I thought I'd better get those referrals now, so I don't have to keep calling your office. And while I'm here, I was also wondering if you could recommend a good specialist for my stomach?

How would you feel if you were this patient's primary care provider? The patient is acting as if the clinician were a clerk whose sole function is to handle the paperwork to give him access to an array of specialists. This PCP—to use today's jargon for the patient's primary care physician—is bound to feel unappreciated and perhaps angry, and might be tempted to reply, "Wait a second, that's not how things work here. I'm the one who decides what referrals you need." This response would almost certainly lead to a needless confrontation. The problem, of course, is that the patient and clinician here have radically different agendas: the clinician sees herself as taking care of the patient and addressing his illness, whereas the patient views her as an administrative cog.

Direct Approach

Dueling agendas demand a direct approach. Unlike the coerced change example, it is unlikely that simple facilitative responses will encourage the patient to accept the clinician's care. The issue here is a radical misunderstanding of (or disagreement with) the nature of primary care. If the clinician tried a simple interchangeable response such as, "Well, Mr. C., it sounds as if you have quite a few medical problems," the patient is likely to agree and indicate that that is precisely why he needs so many doctors. What is required here is a clear and relatively complete educational statement, using skills similar to the transparency employed in orienting patients to the flow of the encounter.

Clinician	**Well, Mr. C., it sounds as though you've needed quite a few specialists, and certainly if you have an appointment with Dr. Nephron on Tuesday, I agree that we should arrange a referral for you. But today we're scheduled for a new patient visit–that means a complete checkup–so I think we should get started so I can understand your problems better. Did you have a primary care doctor before you joined Magna Care?**
Patient	Not really. I used to go to Dr. Smith for colds and things, you know, maybe once a year, but he never did any testing, just wrote me a prescription for antibiotics or something.
	OK, then, let me start by explaining how I view my role. I'd like to be your main doctor and coordinate all your medical care. And I'd like to get to know you better, so that maybe together we can work on improving your health. If we decide that you

> need to see a specialist, then he or she will report back to me
> and we can talk about it. Now first, I'd like to understand your
> health problems. So can we start from what's bothering you
> right now, your stomach, and then we can talk about your
> sugar and your heart and so forth. How's that?
> Well OK, but it's a long story.

This approach, of course, is not a miraculous resolution to dueling agendas: there will probably be continued tension over referrals, the need for additional education, and, possibly, confrontation. Note, however, four aspects of this clinician's approach.

- She immediately acknowledges the patient's most pressing request: the appointment with Dr. Nephron. Whether or not a nephrologist is required, the PCP minimizes the disruption to the patient's expectations by acceding to that referral. At the least, the referral buys her some time to establish a relationship based on education and negotiation and, ultimately, trust.
- She begins to establish the ground rules, including the fact that she views herself as the patient's major care provider. The message to Mr. C. is clear, although not yet fully detailed.
- She states her case without reference to Magna Care rules or expectations; good medical care is justified on its own merits. If she had said, "You're in Magna Care now, so let me explain the restrictions they have on referrals to specialists," she would, to some extent, be opting out of the therapeutic role by engaging in a game of "us versus them."
- She is reasonable and friendly in her explanation. She speaks firmly, but does not yield to the understandable impulse to begin with, "What do you think this is, a supermarket where you can come in and pick out anything you want?"

Dueling agendas are often obvious in managed care arrangements, but this dynamic is important in all forms of clinical practice—for example, the patient who demands an antibiotic for a viral illness or insists upon a 2-week work excuse for a minor injury or the patient who can't understand your hesitation when she comes to your office (after a 6-month interval) demanding, "I want to see a specialist because this never really went away—the cold I had in January—and it's now August."

We present additional examples in the section on "Papers, Forms, and Clearances" later in this chapter and consider the subject in more detail in Chapter 18, Education and Negotiation.

E-mail Communication with Patients

Electronic mail has the potential to add an important new dimension to clinician-patient communication. For example, patients' use of e-mail might well alleviate such chronic problems as gaining easy access to their clinicians to ask health-related questions, or providing an efficient way to transmit additional information, or obtaining lab reports promptly. Clinicians might use e-mail as way of responding to non-urgent patient messages, or of providing patients with important health education updates. Patients expect to participate in a process of shared decision making regarding their health care; yet geographic and temporal barriers between patient and clinician often prevent the flow of information that would allow such a process to occur. We can take a big step toward eliminating such barriers through the intelligent use of e-mail. Nonetheless, as anyone who has ever received a "spam" message well knows, e-mail also has great potential for unethical and inappropriate use.

Although e-mail has become almost universal in our culture, we have no idea how this age of virtual messaging will affect clinical practice in 10 or 20 years. However, there is every indication that electronic messaging will rapidly grow here as elsewhere. Studies have shown that between 6% and 16% of adults engage in some form of e-mail communication with their clinicians, most frequently to obtain laboratory results or request prescription refills. Other common message types include feedback to the clinician regarding home health monitoring (e.g., blood pressure, blood sugar), specific health questions, and queries for office staff (e.g., appointments, billing). Patients surveyed in these studies agree that e-mail is more efficient and satisfying than telephone contact, even though it lacks the synchronicity and spontaneity of verbal interaction. In fact, Medicare (in the 2005 Healthcare Common Procedure Coding System Update) lists a procedure code for electronic patient-clinician interaction: "online evaluation and management service, per encounter, provided by a physician, using the Internet or similar electronic communications network, in response to a patient request, established patient."

Patient-to-Clinician Electronic Messaging

In this text we presuppose that the appropriate way to initiate a clinician-patient relationship is by conducting a medical interview, which is ordinarily a live interactive process in which the participants speak face to face (and, hopefully, heart to heart as well). Although there may be unusual circumstances in which it is necessary to conduct a medical interview over the phone or by means of interactive video technology, we do not consider e-mail in any form as a viable replacement for a live medical interview, either in establishing an initial database or in developing a relationship.

◆ PRACTICE POINT
E-mail can be an effective tool to improve communication with patients. Like any other tool, e-mail is most effective when used with specific, limited, and well-defined goals in mind.

However, e-mail may serve a useful purpose by filling in needed details of the medical history, enhancing accuracy of data already provided, or providing a mechanism to "reopen" the clinical history for new material, if necessary, long after the clinician-patient encounter is over. Consider the following e-mail messages:

> Yesterday I couldn't remember how my grandparents died. I just asked my sister and she said grandpa died of a heart attack when he was 72 or 73 years old; and grandma evidently had leukemia.

> About my colectomy, it was done at Good Samaritan Hospital in 1984, not at St. Charles like I said when I saw you last week.

> I don't know why, but I forgot to mention my anemia. I've always had a low blood count. My old doctor said it was hereditary.

In each case the patient provides useful information that might have been lost if he or she had to deliver the message over the phone ("Is this something worth calling the doctor about?") or wait until a subsequent appointment.

Information transfer is an ongoing process, which continues—ideally, with more and more efficiency—as the relationship progresses over time. Later in the relationship, a patient might send her clinician messages like these:

> I'm coming in on the 28th, 2 PM. Before I forget, here are 4 things we need to talk about: Henry's ulcer, that new cream for my psoriasis, osteoporosis, and my shoulder—the exercises seem to make it worse.

> Doc, I've attached a list of my blood pressures for the last 2 weeks—checked it once before work each day and once before supper, like you said.

In the first message, the patient establishes her agenda for the upcoming office visit, thus providing an important "heads up" to the clinician, who could begin negotiating priorities for the visit by referring to the message in the patient's chart. Likewise, the second message provides a convenient way of transmitting (as well as documenting) useful clinical data.

Clinician-to-Patient Electronic Messaging

The most obvious, and evidently most frequent, role for e-mail communication in clinical practice at present is to enhance the patient's access to information: to obtain lab results more quickly, or to provide an easy way to ask questions, for example. Telephone contact with clinicians' offices is notoriously unreliable and frustrating: "Dr. X never returns my calls;" "Dr. Y's receptionist puts me on hold and then 10 minutes later the line goes dead and I get a dial tone;" "My kids' pediatrician says to call during her telephone hour, but the line is always busy, so what good is that?" E-mail empowers the patient to circumvent these problems and get the job done—*as long as the clinician is committed to making it work*. We cannot suggest the range of possibilities of clinician-to-patient e-mail in this short section, but in developing your own approach to using this form of communication with patients, there are two major considerations to keep in mind:

- **Identify and explain the potential use of e-mail in your relationship with the patient.** As with any aspect of clinician-patient contract, the role of e-mail in your relationship with your patient should be clarified from the outset. Do you consider e-mail contact appropriate in your clinical practice? Under what circumstances? What procedure should the patient follow in contacting you? What type of response from you should the patient expect? And in what timeframe? This type of information may be included as part of a brochure or flyer provided to all new patients who enter your practice.
- **Privacy considerations.** When using e-mail to respond to patients' comments or queries, clinicians are subject to the same standards of respect, confidentiality, and professionalism as when interacting in person or by phone. It is especially important to warn patients about possible threats to their privacy in transmitting personal health information over the Internet. Patients may dismiss or minimize these concerns, but clinicians should describe and explain the extent of their own willingness to transmit information to patients, consistent with Health Insurance Portability and Accountability Act (HIPAA) guidelines and ethical patient care. For example, it might be reasonable for a clinician to indicate her willingness to transmit laboratory results of interest to the

patient, thus providing more efficient (and probably more private) feedback than playing telephone tag or leaving a message on an answering machine. However, at the same time the clinician might make it clear that he or she does not e-mail complex reports that require interpretation or discussion, or imply significant changes in therapy. In such cases it is necessary to arrange an office appointment.

Health Information on the Internet

Tens of thousands of medical Web sites can be accessed with a click of the mouse, but health "information" on the Internet is often overly simplified or incomplete, not to mention sometimes downright inaccurate. The opportunity for patients to research their questions easily may transform their interactions with clinicians. The patient who feels intimidated or has not had his or her concerns addressed completely may go to the Internet, where medical myths flourish and cures are easy to come by, for information. And it may happen that the clinician is the party who ends up feeling intimidated when the patient returns with a wealth of information (or misinformation) perhaps unknown to the clinician. Some useful techniques for dealing with this situation include:

- Encourage your patients to become knowledgeable about their health concerns and problems.
- Guide them to high-quality Web sites.
- Ask them to bring you a copy of the information so you can respond and clarify.
- Acknowledge the patient's "expertise" and partner with patients in their pursuit of better health.
- If the patient has misinformation, explain why you think it is inaccurate in a clear and nonjudgmental manner.

COMMUNICATING ABOUT PREVENTION AND HEALTH PROMOTION

Many patients expect health care professionals to address prevention and health maintenance, and they actively seek out clinicians who address these issues. Good clinician-patient communication is central to prevention and health promotion. The medical interview allows you to identify the patient's risk-related behaviors, personal preferences, and needed preventive services. Interviewing skills also facilitate health education, negotiation, and counseling regarding healthy lifestyles. In these ways the

TABLE 9–1

PREVENTIVE HEALTH ASSESSMENT

Introduction

- "Now I'd like to ask you a few questions about keeping healthy."

Immunization status

- "Can you recall anything about your immunizations?"
  - Basic immunizations: "Did you get the regular shots as a child?"
  - Boosters: "When was your last tetanus shot? Flu shot? Pneumonia shot?"

Screening

- "Have you ever had your cholesterol checked?"
  - Age- and gender-specific screening tests: "When was your last Pap smear?"
  - Appropriate screening intervals
  - Screening behaviors (breast self-exam, testicular self-exam)

Family history

- "Are you concerned about anything in your family that might put you at risk?"
  - Diseases and disorders predisposing to high risk: "Has anyone in your family had colon cancer? Breast cancer?"

Specific risk factors

- "I'd like to ask you some questions about things that might put you at risk for certain diseases."
  - Behaviors: cigarette smoking, abuse of alcohol and other drugs
  - Exposures: occupational and environmental factors, multiple sexual partners, unprotected intercourse
  - Clinical findings: obesity, hypertension, diabetes

Lifestyle issues (see Chapter 5, The Patient Profile)

- Nutrition: "Tell me about your diet."
- Exercise: "Do you exercise regularly? Tell me what you do for exercise."
- Stress management: "What do you do to prevent stress in your life? How do you cope with stress in your life?"

Health beliefs

- See Chapter 12, Cultural Competence in the Interview

interview is a powerful tool for promoting better health. Table 9–1 outlines the components of a preventive health assessment that are often embedded in the initial outpatient interview.

Questions about health-related behaviors, immunizations, and early detection (screening tests) are easy to neglect in ambulatory medicine because office visits are commonly short and highly focused. As a matter of fact, studies show that primary care physicians often miss important prevention items in their ongoing care of patients. Unless such questions are included in a structured database approach at the initial interview, or during routine periodic checkups, they are likely to be forgotten, or remembered only intermittently and not well documented.

◈ PRACTICE POINT
Preventive care questions should be systematically integrated into the initial interview.

Begin your segment about prevention and screening tests with a brief introduction, such as "Now I'd like to ask a few questions about preventive care" or "I'd like to ask about things that keep you healthy." As part of the initial medical history, the patient profile (see Chapter 5, The Patient Profile) should also provide you with information about major cardiovascular and cancer risk factors. Other risk factors may be identified in the past medical history and family history. This information-gathering phase of the clinical interview sets the stage for later negotiation with patients (see Chapter 18, Education and Negotiation) to alter their risks.

TRUTHFULNESS AND CONFIDENTIALITY IN AMBULATORY CARE

Maintaining Confidentiality

Confidentiality is not only an ethical precept; it is also a legal precept following the passage of the Health Insurance Portability and Accountability Act, compliance required as of April 2003, which mandates protecting the security and confidentiality of personal health information.

◈ PRACTICE POINT
Confidentiality does not simply mean keeping an occasional secret, but rather indicates a daily pattern of respect for the privacy of patients and their stories.

Appropriate Talking

Discussing cases with friends, roommates, or spouse is inappropriate, even when the information in question is interesting and not strictly personal. Of course, some people do have a right to know. Health care is a collegial enterprise. Clinicians function as members of teams, so we often need to discuss patients with our peers, consultants, and other professionals. As a learner, you have a particular obligation to discuss patients with teachers; even in these situations; however, discretion is important. It is never justifiable to talk about patients on crowded elevators or in other public settings. In the hospital, presenting patients at the bedside is a good teaching technique, but it may infringe on confidentiality if a roommate can hear the discussion of a patient's illness and personal life. Likewise, discussing a patient's personal information in a busy office setting, where patients in other examining rooms or people sitting in the waiting room might overhear, is always a concern.

◆ PRACTICE POINT

Always be circumspect when sharing a patient's personal health information with colleagues, consultants, students, and teachers. Consider the time and setting. Share only as much information as you need to under the circumstances, but in clear and appropriate detail.

Appropriate Writing

Another important aspect of maintaining confidentiality is to write only appropriate information in the patient's clinical record (see Chapter 8, The Clinical Narrative). You should approach the record as a document that the patient has the right to review at any time and that others (e.g., office staff) will inevitably have access to. Under HIPAA, patients have the right to see and obtain copies of their medical records and to request corrections if they identify errors. Especially with regard to sensitive information, you should always ask yourself whether writing a particular item in the chart is important to your patient's care. Some examples of sensitive information include details of sexual practices, criminal records, marital conflict, and financial difficulties. Mental illness, suicide attempts, and substance abuse constitute sensitive information that ought to be recorded but should be handled sensitively and with an eye toward minimizing invasiveness. In some cases, it might be possible to write a brief "neutral" note to jog your memory, without detailing lurid details. Computerized records and e-mail communication present additional challenges to office confidentiality; these are discussed briefly in Chapter 16, Ethics and the Law.

Confidentiality in the Face of Specific Threats

Confidentiality is challenged in small, and not-so-small, ways every day in practice. Consider this example of a 58-year-old woman who comes to you for follow-up of hypertension:

Clinician **So, how have you been?**

Patient   Well, I'm fine; it's my daughter I'm worried about. [Her 28-year-old daughter is also your patient.] I don't know if it's stress or she's just taken on too much or she's got something wrong with her. I know she's talked to you.

Actually, the daughter has not talked to you. But do you say that you haven't seen her daughter for months? Even though the patient seems to assume that you have recently dealt with her daughter's problem ("and why aren't you doing anything about it?"), it is best to reply:

Clinician **Well, I know you appreciate that Jane's relationship with me is confidential.**

Ideally, the patient agrees and says:

Patient   Of course, I know I can talk and you can listen and that you can't say anything. I know. I wouldn't want it any other way.

If, on the other hand, she may persist in asking about Jane's condition:

Patient   But you know how Jane is. She doesn't take care of herself. If you just let me know what her problem is, I'll make sure she follows your instructions.

Clinician **I can hear that you're really concerned about her. And I'm sure she doesn't want you to worry. So the best thing would be for you to sit down with her and explain how you feel and encourage her to follow up with me.**

Limits and Exceptions to Confidentiality

Confidentiality is a qualified duty, not an absolute one. In Chapter 16 (see Exceptions to Clinician-Patient Confidentiality) we list and discuss standard exceptions to the rule of confidentiality.

These exceptions may be easier to deal with in hospital practice because the threat is immediate and the patient may be relatively anonymous; for example, the law may require hospital clinicians to report knife and gunshot wounds or new cases of certain communicable diseases. However, in office practice such situations may arise in the context of long-term clinician-patient relationships, which may make it more emotionally difficult for the clinician to comply with the duty. In addition, the potential risk to others may be perceived as smaller or less probable. For example, a patient develops a seizure disorder. The law may require that the diagnosis be reported to the state motor vehicle licensing agency, which could lead to license suspension until the patient is certified as medically stable for a specified period. Such laws are designed to prevent motor vehicle accidents and protect the public, but they may also cause hardship for the person whose license is suspended. If the person is your patient, he or she may beg you not to report the situation, or bargain with you ("I won't drive unless I absolutely have to"). You may conclude, based on the neurologist's report, that the likelihood of another seizure is small. What do you do in such a situation?

You must obey the law, although if the question involves expert medical judgment, it is often best to refer the question to a more knowledgeable specialist—in this case, the neurologist. However, if breach of confidentiality becomes necessary, you have a duty to inform your patient. When such a situation arises, notify the patient and attempt to secure his or her permission. Failing that, be truthful about what is required and what you intend to do. If you diagnose syphilis, tuberculosis, or HIV/AIDS, for example, explain that the law requires you to submit a report to the health department. While describing the public health reasons for this requirement, you are also giving the patient crucial information about communicability and its implications for his or her behavior. For example:

- "I'm required by law to let the state health department know so they can follow up and make sure your contacts are identified and treated."
- "You had a seizure, and I'm not permitted to let you drive because you could hurt someone if you had a seizure while you were driving."

There are special problems and considerations regarding confidentiality in the care of adolescent patients, whose privacy ought to be respected even though they are legally minors (see Chapter 10, Pediatric and Adolescent Interviewing), and geriatric patients, who may in some cases no longer have decision-making capacity (see Chapter 11, Interviewing the Geriatric Patient).

Paperwork and Telling the Truth

Paperwork is the bane of modern clinical practice. Individuals need medical forms completed for jobs, school, insurance, public assistance, nursing homes, social programs, driver's licenses, and more. Likewise, health insurers require the proper paperwork to justify payment for medical or laboratory services, referrals to specialists, and so on. Truthfulness in everyday medical practice requires honesty in the way we handle these bureaucratic headaches, even though we may not be inclined to devote our finest literary efforts to grinding out such administrative fodder. Truthfulness is also a prerequisite for informed consent (see Chapter 16, Ethics and the Law).

Suppressing Information

Two issues frequently arise with regard to clearances and certifications in primary care. In one case, the patient asks that information be suppressed:

- "Don't put down that I'm a diabetic. After all, my diabetes is in good control. And it'll cost me plenty in extra insurance premiums."
- "Listen, that nervous breakdown was 3 years ago. It won't happen again. I'm all right now."

What should you do, given that telling the truth might well result in significant adverse consequences for your patient?

Because you must be *honest* in answering explicit questions on a particular form, explain to the patient beforehand what the medical record contains to avoid false expectations when giving consent for you to share medical information. Patients do not realize what is in their medical records, and they often give permission to share these records without knowing what information lies therein. For example, many patients decline to have their psychiatric records released but do not realize that their clinician's record will list their psychiatric medications or hospitalizations. It is best to inform your patient what is in the record and allow the patient to decide whether or not to release it. For example, in response to one of the requests above:

- "It would be great if I could leave out your diabetes, but I have to be honest. Besides, how we are treating your diabetes is all over your records. If the company requests your chart, and sometimes they do, they'll see that you and I lied, which won't be much help to you."

However, you can certainly take the time to *write additional explanatory material* if you believe that it will benefit the patient. You might indicate, for example, that the diabetes is in excellent control or that the episode of depression has completely resolved with no residual symptoms.

On the other hand, *don't volunteer information* unless you have reason to believe it is relevant. Often, a final question will be something like, "Are there any other significant medical problems or conditions?" There is no need here to detail the patient's medical history; simply put what might, in your clinical judgment, be significant to the insurance or job or program in question.

Providing Misinformation

A different problem arises when patients ask you to make false or unsupported assertions about their illness or disability. The patient's insurance carrier or the state welfare department might ask if, in your opinion, the patient is "totally disabled." This type of determination can be made only on the basis of a thorough functional assessment, along with a clear understanding of job-related skills and requirements. Perhaps the evidence of functional impairment is limited or ambiguous. Although you have a duty to advocate for your patient, the duty does not extend to lying in order to gain benefits for the patient. In this case you should provide a truthful assessment based on your clinical observations. For example:

- "Yes, Mr. X does have diabetes controlled with diet and medication. He reports occasional symptoms, but no long-term sequelae are present."
- "Yes, Mrs. Y does have degenerative joint disease but this, in my opinion, does not in itself explain her chronic pain syndrome." (Of course, chronic pain is in itself a severe disability, whether or not a disease-based cause can be identified.)

You should never make assessments of disability that are not warranted by your clinical judgment. Often the clinician will be asked only to provide data, which a disability specialist will subsequently interpret to determine the patient's disability, based on criteria utilized by the relevant governmental agency. You can, of course, decline to complete a disability (or any other) form if you feel that your opinion would not serve the patient's best interest.

SUMMARY—Communication in the Office Setting

Office practice can be a source of great professional satisfaction; it also presents challenges to clinician-patient communication. New institutional and insurance arrangements exacerbate these interactive concerns and present new concerns. In this chapter we reviewed skills that will help you achieve efficiency and focus in the encounter, thereby improving your ability to help the patient and enhance satisfaction. You should:

- Allow the patient time to state his or her concerns (doing so always saves time in the long run, and sometimes immediately)
- Negotiate priorities, then set the agenda
- Explain the issues in plain language and check for understanding
- Confront coerced change directly; empathize with the patient and indicate a willingness to work together
- Confront dueling agendas directly; explain the options, while respecting the patient's experience and expectations

Other issues pertinent to office interviewing include:

- Health promotion and prevention. The interview is important both diagnostically (establishing the patient's risk factors) and therapeutically (laying the groundwork for behavior change).
- Confidentiality in day-to-day clinical practice. Confidentiality is a primary value, but not an absolute one.
- Truthfulness in day-to-day practice. Patient advocacy is an important part of primary care practice, but it must be based on truthful assessments.

CHAPTER 10

Pediatric and Adolescent Interviewing

Headed in the Right Direction

Stuart rose from the ditch, climbed into his car,
and started up the road that led toward the north.
The sun was just coming up over the hills on his
right. As he peered ahead into the great land that
stretched before him, the way seemed long. But
the sky was bright, and he somehow felt he was
headed in the right direction.

E. B. White, *Stuart Little*

UNDERSTANDING THE PEDIATRIC AND ADOLESCENT INTERVIEW

Why devote a separate chapter to pediatric and adolescent interviewing? Are the medical histories of children and adolescents that different from those of adults? In the following pages, we take the perspective that children and adolescents are not merely "miniature adults." Not only is the style of a pediatric interview different from the style of an interview with an adult, but the style of the pediatric interview also varies dynamically from one developmental stage of childhood to the next.

CHILDREN VERSUS ADULTS: SIMILARITIES AND DIFFERENCES

There are, of course, many similarities between pediatric and adult medical interviews. For example, the basic organization of a clinical history is the same for patients of all ages: chief complaint, history of present illness, past medical history, family history, patient profile, and review of systems. Similarly, skills and values that facilitate good adult interactions—

such as empathy, respect, and genuineness—are equally important in pediatric patients.

There are, however, important differences between the adult and pediatric interview; these differences include the individuals who participate in the conversation and the topics emphasized at different stages of development. Parents or other family members often provide much of the information. Although this need is obvious in the case of a young child, the precise point at which a child has the skill to contribute his or her own story is not always easy to determine. With regard to topics, the prenatal history, for example, is vitally important in the case of a neonate but less so in the case of an adolescent. And the achievement of developmental milestones, which is critical to the routine assessment of a 6-month-old infant, is of minimal significance in the evaluation of a "straight A" second grader who presents with a sore throat. Trying to sort through the requirements of different developmental stages and the demands related to the reason for the visit can be confusing if not downright overwhelming. What do I need to know about this child today? (Fortunately, you can maintain the same open-ended approach to the interview as you do with your adult patients and let the child and person[s] accompanying the child be your guide.)

◆ PRACTICE POINT

Open-ended questions allow you to sit back and size up the situation—the reason for the visit, the child's behavior, the parent or guardian's level of concern—while you plan your approach to the interview.

SETTING THE STAGE FOR EFFECTIVE COMMUNICATION

Comfort and Privacy

A private and comfortable environment is essential to the pediatric interview. If the patient is in a hospital room with several beds and the neighbor's television is turned on, visitors are chatting, and medical personnel are performing procedures, then families will feel uncomfortable talking about even mundane historical items, much less about giving thoughtful observations of behavior or potentially embarrassing details. Before starting, suggest that the television and radio be turned off and, if possible, roommates be taken elsewhere by their parents or by staff members. Otherwise, draw curtains around the child's bed to provide at least the illusion of privacy. Similarly, you should see that an infant is comfortable and quiet (usually in a loved one's lap) before expecting the parents to be relaxed enough to provide you with detailed information.

Establishing Rapport

In the case of a preschool child, offering the patient a toy to play with may well improve the efficiency of an interview. At the beginning of an interview, establish rapport with the patient and family members. For example, with a newborn's parents, spend a few moments admiring the baby; with the a 2-year-old toddler, try to charm him or her before interviewing the mother; with the school-age child, ask him or her about a favorite television show or after-school activity.

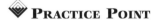 **PRACTICE POINT**

With children it is often easier to establish rapport *indirectly* by admiring a toy or a pair of new shoes rather than greeting the child too enthusiastically.

Spend a few moments talking to the parent or guardian to give the child time to size you up (while you size up the child as well). Here's how one clinician observes his 4-year-old patient.

Clinician	**[Entering quietly and looking first at the child's mother]: Hi there. So how's he doing?**
Patient	[Mother]: He seems fine. He did really well with the medicine. [Mother is sitting on the examination table and the child is walking around the room.]
	[Child]: I want you to look at mommy's ears.
	That's a good idea. Would you like to help me?
	[Child]: Okay.
	You can hold my stethoscope [handing it to child] while I get the light [reaching for otoscope]. [Looking in mother's ears] These look good. What about your friend Winnie the Pooh–can I look in his ears next? [Child hands stuffed toy bear to clinician.] They look good, too. Do you want to see? Now I can look in your ears, they look excellent. Very good. You did a very good job.

Notice how the clinician gives this child time to size up the situation and provides an opportunity for the child to become familiar with potentially scary maneuvers. Sometimes the examination room becomes a three-ring circus when parents bring more than one child. In these situations, do the best you can to maintain your focus and use the opportunity to observe how the parent or guardian sets boundaries and expectations for the children. These observations take no additional time and become a part of your assessment of the child.

Understanding Relationships

Make no assumptions about the relationship of the caretaking adults to the child patient. The parents of an infant may not necessarily bear the same married name. Thus, the term "his father" rather than "your husband" or "the baby's mother" rather than "your wife" might be more appropriate until the parental relationship is better understood. Similarly, an infant and his or her parent may not carry the same surname. A brief glance at the registration form might reveal that the infant's name is Doe, while the mother's and father's name is Smith. Because you need to understand the relationship for the benefit of the child, it is best to ask, simply and nonjudgmentally, "I notice that your name is Smith and William's name is Doe. Can you explain the relationship to me?"

Finding the Right Words

Finally, tailor your vocabulary to the level of understanding of the family members with whom you are speaking, although discernment of their verbal and clinical sophistication is subject to bias and may at times be difficult. Consider this aspect, too, in speaking with the child, who will understand more than you may expect if you use appropriate words. For example, you could say to a parent, "Tell me about this rash." But you can say to a child, "Do you have any spots?"

TALKING WITH PATIENTS OF DIFFERENT AGES

The style and content of a medical interview vary enormously with the child's age as well. The questions you ask new parents about their baby will be different from those you ask a teenager. The content of the medical history changes with age, just as the style and dynamics change. Topics that are obviously important in the prenatal visit or in the newborn interview become distinctly less important as the child matures and, indeed, may not be mentioned at all in the medical conversation with an adolescent. For convenience, we distinguish four types of pediatric interviews: the prenatal visit, the infant or toddler visit, the school-age child visit, and, finally, the adolescent visit.

The Prenatal Visit

Ideally, the clinician responsible for the medical care of a newborn should meet with prospective parents before the birth. This **prenatal visit** allows the caregiver to obtain important medical information and establishes a partnership of mutual trust and respect. The diminished role of extended, multigenerational families means that in many cases the primary emotional and educational support for new parents may come from a clinician, rather than from family members. A brief, informal meeting initiates such a support system and dispels myths and misconceptions that the new parents might have. The information you acquire during this prenatal visit includes a detailed family history, the parents' knowledge about child care, and their plans for feeding the baby (breast versus bottle) and for circumcision (yes or no). Practical issues such as the schedule for well-child office visits, clinical fees, and telephone access can also be presented at this time.

During your meeting with prospective parents, obtain information about the family history: familial disease, previous histories of birth defects, and perinatal deaths. The purpose of this family history is twofold:

- To alert you to possible genetic disease in the infant as well as the parents' fears about such disease
- To reassure or inform parents concerned about implications for their child of certain familial illnesses or tendencies

Listen especially for details of miscarriages and neonatal or childhood illness or death; such tragedies have lifelong impact on families. The parents' health and their past medical history should be outlined in some detail, especially with respect to disease states that might endanger the life or health of the fetus during pregnancy. In this way, you are able to pay attention to the physical, social, and emotional environment into which the child will be born. Parents' discussion of their plans for feeding the baby and their knowledge of child care inform your educational efforts not only at the prenatal visit but also at subsequent well-baby visits.

◈ PRACTICE POINT

The prenatal interview provides an opportunity to lay the groundwork for anticipatory guidance, which is the critical educational aspect of caring for children.

For example, take the opportunity to discuss issues such as:

- The parents' perceptions of changes that will occur in their lives with the newborn's arrival
- Identification of support persons for the mother and father when the infant goes home
- The parents' knowledge of safety for the infant at home and in the automobile
- How the parents view preparation of siblings for the new addition to their family

Sample Screening Questions at the Prenatal Interview, below, provides some typical screening questions that are useful at the prenatal visit.

WHAT TO SAY
Sample Screening Questions at the Prenatal Interview

- Have you had any problems with your pregnancy? Any extra doctor visits or special tests? Everything going normally?
- Do you have any special concerns or questions about having this baby?
- In your family, and in the baby's father's family, have there been any babies or children with problems or illnesses?
- Who is going to help you out at home when the baby arrives? Tell me what you're thinking about going back to work.
- Lots of new parents are pretty nervous about caring for their first baby. How are you dealing with that?

The Infant and Toddler Visit

During infancy and the preschool years, the child is the focus of the interview but is usually not a participant. Although the patient may add little to the actual conversation, the interview is usually conducted while the infant or toddler is present. This small but important person serves as a catalyst to aid parents' recall of historical details. Also, parents are likely to be more comfortable if they are with their child, and certainly the child will be more comfortable with the parents. And when the child sees you interacting with the mother or father, the child is more likely to develop a (very tentative) feeling of trust.

A child who is fussy or in pain will only distract both you and the parents, however. The situation can be remedied with a pacifier or bottle for the infant or a familiar toy for the toddler. It is useful to carry around a colorful item or two to interest your preschool patients. Sometimes inexperienced clinicians either ignore the patient completely (to the consternation of parents) or try to become instant "buddies" with the child, forgetting that by age 1 most children are quite wary or even frightened of strangers. Moreover, illness may make the toddler irritable, and the clinical setting may be terrifying.

 PRACTICE POINT

A good compromise during the infant/toddler visit is to begin the encounter with a simple, friendly greeting, followed by the enthusiastic but brief examination of one of the child's toys.

The medical history information about the perinatal period should include:

- Complications and problems during the pregnancy and labor (e.g., "Did you have any problems during your pregnancy or with your labor and delivery?")
- Problems during the first days of life (e.g., "Did Zack have any problems when he was born?")

If it has not already been obtained, you should take a careful family history as well. Ask about the child's crying, sleeping, and bowel and bladder function. Ascertain the child's immunization status, including reactions to the immunizations. Carefully review developmental stages, focusing on different milestones depending on the age of the child, and try to get a sense of the child's temperament (e.g., regular versus irregular habits, mellow versus intense reactions).

Here's how one clinician performs a quick developmental screening of a 6-month-old:

Clinician	**So. It's good to see you. You look as if motherhood is agreeing with you, but I know it's hard work. How's Jacob doing?**
Patient	[Parent]: He's doing really well. He's easier than Elizabeth was. He's very predictable, although sometimes in the middle of the night he wants to play.
	He looks like a playful character and he clearly loves his mommy, and I can see he's not too sure about me. What's he doing for you?

[Parent]: Well he's rolling over both ways and if I sit him up he can stay there. Everything goes in his mouth.
That all sounds very normal. Have you ever seen him pass something from one hand to his other hand?

Notice how the clinician provides the parent with support and positive feedback and progresses from open-ended to more specific questions, building opportunities for anticipatory guidance even during this information-gathering phase of the encounter.

◆ PRACTICE POINT
Avoid leading questions, such as "Doesn't he sit up yet?" that create needless anxiety (if he's *not* sitting up yet) and inhibit true answers and sharing of concerns.

Sometimes a developmental history can be accomplished with a single question when there is an older normal sibling: "Tell me how Jacob has been for you compared to Elizabeth."

Nutrition questions are also important in your clinical history. A few screening questions often suffice:

- "How many ounces of formula [or, for older children, milk] does your baby take each day?" For breast-fed babies, "How many times does the baby nurse in 24 hours?" and "What's the longest he or she goes between feedings?"
- For older infants and toddlers, "Are there any foods your child refuses to eat?"
- "Does your child get much in the way of sweets and fast food?"

◆ PRACTICE POINT
Because anticipatory guidance plays an important role in every interaction in this age group, try to obtain enough information to anticipate later discussions of accident prevention, feeding, toilet training, teething, and acquisition of normal speech patterns.

Here's how one clinician began her closure of a newborn well-visit by summing up her findings, showing her appreciation of the infant, and receiving back from the baby's mother a statement which, despite its brevity, indicates much about the family's culture and point of view:

Clinician [Admiring the infant] **He's perfect. How did you get so lucky?**
Patient   I'm blessed.

The content of the interview varies with the reason for the visit: well-child care, an office visit for illness, a sick child in the hospital, or a child about to have a surgical procedure. The child's demeanor and the parents' level of anxiety and ability to provide precise information about the child's illness will vary. Parents may be extremely focused on whether they have cared for their child correctly or have done anything to provoke or worsen an illness.

◆ PRACTICE POINT
During the interview with a pediatric patient, convey that the parent is a good parent.

When the clinician asks about the child's behavior and milestones, parents may see their skills being challenged. If so, they may give "ideal" answers, even though they would like to share their fears and worries. Sometimes, especially early in the interview, you may be unable to provide such reassurance and may need to say:

Clinician   I understand your concern about whether you should have given Molly that cold medicine, but I'd like to leave that aside for the moment and get back to how she's been acting over the last few days. When did you first notice that she wasn't her usual self?

Once you have established the history, you will be able to reassure the parents that they have not hurt their child or, alternatively, to educate them in the proper care of a sick child.

◆ PRACTICE POINT
The symptoms of pediatric illness, particularly in the preverbal child, are often nonspecific and tell us more about how sick the child is than about precisely what the illness is.

A 15-month-old cannot tell us that his or her left ear hurts; rather, he or she will cry, be irritable, have a fever, and possibly have a loss of appetite or even vomiting and diarrhea. If we are lucky, the child may tug at the affected ear, but many children with healthy ears do that as well.

We have to rely on our physical examination to make the diagnosis of left otitis media. But if the child is exceedingly irritable, refuses to play, and refuses liquids, we may need additional diagnostic studies to rule out more serious illness such as meningitis. Table 10–1 lists the key information required in the infant and toddler interview.

Typical Screening Questions at the Infant and Toddler Visit, page 203, provides some typical screening questions that are useful at infant and toddler visits.

TABLE 10–1

CONTENT OF THE INFANT AND TODDLER INTERVIEW	
Reason for Visit	*Topics Discussed*
Well-Child Visit	• Parental concerns
	• Prenatal and birth history
	• Developmental milestones achieved
	• Dates of prior immunizations. Is child current?
	• Eruption of teeth
	• Habits: sleeping, crying, and bowel and bladder function
	• Intercurrent illness and other illnesses
	• Nutrition history
	• Cultural and family practices (feeding, taping umbilical hernias, keeping face covered to prevent colic)
Sick Visit or Admission to Hospital	• All of the topics discussed in a well-child visit
	• History of Present Illness (see Chapter 3, Chief Complaint and Present Illness) with special emphasis on time of onset, initial symptoms, and subsequent symptoms
	• Difficulty feeding—too slow, not at all, refusal of liquids or solids, or preference for water or juice as opposed to milk or formula
	• State of hydration. When was the last wet diaper and how wet was it?
	• Does the infant or child seem himself or herself? Playful, alert, pleasant, or acting sick?
	• Temperature taken at home? (Rectal? Axillary?)
	• Medications (including over-the-counter) already given and dosages?
	• What concerns the parents most? What do they think is causing the illness?
	• History of recent similar illnesses in patient or family?

WHAT TO SAY
Typical Screening Questions at the Infant and Toddler Visit

Ask the screening questions related to the prenatal visit if not previously done.

- Did you have any problems with your pregnancy or with your labor and delivery (getting this baby born)?
- Did the baby have any problems when he was born? Go home with you at the usual time?
- (To screen for temperament) Tell me what kind of baby she is.
- (To screen for developmental milestones) What's she doing for you?
- Tell me what a typical day is for him, with eating, sleeping, wet and dirty diapers.

The School-Age Child Visit

When a child reaches age 5 or 6, the interactive balance in the interview begins to change. Children are now more able to contribute substantially to the collection of data, but their reports are usually broad and sometimes difficult to interpret. Thus, you must turn to parents to provide accuracy and precision, while always trying to confirm the data with the small patient insofar as is possible. An enormous maturational range is found in elementary school–age children. You can expect to find behaviors ranging from shy, sullen, and silent to that of the garrulous child who cannot be stopped.

◆ PRACTICE POINT
As a sensitive interviewer, you must take your cues from observing the patient before deciding whether and how much to involve the child in actual history taking.

In general, the school-age child is a healthy child. Well-child visits emphasize historical information concerning immunizations, development, and nutrition, as well as the psychosocial aspects of a child's environment. Knowledge of the child's school performance and friends is necessary for the global understanding of a school-aged child's well-being. Anticipatory guidance at this age emphasizes accident prevention,

TABLE 10–2

CONTENT OF THE SCHOOL–AGE CHILD INTERVIEW	
Reason for Visit	*Topics Discussed*
Well-Child Visit	• Parental concerns
	• School progress, school readiness, relationships with peers
	• Developmental milestones achieved? At what age?
	• Habits (eating, sleeping, continence)
	• Age-appropriate play?
	• Similarities to and differences from peers
	• Significant past and birth history
	• Illnesses since last visit
	• Nutrition
	• Dates of prior immunizations
Sick Visit or Admission to Hospital	• All of the topics discussed in a well-child visit
	• History of Present Illness (see Chapter 3, Chief Complaint and Present Illness) with special emphasis on parents' observations
	• Child's description of symptoms
	• Medications (including over-the-counter) already tried
	• Similar illnesses in household or peer group

both in the home and at school, and good nutrition. Special aspects of the content of the school-age child interview are indicated in Table 10–2.

Typical Screening Questions for the School-Age Child, below, provides some typical questions that are useful for the school-age child.

WHAT TO SAY

Typical Screening Questions for the School-Age Child

- Tell me how school is going for you.
- What's your favorite subject? Do you think your teachers like you?
- What do you do after school?
- (To the parent or guardian) Do you think she is at the same level as her classmates and friends?
- (For a sick visit) Anyone else at home or at school have any symptoms like this?

The Adolescent Visit

Your interactions with teenagers are potentially the most complicated and difficult of any interviews you will conduct. Because the adolescent person is frequently ambivalent or confused by his or her own feelings and resists talking about them, you will likely notice a lot of silence during these interactions.

 PRACTICE POINT

In the patient interview with an adolescent, the yes/no and other types of closed-ended questions will yield extremely brief answers that leave you struggling to come up with more questions.

Moreover, during the adolescent years, patients take an increasingly active role in their own health care, while their parents move progressively into the background. This is a change that many mothers and fathers, as well as their teenage children, find difficult.

You may initiate the interview with an unfamiliar teenager with a direct, unaffected introduction:

Clinician   Hi, I'm Dr. Smith and I'm glad to meet you. Tell me what made you decide to come to see me or why your parents made you come in.

Sit down and meet the teenager at his or her level with eye contact that allows for natural breaks.

 PRACTICE POINT

Remember that initially you are a stranger and must establish a basis for trust.

Many clinicians try to become instant friends with teenagers, succeeding only in confusing or antagonizing them. It is important to be the person you are (see "Genuineness" in Chapter 2): if you are not "cool," don't try to be. It is appropriate to talk with adolescents alone for part of the interview, if not for the whole interaction. Most parents are cooperative and will leave the examination room without difficulty when you explain why, for example:

Clinician   You know how important it is for you to feel that you have a private and confidential relationship with your doctor? Most of

> **my young patients feel the same way. So I'm going to ask you to leave while I talk with Jamie. Is there anything you'd like to tell me before you go?**

When speaking with an adolescent, establish that your conversation is confidential. Whether the information is potentially embarrassing or not, build trust by assuring the patient. For example:

Clinician   **I always want to make it clear to all my patients that what they tell me is private. I will not repeat anything you say unless you give me permission to do so or I'm worried about you and we need to tell a responsible adult, like if you get very sick or something. But you know, your Mom cares about you and may have some concerns about what we do today. If she asks me anything, in order to protect your privacy, I'm going to tell her that she needs to ask you. So you might want to think about what you'd like to tell her, and we can talk about that some more at the end of our visit.**

The statement above not only nourishes the adolescent's desire for autonomy, but it also acknowledges the parent or guardian's rightful interest in the child who has not yet achieved full adult status. It also implies that parents and their children should talk about important topics, even those that are difficult, such as sexuality.

Important information to obtain from the teenager centers around the teenager's interaction with his or her environment and social world. In a sense, the patient profile or social history is *the* history in the adolescent. Tactfully posed questions dealing with drugs and alcohol, safety, sexuality, contraception, and sexually transmitted diseases are an important part of a medical history in this age group. But even the most tactful interviewer often has difficulty breaking through the outward reserve that many adolescents display. If this is the case, posing sensitive questions in the past tense is sometimes helpful. For example, rather than asking, "Do you smoke cigarettes?" you might ask, "Were you smoking cigarettes 6 months ago?" This avoids direct confrontation. Here is another example of how you might "open up" a silent and possibly angry adolescent interview.

Clinician   **I'm sorry that your father dragged you in here against your will. I know if I were in your shoes I'd be pretty angry. But since we have this time together, do you think we could talk about some**

of the things that have been going on in your life? None of this is any of my business unless it's okay with you for me to get to know you better. I'd like to hear more about how you've been feeling.

Other important issues to discover during the interview include:

- School performance
- The presence or absence of close friends
- Behavioral difficulties both at home and at school
- Stress and stressors, and symptoms such as anxiety or depression.

Ideally, you should obtain most of this information directly from the adolescent rather than from a parent or guardian. Topics important to review during the visit with the adolescent patient are listed in Table 10–3, and *Typical Questions and Statements to Engage the Adolescent,* page 208, provides some helpful screening questions and statements to engage this patient.

TABLE 10–3

CONTENT OF THE ADOLESCENT INTERVIEW	
Reason for Visit	*Topics Discussed*
Well Visit	• Parental concerns and confidentiality in the clinician-patient relationship
	• School progress and peer relationships
	• Habits (eating, sleeping, physical activity)
	• Smoking, alcohol, and drug use
	• Sexuality and sexual activity
	• Past history (illnesses, medications, allergies)
	• Interval history (any illness or symptoms since last visit)
	• Immunizations (and related childhood diseases)
Lay the groundwork for anticipatory guidance:	
	• Diet and exercise
	• Injury prevention (bicycle, motor vehicle, firearms)

(continued on following page)

TABLE 10–3 *(Continued)*

CONTENT OF THE ADOLESCENT INTERVIEW	
Reason for Visit	*Topics Discussed*
	• Smoking, alcohol and drug use
	• Sexuality, contraception, unintended pregnancies, sexually transmitted diseases
	• Stress, depression, hopelessness
Sick Visit	• Reason for coming (parents' view, adolescent's view)
	• History of Present Illness and related Review of Systems
	• Boundaries of confidentiality (what parent needs to know when adolescent is sick)
	• Possible relationship of sexual activity and substance use to current symptoms
	• An abbreviated review of well-visit topics if the sick visit is also a first visit to the office

---

WHAT TO SAY
Typical Questions and Statements to Engage the Adolescent

■ (With parent, at first, in the room) I like to have a private relationship with my young patients unless, of course, there is something that parents need to know. Do you have any questions or concerns about that?

■ (To the parent) Are you okay with stepping out while we talk and I do my exam? Then I can have you come back when we're done.

■ Here comes the sex and drugs. It's my job to ask you those hard questions about smoking and sex and drugs and your safety. Are you doing any of that? Tell me more about that.

■ The reason I ask is that these things are important to your health and I want you to take responsibility for being healthy. And if you have any questions, you can ask me. Like I know you're not having sex now, and I will tell you that having sex is not a good idea. But if you do have sex I want to make sure you don't get pregnant or get sick, like with AIDS or something.

The Adolescent Sexual History

The sexual history is a critical but particularly difficult topic for adolescents, which must be covered when there are genitourinary or gynecologic symptoms. It is also part of preventing and screening for sexually transmitted diseases and pregnancy. As with patients in any other age group, you should use clear language that the patient understands and proceed from less intimate questions ("Tell me about your family and friends." "Do you have any special friends?" "How about boyfriends or girlfriends?") to more intimate questions ("Do your friends go on dates?" "How do they feel about having sex?" "How do you feel?" "Are you sexually active now?"). If you are uncomfortable with these issues, it is okay to say so. Useful approaches include:

- "It may be an uncomfortable topic, but as your clinician I need to find out if you're at risk for HIV and other illnesses."
- "Do you have any questions about your body? About sex? About how not to get pregnant? Have you thought about birth control?"
- "Are your friends (or the kids at school) having sex? How about you?"
- "Some kids your age get pretty serious about relationships and start having sex. How about you?"

◆ PRACTICE POINT
Adolescent patients should be given time to respond and allowed to answer in their own way with your assurance that the information is confidential.

Teenage males should be queried about their risk of getting someone pregnant, just as teenage females should be asked about their personal risk of pregnancy.

One problem, of course, is making sure that, when you use a term such as "sexually active," the patient understands what you mean. Young teenagers vary widely in their sexual knowledge and experience; among 14-year-old girls, you will find those who have already been pregnant and others who will look wide-eyed and disbelieving that you could even think of asking such questions. For this reason, questions about their peer group as well as questions that do not imply any right answer or particular level of experience are useful. For example:

Clinician	**Some girls your age who are late with their period will worry that they may have gotten pregnant. Have you had any worries like that?**
Patient	No, because I know I can't be.
	You can't be. Tell me more.
	Well, I didn't have sex. I don't even go with boys; none of my friends do.
	Sometimes the conversation takes a different turn:
Clinician	**Some girls your age who are late with their period will worry that they may have gotten pregnant. Have you had any worries like that?**
Patient	Well, I thought about it.
	Tell me more.
	Well, I don't really think I can be.
	Did he touch you or did he put his penis near you or inside you?

◆ **PRACTICE POINT**

It's important to be simple and precise in your language so that you can be sure that you are obtaining accurate information.

SUMMARY—Pediatric and Adolescent Interviewing

Even the toddler can provide important data in the history, and many older children do not require intermediaries to transmit their stories.

To make the most of your interactions with pediatric patients, be sure you:

- Approach the young child indirectly by first admiring a toy or item of clothing
- Understand the parent or guardian's view of the illness to lay the groundwork for assuring them that they did not cause it
- As children get older, involve them more and more in the interview, choosing words they understand
- Help families understand common problems and developmental milestones, laying the groundwork for anticipatory guidance

To make the most of your interactions with adolescents, be sure you:

- Establish the confidential nature of your relationship, as well as its limits and boundaries
- Avoid yes/no type questions that tend to produce brief responses ending, ultimately, in silence
- Address topics such as drug and alcohol use, sexuality, and safety

CHAPTER 11

Interviewing the Geriatric Patient

A Different Silhouette

A human being sheds its leaves like a tree. Sickness prunes it down; and it no longer offers the same silhouette to the eyes which loved it, to the people to whom it afforded shade and comfort.
Edmond and Jules deGoncourt, *Journal*, July 22, 1862

WHO IS THE GERIATRIC PATIENT?

In this chapter, we consider special sensitivities and skills required for interviewing older or geriatric patients. Who are these "older" patients? Consider this opening exchange between a physician and a woman in the office for follow-up of hypertension and chronic diarrhea:

Clinician	**So how are you?**
Patient	Okay, I guess. I guess it's just old age.
	What about old age?

When does old age begin? This patient was 88 years old; but what if she had been only 78, 68, or 58? Although you would have special concerns if a 58-year-old patient complains of "old age," you will find it difficult to have any hard and fast rules about when an "older person" has become "old." (One older patient with a sense of humor describes old age as that time of life when the word "doctor" becomes a verb!) The 68-year-old chief executive with neither health problems nor plans to retire is certainly not the same kind of older person as the 68-year-old retired mill worker with oxygen-dependent chronic lung disease and recent memory loss. The former would find questions about his ability to perform routine activities of daily living insulting if not bizarre; the latter would find such questions very relevant to his overall management.

◈ **PRACTICE POINT**

The approach to older persons is individualized and geared to the patient's life experience, without making rigid classifications based on chronologic age.

THE STYLE OF THE INTERVIEW

The short vignette in the introduction illustrates the way in which many older persons attribute their symptoms to normal aging and may require open-ended prompting ("What do you mean by old age?") to discuss symptoms that could indicate a specific disease process as opposed to normal physiological processes. Patients may attribute nocturia or joint pain, for example, to aging, even though the symptoms may, in fact, indicate pathological conditions such as congestive heart failure or rheumatoid arthritis. Moreover, vague symptoms may have special implications in elderly patients, as in the case of a 90-year-old man who experiences loss of appetite and feelings of malaise as symptoms of pneumonia, rather than the more typical fever and cough. Likewise, chronic symptoms must be distinguished from acute or unstable symptoms. For example, the sudden onset of urinary incontinence requires a different approach than does incontinence of many years' duration. You also will notice that the pace of the interview is often slower with older patients and that they infuse their medical stories with a lifetime of experience that demands our respect.

Consider this example of a 77-year-old woman with end-stage renal disease:

Clinician **So, hi, it's nice to see you back. How've you been feeling since you left the hospital?**

Patient   Well, each day is a little better and with that new fluid pill I'm not gaining any weight. But I'm very tired, more tired than I used to be. You know, my husband—he's 95 years old—just got out of the hospital, too. I'm taking care of him and I'm taking care of myself. But it's in the Lord's hands and I have a family in my church. They bring food, they help out. I used to be the choir director.

Notice how the clinician gives the patient time to respond, in the process learning much about not only the patient's illness but also how she's managing with it. It is clear, too, from her response that this patient's cognitive skills are intact.

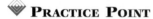 **PRACTICE POINT**

In interviewing older patients, the pace of the interview is often slower, and it is necessary to differentiate not only acute from chronic, but also natural features of aging from symptoms that signify specific disorders.

THE CONTENT OF THE INTERVIEW

In addition to differences in style, the geriatric history emphasizes distinct content areas as well. For example, remote events, such as childhood history, are usually not relevant and may be obtained with a minimum of detail, with such questions as "Any unusual illnesses when you were a child?" The family history is also less important because most familial diseases will have expressed themselves by the time a person reaches old age. Family history also takes on a different twist because you are now looking not only at the preceding generation but at the patient's children

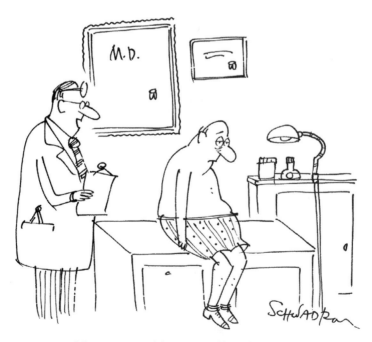

"Mr. Haroldson, I'm taking you off trying to stay young."
©2000 Harley Schwadron

and grandchildren as well. For example, an older woman whose daughter has breast cancer may herself be at increased risk for the disease and may be unaware that, in fact, it was breast cancer that took the life of her mother 40 years earlier. Moreover, older persons may worry about the health of their children and grandchildren, and your interest in their families provides an opportunity to explore those concerns.

 PRACTICE POINT

Perhaps the most striking difference in interviewing older patients is the need to assess their functional status in terms of everyday activities and their abilities to do those activities necessary to sustain and enjoy life.

The patient profile (see Chapter 5) includes most basic activities of daily living, including the ability to eat (chew and swallow), sleep, bathe, dress, walk or move about unaided, and maintain continence. The ability to cook and to perform simple household chores must also be assessed. Several useful rating scales are available for measuring functional status or activities of daily living; *Special Aspects of the History in the Elderly Patient,* below, presents useful screening questions.

WHAT TO SAY
Special Aspects of the History in the Elderly Patient

Topic	Sample Questions
Normal sleep-wake cycle	"Are you able to sleep when you want to sleep and not sleep when you don't want to?"
Continence of bowel and bladder	"Can you manage by yourself in the bathroom? Can you get there in time?"
Dietary habits	"Who helps you with the shopping and cooking? Let's go through what you eat on a typical day so I can see whether you're getting everything you need."
Mobility	"Do you have any trouble getting around? Going up or down stairs? Have you had any falls?"
Medications	"Let's go through all the pills you brought with you. Tell me how you take each one."
Alcohol use	"Tell me how much alcohol you drink on a typical day. What about other days?"

(continued on following page)

Support system	"Do you have family or friends or neighbors you can call when you need help?"
Vision/hearing	"Are you able to see what you want to see? Hear what you want to hear?"
Memory	"Have you been having any problems with your memory?"
Depression	"How have your spirits been?"
Sexuality	"Have you had any change in your interest in sex?"

Nutrition

Details about the patient's diet include consideration of specific nutrients such as calcium (to prevent osteoporosis) and fiber (to help prevent constipation and treat diverticular disease or hemorrhoids). Many older adults also take multiple vitamins and pills that contain iron and other minerals. Elderly patients are not necessarily immune from food fads and novelty diets—"Lose weight fast! Low-carb, low-fat, low-protein!"—which may be heavily promoted, especially on television.

Medications

Another content area of special importance for elderly adults is the detailed review of all medications they are taking, including over-the-counter as well as prescription drugs. This review is often best accomplished by asking patients to bring all their pill containers to the office with them, even containers of medications they are no longer using. Polypharmacy (using many different medications at the same time) can be an important cause of symptoms in patients who take multiple medications for multiple health problems, even though each individual drug is an appropriate treatment for its target disorder. When older patients report new symptoms, it is important to ascertain any recent changes in their medication regimen. For example, the 82-year-old woman who has been stable on six prescriptions for diabetes, hypothyroidism, and heart failure suddenly develops severe "heartburn." An Urgent Care doctor prescribes a proton pump inhibitor and refers her to a gastroenterologist. However, her family physician reviews the medication list and learns that her cardiologist has recently prescribed a nonsteroidal anti-inflammatory drug—which can cause gastritis—when the patient complained of aching in her joints. By discontinuing the drug, the family physician eliminates his patient's "heartburn."

At times, drug interactions can be dangerous and should be carefully looked for. Nowadays, many older men routinely take medications to enhance sexual performance. Because some men may be embarrassed at needing these drugs, they may not readily report using them to physicians other than their urologists. However, Viagra and related drugs are quite dangerous when taken with nitrates, which are commonly used to treat coronary artery disease. Thus, in the case of an older man with heart disease, it is important to ask specifically if he is taking such a drug, and to explain this serious drug interaction.

Alcohol and Substance Use

Questions about alcohol intake should not be neglected, but the CAGE questions (see *Screening Your Patients for Problem Drinking* in Chapter 5), though useful, may not be as sensitive in elderly patients. Additional questions about the frequency and quantity of alcohol consumed increase your ability to detect abuse or dependence in this age group. Abuse of prescription drugs, such as opioids and benzodiazepines, may also occur; alternatively, the recent prescription of an opioid to treat severe pain (e.g., a fractured hip) or a benzodiazepine to treat anxiety (e.g., over a major life change) may be responsible for the acute onset of such symptoms as confusion, unsteadiness, falling, or constipation. Standard inquiries about cigarette smoking maintain their relevance in taking older persons' histories, and stopping smoking may lead to health benefits even in older patients. In addition to the decreased risk of cardiovascular disease and cancers, a patient can decrease the risk of getting burnt by a cigarette or starting a fire, as is especially possible with older patients, who might be extremely frail or confused.

Immunizations

Immunization status is an important part of the geriatric medical history that is often given insufficient attention. Immunization history should include diphtheria-tetanus vaccine (booster every 10 years), influenza vaccine (annually), and pneumococcal vaccine (once at age 65).

Sexuality

Finally, you should also assess sexual feelings and function, but this must be done sensitively and in context. Frail, sick, or widowed elderly patients may find questions like "Are you sexually active?" or "Are you having any sexual problems?" surprising, if not downright inappropriate. It is better to give the patient plenty of leeway, based on his or her own situation. For example: "As people get older they sometimes find that their marriage changes. How has it been for you?" and then "Has anything changed in your sexual relationship?" Change in sexual function may also be related to specific illness, rather than to age per se. For example: "I can see that you're having problems with the circulation in your legs. Sometimes when men have this problem, they also notice problems getting an erection. Have you noticed anything like that?" The technique of laying the groundwork with an introductory statement that normalizes potential sexual problems and allows the patient to understand the context of the question (as discussed in Chapter 6, The Sexual History) is effective with elderly patients as well.

MENTAL STATUS ASSESSMENT

The Informal Assessment

The interviewer must facilitate a technically competent interview with patients who may be frail, hard of hearing, visually impaired, or suffering from memory loss.

◆ **PRACTICE POINT**
You can quickly and inconspicuously assess cognitive function in the opening moments of the interview with the elderly patient, usually without performing a formal mental status examination.

The purpose of the informal assessment is to determine whether the patient is competent to give his or her own history and what assistance might be needed to help ensure accuracy and precision of medical data. How is this informal assessment accomplished? First, clues about mental status arise even before the examination, as you observe the interaction between the patient and family members or caregivers. For example:

- Does the patient himself or herself call to make an appointment or to report symptoms?
- Does he or she arrive in the office alone, having driven a car or taken a bus or taxi?
- Does the patient forget an appointment even when reminded with a postcard or phone call?

Patients who cannot remember having made appointments may also be unable to remember medications or to recall and report symptoms that they experience.

Next, as you enter the examination room or the patient's hospital room, pay careful attention to the patient's level of alertness, such as whether he or she is awake or drowsy. The patient sedated with a narcotic to alleviate renal colic may not be able to tell you much (other than that he or she is feeling better now) until the medication wears off. Is the patient alert enough to focus attention on you and follow you from one question or statement to the next? Problems with alertness are common in hospitals and tend to be under-recognized. You should also note the patient's general appearance and behavior. For example:

- Does he or she appear socially appropriate?
- Is the patient clean and quiet, or disheveled and agitated?
- Is the patient physically active or slow and retarded?

As you begin the interview, you next assess the patient's verbal output or speech. Is it relevant or irrelevant? Rambling or reticent? Repetitious or almost mute? Coherent or incoherent? These characteristics, in turn, tell you a great deal about the patient's thought process and content. Is the pattern of thought logical or tangential? Is the patient preoccupied with thoughts of death? Is there an obvious delusional system?

Here is an example of the opening moments of a follow-up visit with a 76-year-old woman who was brought in by her family because of weight loss and abdominal pain:

Clinician **You said you've been feeling sad.**

Patient   Yeah, my mother died before the baby was born, and I just started talking to the women about it and all of a sudden I said I couldn't. It's just sad. Well, I raised a boy, his name was Andy, and he stayed in Europe and he couldn't get out there and he was about 10 years or something like that. And then my sister, you know, wanted to come back and I went to look for the money we were trying to collect for. So I went up and—you know how it is—and on a Sunday I went over there and the baby was born.

How would you describe this patient's thought process? Although her statement does seem vaguely related to the issue of sadness, it is difficult to follow the thread of her story, and it is certainly not a response to the question. We would describe it as rambling, tangential, and probably incoherent. It is typical of this patient, who could not actually remember how she had been feeling. This is dementia, not psychosis.

In observing the patient, you will also notice mood and affect. Is the patient flat or sad? Anxious or inappropriately merry? Cooperative or combative? Although orientation to time, place, and person may be obvious in the opening moments of your interview as you engage in social "chit chat" with your patient, be aware that many mildly and even moderately demented older persons retain excellent social skills that belie their cognitive deficit. We are reminded of two elderly women, both age 93, who came to the office one day for back-to-back appointments. The nursing and reception staff commented, "Aren't they doing well!" In reality, however, one was doing well and the other was not. Each exhibited the social amenities of saying hello, observing how much she liked her clinician and commenting on the weather. One patient then went on to give a detailed account of her arthritic symptoms over the past month. The other, despite enthusiastically greeting her clinician, whom she had seen many times before, replied as follows:

Patient   It's so very nice to see you. You're such a grand person.
Clinician   **Why, thank you. It's nice to see you, too. Do you remember who I am?**
            Well, you look very familiar. What's your name again?

The patient's ability to remember becomes readily apparent as the interview proceeds and you try to gather precise information about symptoms. The elderly gentleman who repeats items in his history at different parts of a brief interview may not remember that he has already told you these details. The patient who says she has been feeling fine despite her family's concern about her repeated complaints of chest pain may not remember these episodes of pain. Indeed, sometimes you encounter factual contradictions, such as a patient with surgical scars on her abdomen who states that she has never had surgery.

In the following encounter, an elderly patient with dementia simply cannot remember his recent symptoms; rather, he is only aware of how he feels at present.

Clinician   **Do you know who I am?**
Patient   Well, I don't know, no.
            I'm Dr. Smith.
            Oh.
            I'm glad to see you today. How have you been feeling?
            Oh, I don't know, just all poured out.
            Weak, are you weak?

I imagine to a certain extent, but it seems just that nothing just seems to be right.

[Taking pulse] Your pulse feels good today.

I'm glad there's something good about me.

Do you feel there's not much good about you?

Oh well, I guess I'm just average.

How's your heart been treating you?

Oh, it never did bother me.

How are you sleeping at night?

No trouble at all.

How's your appetite?

Always with me.

In such situations, we ordinarily dismiss the possibility of a useful interview with the patient and seek information elsewhere. In this example, the clinician spoke with the demented patient's wife, who stated that his appetite was poor, he was having trouble sleeping, and he was frequently short of breath.

 PRACTICE POINT

Be aware that dementia may be mild and variable; you need to listen carefully for inappropriate responses or evidence of confusion. It is useful early in the interview to detect these problems, which will otherwise lead to faulty data collection.

Formal Mental Status Testing

Usually, careful observations during the interview are sufficient to assess your patient's reliability and to rule out significant organic mental problems, such as delirium or dementia. Sometimes, however, it is important to perform a more complete evaluation that includes specific components of mental status, including:

- Appearance and behavior
- Attention and alertness
- Speech and language
- Mood and affect
- Memory and orientation
- Thought process and content
- Judgment and insight
- Abstract thinking, knowledge, and calculation

One semiquantitative tool that is often useful in capturing these mental status factors is the Folstein Mini-Mental Status Exam. Although this widely used tool does not cover all the attributes of a complete mental status examination, it does give a relatively rapid numerical score to estimate cognitive function. In the hospital, the Mini-Mental Status Exam can be used to follow patients with fluctuating mental status by administering it at various times of the day, such as morning and evening. In the outpatient setting, it can be used to evaluate and follow patients' cognitive function over the course of months or years.

The Folstein Mini-Mental Status Exam is shown in Table 11–1. Low scores or scores that change over time suggest neuropsychiatric or neurological disorders such as delirium, dementia, or the so-called pseudodementia of severe depression. False-positive results may occur in patients who cannot concentrate because of extreme anxiety or thought disorder. In highly intelligent patients, the test may not be very sensitive, so that false-negative results may occur. Such problems should be noted during

TABLE 11–1

THE FOLSTEIN MINI-MENTAL STATUS EXAM		
	Score	Maximum Score
Orientation		
What is the (year) _____ (season) _____ (month) _____ (date) _____ (day) _____?	( )	5
Where are we (state) _____ (county) _____ (town) _____ (hosp.) _____ (floor) _____?	( )	5
Registration		
I am going to name three objects and I want you to repeat them after me. (Interviewer, give one point for each correct answer. Repeat the objects until the patient can name them all–six trials maximum.) Number of trials ( ).	( )	3
Attention and Calculation		
I am going to ask you to do some subtraction. Think of the number 7. I want you to subtract 7 from 100. Now subtract 7 from that and keep on going. 100, _____, _____, _____, _____, _____. Stop. Alternative: Spell "world" backwards.	( )	5

	Score	Maximum Score
Recall		
Please name the three objects that I had you repeat after me just a short while ago. (Interviewer, give one point for each correct answer.)	( )	3
Language		
Please name these for me. (Show patient a watch and a pencil.)	( )	2
Now, please repeat the following: " no ifs, ands, or buts."	( )	1
Now I am going to ask you to do something for me. "Take a paper in your right hand, fold it in half, and put it on the floor."	( )	3
Now I want you to read this and do what it says. (Interviewer, hand the patient a card that says "Close your eyes.")	( )	1
Now, please write a sentence for me on this blank piece of paper. (Interviewer, give the patient a blank piece of paper and ask him or her to write a sentence for you. Do not dictate a sentence; it must be written spontaneously. It must contain a subject and verb and be sensible. Correct grammar and punctuation are not necessary.)	( )	1
Visual-Motor Integrity		
Please copy this design. (Interviewer, on a clean piece of paper, draw intersecting pentagons, each side about 1 inch, and ask him or her to copy it exactly as it is. All 10 angles must be present and 2 must intersect to score 1 point.)	( )	1
TOTAL SCORE	( )	30
INTERVIEWER: Assess patient's level of consciousness along continuum.		

Alert	Drowsy	Stupor	Coma

From Folstein MF, Folstein SE, McHugh PR. Mini-mental state: A practical method for grading the cognitive state of patients for the clinician. *J Psychiatr Res* 1975; 12:189–198, with permission of Pergamon Press PLC.

the test; when in doubt, more complete cognitive testing (which is beyond the scope of this chapter) can be done.

Clinicians are often reluctant to perform mental status testing, partly because they find it awkward to incorporate these tests into their interview format. Indeed, the data obtained are not really part of the medical history as such, but, more correctly, are part of the objective database, akin to the physical examination. Patients may also find specific questions about memory or cognition stressful. To ease these tensions, it is best to introduce mental status testing after the history portion of your interaction, either just before or just after your physical examination. By this time, you will already have developed a relationship with your patient as well as an understanding of what some of his or her problems are. Such knowledge allows you to introduce this part of your evaluation in a straightforward and natural way. For example:

Clinician	**I've noticed that as we've been talking there are some things you have trouble remembering. Would it be all right if I test your memory?**
Patient	How do you do that?
	Well, I will ask you questions, some of which will seem silly to you and easy, and others may be hard for you. Would that be okay?

or

Clinician	**Do you ever forget to take your medication?**
Patient	No, I never do.
	How do you remember?
	That's the first thing I do every day. But sometimes my memory is not so good. Sometimes I forget things I'm going to say.
	Is that a new problem for you?
	No, it has been for some time. I guess at 88, what can you expect?
	At 88 I think you're doing fine. Would it be okay for me to test your memory so we can get an idea of how much of a problem it is?

During the examination, patients will be more relaxed if you provide support and encouragement, especially when they struggle with finding the correct answers. For example:

Clinician	**Please name this for me. [Interviewer shows patient a pencil.]**
Patient	Well, it's something for something to say in, I don't know.
	Would you know how to use it?
	No, I don't think so. I couldn't even write my name anymore.
	You couldn't write your name anymore? Do you know what you could use this for?
	I have no idea.
	Okay, well it's a pencil.
	A pencil.

You can write with it, you just do like this and you can write with it. I see that you wrote your name pretty well here.

Notice in this case how the clinician provides information and positive reinforcement to the patient (an 82-year-old man with multi-infarct dementia), who, in fact, made a connection with the object ("I couldn't even write my name anymore") but was unable to name it or to describe its use.

THE THIRD PARTY

No discussion of interviewing elderly patients would be complete without mentioning the issue of autonomy and the role of concerned family members or caregivers. Difficulties arise when the patient and concerned others disagree on the extent of disability caused by dementia or other illness, or when the patient and family disagree about the value of some proposed plan of treatment. In the case of a failing or frail octogenarian with mild dementia, it is often difficult to evaluate medical decision-making capacity or to assess the legitimate interests of family or caregivers. Within the interview, we may hear different histories: for example, the family of an 80-year-old woman reports that she leaves the stove untended and soils herself, but the patient denies these problems. Family members may want to discuss matters with the clinician in private, out of the patient's earshot, and subsequently forbid the clinician to discuss their concerns with the patient. Or a daughter may bring her mother to the office seemingly against the patient's will. How do you respect the daughter's concerns and at the same time nurture the patient's autonomy?

Respect and Autonomy

The preceding sentence contains two words that summarize our approach to the older patient: respect and autonomy. First, you should approach your elderly patient with the same respect and concern that you have for any other patient. Your contract as a clinician includes honesty, privacy, and confidentiality, as discussed fully in Chapter 9, Communication in the Office Setting. Consequently, while being sensitive to the family's concerns about what grandma should or should not be told about her condition, it is important for you to emphasize her right to know and the fact that most elderly patients respond well to being fully apprised of their situation.

Moreover, you should be sensitive to the patient's feelings about privacy and, therefore, minimize the third party's involvement if the patient so wishes. A direct approach with family members is often helpful.

Clinician	**I know you want your father to have a confidential doctor-patient relationship and to know that I respect him. Would it be okay if I speak with him alone?**
Patient	(Patient's daughter responds) Well, he gets confused sometimes. He may not understand what you tell him. I think sometimes he only pays attention to what he agrees with.
	After he and I talk, I'll ask his permission for you to come in so we can discuss this together. The best way to do this is for no one to feel like we are keeping secrets.

In this case the daughter probably has her father's best interest at heart. She believes that he needs help in answering questions accurately and understanding what the clinician says. Nevertheless, these considerations must be weighed against respect for the patient and his right to privacy. Here, the clinician clearly indicates his reasons for interviewing the patient privately, while at the same time he shows respect for the daughter's motivations. When she responds with statements about her father's cognitive limitations (of which the clinician is already aware), the clinician assures her that respecting the patient's privacy need not interfere with a later opportunity to "discuss this together."

Respect for other family members demands that you apprise them at the outset of your clinician-patient contract: you will not collude with them to withhold information or to "help" the patient against his or her competent wishes. Second, insofar as it is possible, nourish the patient's autonomy. Some elderly patients have deficits that render them temporarily or permanently lacking in capacity to make medical decisions. But even if your patient lacks capacity, you continue to have an obligation to respect his or her interests. Sometimes you may disagree with family members about just what the patient's best interests are. For example, optimal medical treatment of an elderly, mildly demented man with heart disease might require a low-salt, cholesterol-lowering diet. This diet may eliminate most of the foods that he has enjoyed eating all his life. The patient's daughter might insist on sticking to "the letter of the law," cooking him only bland food that he doesn't like. Perhaps she believes this is in "Dad's best interest." "He doesn't know what's good for him," she tells you. Doesn't he? It might be far more beneficial to the 80-year-old patient to relish eating his meals than to have a small reduction in his cholesterol level. In this case, the clinician's obligation (nourishing autonomy) might be to counsel the daughter to provide a more enjoyable—though perhaps less medically "correct"—diet for her father.

Summary—Interviewing the Geriatric Patient

To make the most of your interactions with geriatric patients, make sure you:

- Adapt your interview style to a slower pace
- Assess problems with activities of daily living
- Assess nutrition, substance use, immunizations, and sexuality
- Perform a detailed review of all medications, including over-the-counter medications
- Assess mental status through both informal observation and formal testing
- Respect the patient's life experience and nourish his or her autonomy
- Try to get the patient's own story rather than going through an intermediary, however well-meaning

With the ability to adapt your interview in both content and style to different age groups, you have begun the process of building on your basic skills and applying them to different situations and different types of patients.

CHAPTER 12

Cultural Competence in the Interview

For the Moment at Least
I Actually Became Them

... for the moment at least I actually became them;
whoever they should be, so that when I detached
myself from them at the end of a half-hour of
intense concentration over some illness which was
affecting them, it was as though I was awakening
from a sleep.
William Carlos Williams, The Autobiography

EXPLORING CULTURAL COMPETENCE

Cultural competence is the ability to understand, accept, appreciate, and work with individuals of cultures other than one's own. In this context we use the word "culture" very broadly to include ethnicity, sexual orientation, and gender. Thus, to be culturally competent also means to avoid stereotypes, bias, prejudice, classism, racism, ageism, xenophobia, homophobia, and sexism in your everyday interactions with patients. The goal of cultural competence is to deliver the best possible health care to diverse populations in our society. Cultural competence is closely linked to "cultural humility," in that the more you know about a particular culture, the more you realize you don't know. In a very real sense, every patient encounter is a cross-cultural encounter.

Because culture drives the patient's values and beliefs regarding health and illness, as well as expectations regarding therapy, the need to understand culture is fundamental to patient care because it affects such critical processes as adherence to treatment, informed consent, and prevention of errors related to miscommunication. The changing demographics of our society and concerns about culturally based disparities in access to health services have resulted in professional and regulatory mandates to acknowledge and consider the patient's values in order to improve health outcomes.

What are these values and beliefs? By "values" we mean the patient's fundamental moral and existential commitments and, in particular, how those commitments manifest themselves in the patient's attitudes and behavior. "Beliefs" means both general and specific understandings about what causes illness, how it develops, what you can do about it, and what will happen if you don't. Values and beliefs inform expectations. The first section of this chapter deals briefly with the ways that values and beliefs affect patients' decision making and behavior regarding illness. The next section considers the skills of cross-cultural interviewing, including situations in which a translator is required because the patient speaks little or no English. In the remainder of the chapter, we discuss cultural stereotypes and the various elements that contribute to personal health beliefs, and we present a framework for eliciting the patient's interpretation of the illness.

CULTURE, VALUES, AND SELF-AWARENESS

Values lie at the core of any clinician-patient encounter. The patient values life and health, as does the clinician. The patient presumably also values the clinician's help, and we expect the clinician to respect (value) the patient. Although these implicit commitments are important, understanding cultural diversity requires us to explore patient values more explicitly because values may differ. A clear example arises in caring for dying patients: one person may consider life so sacred that it should be preserved at all costs, whereas another places greater value on quality of life. Advance directives are designed to reflect such commitments and the health care decisions that derive from them (see "Advance Directives" in Chapter 14). Similarly, in the care of the chronically ill, you will find that some patients place an extremely high premium on personal independence and self-determination, but other patients are more oriented toward family relationships and interdependence. Specific religious values sometimes significantly inform medical treatment, such as "sanctity of life" beliefs in decisions about withholding or withdrawing life-sustaining therapy, or "purity" in decisions by Jehovah's Witnesses, such as not accepting blood transfusions. In other cases, cultural values play a major role in the process of decision making. Native Americans, for example, value a process of group decision making by the family that appears to conflict with the concept of personal autonomy so valued by other cultures, including the "culture" of American biomedical ethics. How do we become aware of others' values, which are often more implicit than explicit?

Understanding Our Own Attitudes and Values

First, we need to be aware of our own attitudes and values. We tend to assume that medical explanations for illness phenomena and medically indicated forms of treatment are self-evident and represent "reality" rather than beliefs. But they are not necessarily self-evident to all. Western medical beliefs reflect the high value we place on attempting to control the world (and our lives) by using science, and a tendency to devalue ambiguity and unscientific explanations. Some clinicians are more tolerant than others of patients with alternative values.

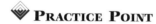 **Practice Point**

A first step toward respecting and understanding patients of different cultures is a commitment to personal self-awareness.

It is also important to understand how our own family, cultural, and religious backgrounds determine, to a large extent, who we are and influence the beliefs and values we bring to our roles as clinicians. Self-awareness also encourages us to acknowledge our limitations in knowledge and experience. The more personal contact we have with a certain group of patients, the less we find ourselves responding to them based on stereotypes we learned from our families or the media.

Culture and Health Beliefs

Once you understand your own values, you are ready to understand those of your patients. Cultural differences are easier to appreciate when your patients have an obviously different ethnic background from your own. In our culturally diverse society, it is common for Anglo clinicians to encounter Hispanic patients; Indian clinicians, Vietnamese patients; Russian clinicians, Haitian patients; and so forth. Language is only the most obvious barrier to communication in these situations. Even when the parties speak each other's language, it may be difficult for them to express deeply held beliefs or complex medical explanations in the nonnative tongue. Moreover, the clinician's understanding of the patient's personal world (e.g., dietary habits, family constellation, and health-related behaviors) may be compromised by cultural ignorance or insensitivity.

Just because patients appear in your clinical setting, they do not necessarily share your belief system regarding the etiology and treatment of illness. *Various Beliefs about Disease Etiology*, below, presents examples of cultural beliefs about causes of disease or illness. In many parts of the world, the concept of bodily imbalance is the basis for traditional understanding of ill health. For example, some Hispanic cultures subscribe to a folk physiology that requires "hot" and "cold" humors to be in proper balance for optimal health. One becomes sick when humors are imbalanced. Moreover, certain diseases are characterized as cold (i.e., having a preponderance of cold humors) and others as hot. Medicines are similarly categorized. To restore the appropriate balance, one normally treats a cold illness with a hot medicine, and vice versa. The non-Hispanic clinician who is unaware of these distinctions and who prescribes hot medicine for hot illness will likely encounter resistance and perhaps noncompliance. Similar notions of illness as imbalance, or disharmony, occur in Chinese (yin/yang), Indian, and Native-American healing systems. In each case, recommended medical therapy may inadvertently be inconsistent with culturally recommended measures. To be effective, the Western clinician must be sufficiently familiar with the patient's belief system to recommend a treatment plan that will be synergistic with those beliefs.

VARIOUS BELIEFS ABOUT DISEASE ETIOLOGY

- Upset in the body's balance or harmony
  - Yin/yang (East Asia)
  - Hot/cold (Central America)
  - Body, mind, spirit [Ayurvedic] (India)
- Soul loss (Native American)
- Spirit possession (Ethiopia)
- The Evil Eye (Mediterranean, Middle East)
- Challenge or punishment from God (Christian fundamentalism)

Culture and Language

Understanding What Words Mean

Cultural differences may lead to other miscues and misunderstandings (see *Cultural Miscues and Misunderstandings*, page 232). For instance,

American phrases or idioms may be taken literally by persons for whom English is a second language; for example, a Korean patient understood a question about preoperative anxiety ("Are you getting cold feet?") as an inquiry about the temperature of his feet. Health care professionals also use medical jargon and "plain" language differently than their patients. One striking example (not as prevalent as it once was) derives from the "high blood–low blood" folk physiology in African-American and rural white populations in the American South. In these cultures, people equate hypertension (high blood pressure) with "high blood," which they interpret as excessive blood thickness or volume. This condition is believed to cause strokes because excess blood backs up in the brain. They use the term "low blood" for anemia, which they believe puts a strain on the heart. Thus, "high blood" and "low blood" are opposite blood conditions and not (as they are in medical terms) diseases of two completely different organ systems. Thus, it is difficult for patients of this cultural tradition to accept the idea that they can have high blood pressure ("high blood") and anemia ("low blood") at the same time.

CULTURAL MISCUES AND MISUNDERSTANDINGS

- Idioms (Using such statements as "To tell you the truth, I think she is getting cold feet.")
- Same language, different meaning (Is "positive" good? Is "negative" bad?)
- Inflammatory words or comments (Using racist or sexist statements or ethnic slurs)
- The polite "yes" (For example, a patient may say "Yes, doctor," but may really mean "No.")
- Eye contact (In some cultures, direct eye contact may be embarrassing or even threatening.)
- Touching (Touching may be therapeutic in itself, a barely tolerated necessity, or culturally inappropriate.)

Another example is the almost universal use of "negative" in medicine as a good finding. For example:

Clinician **You don't have to worry, Mrs. Nguyen, your tests were negative.**

Patient   Oh my God, I knew it. I knew this was coming. What will I do? This is what I was afraid would happen.

This Vietnamese-American patient has understood the word "negative" (quite reasonably) to mean a bad outcome. Thus, the clinician seems—inadvertently—to be confirming her worst fears when, in reality, he was actually trying to deliver good news.

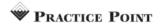 **PRACTICE POINT**

Make sure you check back with the patient to assure he or she understands the meaning of what you say.

Disrespectful Words

Other language miscommunications involve words or expressions that seem neutral to the clinician but are inflammatory or disrespectful from the patient's perspective. Consider the contemporary American woman's feelings of disrespect (based on sexism) when a clinician refers to her as a "girl" or "honey." The use of a patient's first name may have a similarly negative effect. Although middle-class American society revels in the informality of quickly placing relationships on a first-name basis, such a practice may be considered extremely disrespectful to older Americans and in many other cultures.

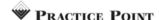 **PRACTICE POINT**

Address the patient formally by title (e.g., Mr., Mrs., Ms., Señora) and surname. Request permission to use the patient's first name only when culturally appropriate.

Nonverbal Miscommunication

Nonverbal behaviors also may lead to cross-cultural misunderstandings, as when the clinician uses direct eye contact (presumably a "good" skill), then discovers that he has insulted his Native-American patient or embarrassed his Asian patient. Likewise, touching, which in secular American culture is considered a positive (perhaps even essential) aspect of a clinician-patient encounter, may be problematic in certain cross-cultural situations, especially when the clinician and patient are of different genders; for example, it is inappropriate for a man to shake hands with (or otherwise touch) a Muslim or Orthodox Jewish woman. This prohibition may at times be set aside for the necessary touching of physical examination, but modesty remains an extremely important consideration. Therefore, expressions of warmth or compassion that might seem natural to an American clinician (e.g., touching an arm or sitting on the patient's bed) may be perceived as disrespectful. Although some patients will politely describe the reasons for their discomfort, others may simply show their discomfort in their body language and apparent reluctance to continue the interview.

Language Translation

In many cross-cultural encounters, the patient does not speak English, or speaks English poorly, and the clinician needs a translator to assist in the interview. Clinical translation services should be widely available, efficient, reliable, and of high quality. Translators should have training in clinical translation because, besides mastery of both languages, they need to be familiar with health care concepts and situations, and knowledgeable about the cultural issues raised in this chapter. Often, however, a trained translator is not available, and nonclinical staff members, or even family members or friends, serve as translators.

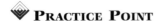 **PRACTICE POINT**

If at all possible, avoid relying on a friend or family member to translate.

A friend or family member may not be able to provide accurate (and thorough) translation for several reasons:

- Lack of sufficient fluency in English
- Lack of clinical knowledge and experience
- Reluctance to ask probing personal or intimate questions
- Reluctance of the patient to reveal personal or intimate information in this person's presence

Sometimes, however, there is no alternative but to speak through a family member in the acute situation. This may not cause a problem for simple, nonthreatening communication, but with more complex issues, the clinician should arrange for a professional interpreter. One highly accessible method of doing this is by telephone through medical translation services provided by long-distance telephone companies. These services are available, by arrangement, to hospitals and other health care settings. They provide the assurance of translation from almost any language to English and back, but they do have drawbacks, including the need to schedule interviews in advance and the loss of spontaneity and nonverbal communication that would have been present in a face-to-face encounter.

Cultural Translation

Even though your patient may be able to speak English adequately to provide basic clinical information, however, language commonly proves to be a barrier to discussing more complex topics or personal matters. Sometimes it is unclear whether language itself is the barrier, or whether the barrier may be cultural practices that prohibit discussing certain topics or revealing certain categories of information. (See *Technical Guidelines for Cross-Cultural Interviewing*, below.) If it appears that the patient would be more comfortable conversing in his or her own language, it may be helpful to use an interpreter even though the patient is ostensibly competent in English. Table 12–1 gives some examples of English terms that may pose problems in translation to the equivalent medically relevant concepts in other languages.

WHAT TO SAY
Technical Guidelines for Cross-Cultural Interviewing

- Determine the patient's level of fluency in English and arrange for a translator, if needed. "Do you speak English?" "Do you understand?"
- Ask the patient how he or she prefers to be addressed. "May I call you by your first name?" "May I call you Dorothy, or do you prefer Mrs. Kaufmann?"
- Avoid shaking hands if cultural prohibition exists. "May I shake hands?"
- Assure the patient of confidentiality. "Everything we discuss is between us unless you want me to share it with someone else. Do you understand?"
- Employ a speech rate, tone, and style that promote understanding and show respect for the patient. "Let me know if I go too fast or if there is something that you do not understand."
- Allow the patient to describe the problem in his or her own terms, then use the patient's terminology to frame more specific descriptive questions. "Tell me in your own words what happened first and what happened next." "You say you 'prayed to God' when you had this pain in your chest. Was that because it was so bad that you felt like you were going to die?"
- Avoid culturally or personally sensitive topics until later in the interview when both parties are more comfortable. "You said that you have this pain

down below. May I ask you some questions about your menstrual periods and sexual relations to help me figure out what is causing it?"

■ Check frequently to determine patient understanding and acceptance, recognizing that "Yes" may often indicate a desire to please, rather than actual understanding. "This is a liquid medicine for your child's ear. But it goes in her mouth, not in her ear. Do you understand?"

TABLE 12–1

FREQUENTLY MISTRANSLATED MEDICAL TERMS	
Term	How to Avoid Misunderstanding
Allergy	Often a question about allergies is interpreted as meaning, "Does the medicine make you sick?" To distinguish side effects or ineffectiveness from true allergy, ask about specific allergic manifestations (e.g., "Does it cause a rash?").
Anxiety, nervousness	Use a variety of terms referring to both physical and psychological manifestations to elicit a history of anxiety. Ask about fears, racing heartbeat, sweating, and so on.
Blood tests	"Taking some blood" may be frightening and difficult to understand. Be explicit about the amount (expressed in teaspoons, rather than "tubes") and the purpose of the tests.
Dizziness	Distinguishing lightheadedness from vertigo can be challenging in translation. Make sure that the interpreter (or patient) understands the distinction between "unsteadiness" or "drunkenness" and the sensation that the room is spinning.
Fever	In cultures that divide illnesses into "hot" and "cold," the word "fever" may be used to refer to any hot disease, even in the absence of measured variation in body temperature.
Sensation of "pins and needles"	The literal translation of this term would be meaningless in languages other than English. Many Mexicans refer to *hormingas* (ants) crawling on the skin. This example illustrates the importance of avoiding idioms or metaphors when translating to a different language (or culture), or making sure that the interpreter understands the English idiom.

Adapted from Rothschild SK. Cross-cultural issues in primary care medicine. *Dis Mon* 1998; 44: 293–319, at 312.

HEALTH BELIEFS IN THE INTERVIEW

Stereotyping

Cultural values and beliefs are not the only factors that influence how persons understand health and illness or conceptualize health care. Religious, gender-based, socioeconomic, educational, environmental, familial, and personal factors also play roles. Thus, although cultural generalizations provide us with useful information, they should not be used to *stereotype* the attitudes or behavior of individual patients. Consider the following global statement: "In Hispanic cultures people tend to believe that they have little or no control over natural forces in the world." Such a statement might be helpful to clinicians insofar as it provides a context for understanding expressions of fatalism among Hispanic patients; but such a generalization is harmful if used to stereotype an individual, or to rationalize not educating and engaging the patient in his or her own health care. Likewise, the statement that women in traditional Arab or Italian cultures tend to express their pain loudly and dramatically may be true from a broad anthropological perspective. However, a clinician who uses this generalization to discount or minimize an individual patient's expression of pain is engaging in cultural stereotyping.

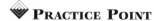 **PRACTICE POINT**

In clinical practice we encounter unique individual patients—not generic cultural representatives.

A Multiplicity of Cultures

Sometimes using the concept of "culture" helps us to understand the common experience of groups of people who may not at first blush appear to constitute cultures. Take, for example, the community of persons who were born deaf. The deaf community has its own language, traditions, and rules of social contact. The life experience of deaf people may foster negative attitudes toward health care professionals who focus on deafness solely as a disability, rather than as an alternative (and extremely rich) way of being in the world. The term "hearing impaired" has clinical usefulness, but in no way does it capture the self-image of persons born into the deaf world. In taking care of a deaf person, the culturally competent clinician must be sensitive to cross-cultural aspects of the encounter. Here are a few examples:

- Deaf persons rely on touch and vision rather than on sound to get another's attention. Touching that is considered appropriate in deaf culture might seem aggressive or uncomfortable in the hearing community. Likewise, exaggerated hand waving or stomping of feet (which produces vibration) to attract attention is normal behavior.
- Because deaf persons value face-to-face encounters (which are essential for signing), leave taking is often an extended process, rather than an abrupt "goodbye."
- American Sign Language (ASL) is the native language of deaf Americans; spoken English is their second language. Thus, miscommunication is likely to occur, especially with sensitive or complex topics, even when the patient reads lips well or the communication is in writing. It is often desirable to enlist an ASL–English translator.

Likewise, we might view the medically underserved population as a separate, identifiable culture, even though underserved communities in the United States may include individuals from various ethnic identities. These communities are generally characterized by low socioeconomic status, multiple social problems, poor access to needed services, and skepticism or distrust of the health care system. One benefit of conceptualizing the underserved as a separate culture (or "subculture") is that, by doing so, one establishes a context for understanding how difficult it is for some patients to think and act "like we do" regarding the benefits of health care or the beneficence of health care institutions. *Elements in Interviewing Patients from Underserved Populations,* below, summarizes skills that assist you in reaching across the cultural divide to make a therapeutic connection with patients from underserved and disadvan-

---

WHAT TO SAY
Elements in Interviewing Patients from Underserved Populations

Empathize

- Listen to the patient's expressions of frustration, failure, and anger.
  - "I can hear how frustrating it must be to have worked so hard and be unable to pay for your medication."
- Elicit a detailed patient profile, including health concerns and beliefs.

- "Tell me how this problem is affecting your life."
- Express solidarity and a commitment to serve.
    - "I want to help you get what you need to get better."

Enlist

- Frame the medical problem in a language and a belief system that the patient understands.
    - "Let me explain what happened to make your leg swell up and hurt. It's a blood clot in your vein. I think the blood clot developed because ..."
- Recognize and validate the patient's priorities.
    - "I understand that your main concern is being able to continue working."
- Inform the patient of the problem's importance and the value of addressing it.
    - "It's important to treat your blood clot, not only so you can get back to work now, but also to prevent more serious blood clots in the future."

Explain

- Avoid medical jargon and probabilistic explanations.
    - "This is what we call a pre-cancerous condition. That means it can turn into cancer, but it isn't cancer now. The reason for treating it now is to prevent cancer."
- Be specific; give explicit, concrete instructions.
    - "Now I want you to take two medications when you go home. Both are to lower your blood pressure, but they work in different ways. The first one is a water pill ..."
- Provide low-literacy instructional materials in the patient's native language.
    - "Here is a brochure that explains your condition and treatment. Why don't you take this Spanish version, too, just in case the English one isn't clear?"

Empower

- Give positive feedback regarding the patient's successes.
    - "I'm so happy you've stopped smoking. That's a real accomplishment!"
- Elicit the patient's concerns about cooperation with the treatment program.
    - "Do you have any questions or concerns about the treatment we discussed?"
- Seek the patient's explicit personal commitment to participate.
    - "I'd like you to make a commitment to follow the diet plan and lose 5 pounds before our next visit. What do you think?"

Adapted in part from Rothschild SK. Cross-cultural issues in primary care medicine. *Dis Mon* 1998; 44:293–319, at 334.

taged communities. Before being able to enlist the patient's cooperation, to explain the situation effectively, or to empower the patient to improve his or her health, you must first establish "contact" through empathy. To understand the patient, you must listen carefully to both cognitive (health beliefs) and affective (anger, powerlessness) aspects of the communication and respond with understanding and a commitment to serve.

Personal Health Beliefs

Like most people, health care professionals often look upon culture as a characteristic of people whose appearance or speech is different from their own. We may readily acknowledge that illness-related beliefs make a difference when treating people seemingly of other cultures, but we ignore the wide spectrum of beliefs and healing practices presented by ordinary people who look and talk as we do. We have a cultural blind spot: our own beliefs seem so obviously "true" that we don't realize that they are culturally determined.

◆ PRACTICE POINT

The "obvious truth" about illness against which you compare others' culturally influenced beliefs may, at least in part, be constructed from your own cultural beliefs and values. The inability to recognize the cultural origin of one's own beliefs is called a "cultural blind spot."

Although culture may provide the context for personal beliefs, such beliefs develop from a variety of sources: childhood experience, formal education, interactions with family and friends, television, newspapers, the Internet, and so forth. One's conceptualization of illness, one's threshold for seeking professional assistance, and one's expectation for cure are based on a personal belief system. Most people do not share the same blind faith in medical science that health care professionals often have. As clinicians, we look to physiology, microbiology, and probability for answers. When you are seriously sick, however, it is difficult to believe that your illness is a random event or a matter of probability. If 22% of persons exposed to a certain virus become clinically ill and, of these, 14% develop jaundice, you may ask, "Why me? Why was I one of the small minority who got sick and came down with jaundice? What does my illness signify?"

Beliefs Based on Values

One type of personal meaning derives from the patient's underlying value system and personality. If a patient views her pneumonia as a justified punishment from God for putting her mother into a nursing home, she may continue to experience symptoms and dysfunction even after the infection has cleared up. If another patient attributes his heart attack to personal weakness in the face of business pressure (i.e., "I just don't have what it takes"), he may well deny its seriousness and resist treatment. Another type of personal meaning has to do with concepts of how illness happens; patients may believe, for instance, that high blood pressure is caused by stress, colds are caused by sitting in a draft, and cancer is caused by electromagnetic fields from high-voltage power lines. These beliefs, in turn, may derive from more global, unifying personal values (e.g., internal balance, harmony with the environment, personal purity), which often are not fully articulated, or they may simply be the result of isolated fragments of information.

Info-Fragments

In today's world, beliefs about illness are often fragmented and contradictory, many of them falling into the category of misinformation. People are constantly exposed to health-related "info-fragments" from television, radio, magazines, newspapers, and the Internet. From these, a person may garner a variety of "facts" and opinions, many of which will be inconsistent with others. For instance, a patient may learn in one article that, to prevent heart disease, one should eat a low-fat diet. Another article will stridently argue for a low-carbohydrate diet. A third item (perhaps dealing with kidney disease) will cite studies that "prove" the efficacy of a low-protein diet. But how can a diet be low in fats, carbohydrates, and protein? There is nothing left! This inconsistency may be obvious to someone who understands physiology and nutrition, but to many patients these beliefs about diet are not perceived as inconsistent. They have all three info-fragments floating in their heads, and they apply each of them in different situations. This confusion makes good nutrition difficult and contributes to anxiety—not to mention total paralysis—about diet.

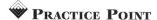 **PRACTICE POINT**
Most patients have a collection of "data" and opinions about health and illness that are fragmentary, inconsistent, and loosely held.

Such info-fragments may be superimposed on more comprehensive and consistent beliefs.

Eliciting Health Beliefs

Cultural Status Exam: The Patient's Interpretation of Illness, below, presents a framework for eliciting patients' beliefs regarding health and illness. This cultural status examination constitutes a kind of screening test to ascertain whether the patient's beliefs and expectations will conflict with medical explanations or treatment and interfere with the clinician-patient relationship. Such beliefs might prevent you from effectively influencing the patient's behavior unless you consider them in your therapeutic plan.

WHAT TO SAY
Cultural Status Exam: The Patient's Interpretation of Illness

Interpretive Level	Examples
Descriptive	How would you describe the problem that has brought you to me?
	What are the main difficulties this condition (sickness, illness, disease, or misfortune) has caused for you?
Conceptual	What does the illness do to you? How does it work?
	Why do you think it started when it did?
	What kind of treatment do you think you need?
	What are the results you hope for? What will happen if you don't get treatment?
	Apart from me, who else can help you get better? How can they help?
Personal	Why did you (in particular) get sick?
	What is most frightening about your sickness?

Adapted in part from Kleinman A, Eisenberg L, Good B. Culture, illness and care: Clinical lessons from anthropological and cross-cultural research. *Ann Intern Med* 1978; 88:251.

The questions at the descriptive level simply recap the characterization of symptoms that we discussed in "Symptom Description," in Chapter 3. It is important to discover precisely what your patient identifies as the major problem for which he or she is seeking help. The ostensible reason for coming, or chief complaint, may not, in fact, be the actual reason for coming or may be only a part of it. Sometimes you must probe further to get the whole story in order to put the chief complaint in context.

The questions at the conceptual level address the patient's understanding of the cause, appropriate treatment, and probable outcome of the illness, as well as the premises and logic that he or she uses as the basis of those concepts. Patients who are aware that they have beliefs that conflict with medical orthodoxy may not feel comfortable explaining them, thinking that you will dismiss them or become angry. Thus, it is necessary to set the stage by developing an empathic connection of trust.

The questions at the personal level deal with the idiosyncratic personal meaning of symptoms. Here again, mutual respect and trust must be present before patients will express their deepest fears or venture their most closely held beliefs (e.g., that the illness is a punishment for past sins).

◆ PRACTICE POINT
The personal and cultural meanings that your patient attributes to his or her illness constitute important clinical data that may greatly influence diagnosis, treatment, and prognosis.

Examples

Consider this segment from a routine follow-up visit by a 65-year-old woman to her primary care provider:

Patient   Green tea. Is it bad? I won't take it if you say not to [holding out a paper to her physician with information about green tea on it]. I take selenium and magnesium and lots of vitamins, but I really have to lose weight. So what do you think?

Clinician   **And what do you want to take this for?**

I'm fat. They say this works, or should I go to Weight Watchers? I don't know.

There's ...

... no magic, I know, I know. What's the matter with me? I just have a healthy appetite. I don't snack, I don't like candy, but I do like to eat. Look at what else I found [produces a handout on tomatoes and lycopenes in prostate health] and it's not written by a cuckoo. How I got this is, a man called in to this doctor who was presenting a report on TV. And he said that his PSA was 30 and he had had biopsies, which were okay, and how to bring his PSA down. And this doctor rec-ommended this. So I'm making my husband take it. [Her husband's PSA is 6 and the biopsies are negative, but she is very worried he has prostate cancer.]

Well, I'm not sure what to say about your husband. But as far as the green tea goes, it won't hurt you. On the other hand, I think you've learned something from the fen-phen experience. I know you were very frightened when all that came out about the side effects. You can lose the weight but the trick is keep-ing it off; you're gonna have to eat less. The way fen-phen took the weight off was that you ate less while you were on it. Green tea or anything else for that matter is no different.

I do want to lose the weight. I promise that when I come back from Florida I will have lost the weight.

Twenty pounds can make a big difference to your health.

The patient first asks about green tea as a weight-loss modality and reveals the source of this info-fragment (a handout from a natural food store). She also indicates that she takes "selenium, magnesium, and lots of vitamins," presumably as a result of other info-fragments about healthy lifestyle or weight loss. At the same time, she acknowledges knowing about a more structured method of losing weight—Weight Watchers. She has obviously heard her clinician's explanations in the past ("There's no magic"), but she cannot bear to abandon the shimmering allure of info-fragments. In fact, she tosses out another one, the use of tomatoes and lycopenes to "promote prostate health," while assuring the clinician that the material from the Internet wasn't written by a "cuckoo," the implica-tion being "so it must be true." The clinician acknowledges the info-fragments without expressing surprise or anger. While indicating a lack of specific knowledge about them, the clinician refocuses the conversation on the basics of nutrition and physiology: to weigh less, you have to eat less. She also refers to the patient's earlier anxiety-producing experience with fen-phen, gently bringing home once again the fact that "there's no magic."

Sometimes health care professionals contribute to misinformation. Consider the following excerpt from a conversation between a clinician and a patient seeking medical care because of epigastric pain and "heart-burn":

Patient   I take shots for allergies and I take two aspirins every day for my blood pressure. ... I don't eat any sugar, any salt.

Clinician Two aspirins for ...
Every morning.
For what, why do you take that?
Trying, trying to thin out my blood to keep my pressure down, I try to keep it around 100.
I see.

Later in the same interview the patient comes back to the issue of aspirin and blood pressure in this way:

But I always take two aspirins; I've taken two aspirins for years.
Clinician **Where did you get into that habit?**
Patient   Ah, when I was in the military in '78 and '79.
Um humm.
A German doctor told me that, ah, if you take two aspirins with milk in the morning, he says, it lowers your blood pressure and thins things out.
Um humm.
And I've always ... my blood pressure is always like 100, 110, it's real low.

If you accept this patient's basic premise, he has a perfectly logical belief regarding aspirin and blood pressure. He assumes that high blood pressure is caused by "thick" blood. If so, and if aspirin thins the blood, it is reasonable to take aspirin to prevent hypertension. In this case the belief is likely to be simply a piece of misinformation, although we do not know if the German doctor actually said that aspirin was good for blood pressure, or the patient misinterpreted. Note, however, that the concept is somewhat similar to the culturally based "high blood–low blood" beliefs described earlier in this chapter. The clinician could easily remedy the misinformation by explaining that blood pressure and blood coagulation involve two entirely different systems. In this case such an explanation would be particularly important if, in fact, the patient has gastritis or gastric ulcer, which may have been caused by the aspirin, or if he subsequently develops hypertension and needs medications to lower his blood pressure.

SUMMARY—Cultural Competence in the Interview
In this chapter we addressed the patient's values, beliefs, and expectations regarding illness and health care as they relate to the medical interview. Clinicians who practice in obviously

cross-cultural settings are usually aware of diversity in health beliefs. However, we must also learn to recognize that "culture" is not simply an attribute of people who appear to be different from us. The dominant American culture and its biomedical subculture fashion our own beliefs and many of our patients' beliefs about illness. The human experience of illness is never free from values or meaning. We also learned that:

- Language is a vehicle of cultural expression. High-quality health care requires expert professional translation when the patient does not speak English. In many cases, translation also improves the quality of communication even when the patient is generally competent in English.
- Cultural competence does not stereotype. Cultural values and beliefs are not the only factors that influence how persons understand health and illness, or conceptualize health care. Religious, gender-based, socioeconomic, educational, environmental, familial, and personal factors also play critical roles.
- The concept of cultural difference helps us to understand patients from diverse communities, such as the deaf community and the medically underserved.
- In eliciting a patient's interpretation of his or her illness, we need to address the descriptive, conceptual, and personal aspects of these beliefs. Knowledge of these factors is essential for us to understand the effects of serious or chronic illnesses, as well as to promote optimal therapy.
- Many beliefs about illness and therapy are fragmented and contradictory, rather than being tightly integrated into a coherent system. To optimize patient care, we must identify and address the effects of these info-fragments.

PART THREE

CHALLENGES IN THE INTERACTIVE PROCESS

CHAPTER 13

Difficult Patient-Clinician Interactions

Seal up the Mouth of Outrage

Seal up the mouth of outrage for a while
Till we can clear these ambiguities
And know their spring, their head, their true
* descent.*
William Shakespeare, *Romeo and Juliet,* Act V, Scene 3

EXPLORING DIFFICULT INTERVIEWS

In our interactive model of the medical interview, both the interviewer and patient play active roles in generating data that are as accurate and precise as possible. Sometimes interviewing is easy: the patient is alert, helpful, concise, and spontaneous; the problem is relatively straightforward; and there are no awkward topics, such as a sexual problem, or conflicted feelings. On other occasions the interviewer—and usually the patient also—becomes aware that the encounter is going poorly. We label particular patients or situations "difficult" when we make such an assessment—something is wrong; "I feel stuck." The problems might arise from the patient, the clinician, the subject matter, or from extraneous events. We have already discussed (Chapter 1, Interviewing as a Clinical Skill, pages 6–10) how observer bias and instrument precision affect the quality of any medical observation, whether it be a gallium scan, cardiac auscultation, or the clinical history. Any of these observations can be improved, but sometimes it takes particular attention, skill, and ingenuity to do so.

When we sense that "stuck" feeling, it is helpful to think of the interaction as a "sick interview"—one that lends itself to appropriate diagnosis and treatment. Although each type of difficulty calls for particular techniques, some general rules apply:

- First, acknowledge that there is a problem.
- Next, try to understand what the problem is.
- Remain calm.
- Finally, address the problem by applying appropriate techniques.

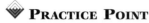 **PRACTICE POINT**

When you feel something is going wrong in the interview, try first to diagnose the problem.

Difficult Patient-Clinician Interactions, below, presents a taxonomy of difficult patient-clinician interactions. Social and cultural issues are covered in our discussions of health beliefs (see Chapter 12), telling bad news (see Chapter 14), complementary and alternative medicine (see Chapter 15), and negotiation (see Chapter 18). In this chapter, we discuss interactive styles, somatization, and the difficult feelings of both patients and clinicians. These categories help us clarify and discuss aspects of the "difficult interview," although we rarely see these problems in pure form and the differential diagnosis of problem interviews is often complex.

DIFFICULT PATIENT-CLINICIAN INTERACTIONS

Process problems

Technical impairments
Organic impairments (delirium or dementia)
Language barrier

Style impairments (see Chapter 3)

Reticence
Rambling
Vagueness

Topical problems (see Chapters 6 and 7)

Sexual functioning
Positive review of systems

Interactive styles

Orderly, controlled
Dramatic
Long-suffering, masochistic
Guarded, paranoid
Superior

Somatization

Difficult feelings

Anxiety
Anger
Depression

Clinician's and patient's feelings about each other

INTERACTIVE STYLES

Occasionally the patient's personality or interactive style interferes with obtaining objective and precise data. Of course, everyone has a personality style, but under stress, such as that which accompanies illness, distinct coping behaviors may become exaggerated or even dysfunctional. Identifying your patient's style gives you important information about how he or she perceives the illness, filters or colors the historic data, and interacts with people in other situations. Kahana and Bibring (1964), in a classic paper, presented observations on personality styles and suggested ways of coping with them during the interview to maximize the clinician's ability to obtain accurate data. These styles are:

- Dependent and demanding
- Orderly and controlled
- Dramatizing or manipulative
- Long-suffering or masochistic
- Guarded or paranoid
- Superior

Although rarely seen in pure form, these styles orient our discussion.

Dependent, Demanding Style

Persons who act dependent and demanding strive to impress the clinician with the urgent quality of their requests. They need special attention, massive reassurance, and constant advice. You may first identify them as optimistic, compliant, and "good" patients, because they often begin by making you feel that you are the only one who has ever cared about them or understood their problems. You soon find, however, that they expect a limitless amount of attention and care. When their need for your constant attention is unmet, they become depressed or withdrawn, or they blame you in a complaining or vengeful way. Trying to fulfill the dependent, demanding patient's every request may drive you to exhaustion.

◈ PRACTICE POINT

Suspect a dependent, demanding style when the patient makes you feel that you are the only clinician who has ever understood him or her.

Dependent tendencies frequently (and temporarily) come to the fore in many acutely ill patients. You should address these needs with respectful, empathic, and generous care directed toward physical and emotional comfort. When this pattern becomes exaggerated or chronic, however, you must set limits. *Setting Limits for Patients with a Dependent, Demanding Style,* below, presents guidelines for resolving some of the difficulties posed by patients with this interactive style.

WHAT TO SAY

Setting Limits for Patients with a Dependent, Demanding Style

- Specify limits of your "contract" with the patient:
    - Provide written instructions. "Let me write down what I expect you to do."
    - Set follow-up appointments. "I want to see you again in 2 weeks."
    - Set limits on phone calls. "I can take your call during my call-in time."
    - Set limits on prescription refills. "The pills should last a month, and I will give you one refill."
- Avoid making promises that you cannot keep, such as solving nursing or insurance problems. "I can't fix the problem with the insurance company, but I can tell you what number to call."
- Emphasize patient responsibility:
    - For understanding the nature and characteristics of health problems: "It's important that you understand this illness."
    - For behavior change and adherence to therapy: "And that you change your eating habits."
    - For fulfilling his or her part of the therapeutic contract: "The pills won't help if you don't take them."
- Remind the patient that available time is limited, despite your interest and concern. Try a statement such as "You certainly have a lot of important

problems, but because our time is so short, I'd like to get back to the reason you came to the office today."

■ Do not take credit for remission in the patient's symptoms, because you will likely be blamed for a relapse. "You got better because of all the hard work you did to follow through on the treatment program."

Orderly and Controlled Style

Some persons cope with their stress by attempting to gain as much knowledge as possible about their situation and to use this knowledge as a way of handling their anxiety. They are punctual for appointments, conscientious in taking medications, and preoccupied with the right and wrong ways of carrying out your instructions. Sickness threatens loss of control for persons who cope in this way. They may present a list of carefully thought-out questions or a precise diary, detailing the frequency and severity of each symptom. They find the scientific approach congenial to their way of thinking and respond well to a professional, systematic sequence of history taking, physical diagnosis, laboratory studies, and therapy. These patients must be permitted to take charge of their own medical care and be given positive feedback about their efforts and abilities.

Because patients with this style are often on the same wavelength as the health care professional, they may not appear to present a difficult situation. But their style suggests that, to minimize anxiety and to optimize health care, you should consider the guidelines presented in *Interviewing the Patient Who Exhibits Rigid, Controlled Behavior,* below. The following transcript is an example of a clinician talking with an orderly, controlled patient:

WHAT TO SAY
Interviewing the Patient Who Exhibits Rigid, Controlled Behavior

■ Take an orderly and systematic approach to your clinical interview, providing frequent "road markers" (indicators of where you are and where you are going).

■ Explain every symptom, disease, laboratory test, or procedure in detail: "These blood tests will check your liver to make sure there are no side effects from the medication."

■ Don't leave any loose ends: "Is there anything else I can explain?"

- Explain the purpose of each maneuver during the physical examination, especially if it appears unusual or prolonged: "I am listening to your heart to make sure there is no murmur."
- Summarize frequently: "Let me make sure I have the story straight."
- Take notes to indicate your interest and thoroughness: "Is it okay if I take notes to make sure I don't forget anything?"
- Avoid mentioning any vague hypotheses, unusual aspects, or jumbled considerations you might have. Keep those to yourself.
- If you don't know, say so, and describe a plan for finding out: "I don't know the answer to that, but here's how we can find out."

Clinician **How have you been?**

Patient   I was trying to remember if I was supposed to call you. I think, I don't remember when I called last and now I couldn't remember if I was supposed to call you again or not.

Well, that's fine. I just was hoping that you hadn't tried and not gotten through or something like that. I understand you got new glasses. Has that helped?

I don't see the slightest difference.

You're not happy because you're having trouble seeing?

I'm not happy because I don't see as well as I would like to see. I can't see numbers well.

Does the eye doctor give you an explanation?

Well, he keeps talking. He talks to me, referring, speaking to me as "your cataract" and I said to him plainly, I said, "You referred to my cataract many times. You have never told me I have a cataract. Do I?" And he said everyone over 30 years old has a cataract. So that's ...

So that's really not an answer. So you don't know whether it's the cataract, whether you have it in both eyes, or whether there's some other problem.

I don't know and I can't get a straight answer.

And later in the interview:

Patient   I wanted to tell you about that and I'm trying to think if there is anything else I should tell you. I don't remember anything. Of course, some of the problems are getting worse but I don't consider that something that wasn't expected. I assume that's what we should expect. Everything else is pretty much under control.

Notice how carefully this patient uses her words. When the clinician says, "You're having trouble seeing?" she corrects this wording with, "I don't see as well as I would like to see." Similarly, she does not say, "There isn't anything else I should tell you"; she says instead, "I don't remember anything" (and this is interesting, because she is elderly and troubled about her recent memory). Notice her concern with doing the right thing, being compliant ("I was trying to remember if I was supposed to call you"). Consider the importance to her of thorough explanation, and how disquieted she is by the ophthalmologist's evasiveness ("I can't get a straight answer"). She accepts the fact that "some of the problems are getting worse," because "I don't consider that something that wasn't expected." Note how the clinician is able to clarify her concerns while avoiding explanations about a problem with which he is unfamiliar (i.e., her eye problem, for which she sees an ophthalmologist).

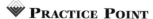 **PRACTICE POINT**

Take an orderly and systematic approach with the controlled patient by explaining what you are doing and not leaving any loose ends.

Dramatic Style

The dramatic style is a pattern of behavior that may charm, fascinate, and frustrate you, and eventually make you angry. The pain is "the worst pain I have ever had ... it's with me all the time, day and night, nothing seems to help ... I haven't been able to sleep in weeks." This person may have a need to be at stage center and may resent your interest in other duties and other patients. Such patients may look upon illness as a drama. At a deeper level, though, the patient may consider sickness a personal defect—a sign of being weak, unattractive, or unsuccessful. Sometimes, particularly when they make us uncomfortable, we describe such patients with judgmental terms, such as histrionic, hysterical, manipulative, or seductive.

Generally, clinicians should allow patients to tell their stories in their own words. We advocate that the interviewer provide direction, but do so without the high-control style that yields inferior data and distant relationships. There are times, however, when the issue of control becomes more central to the interview process, and the dramatic patient's need for control may prevent you from obtaining the information you need. Sometimes the problem permeates the entire history. At other times, it may be limited to a particular facet. For example, a patient who abuses drugs may steer the discussion to a more neutral area every time you approach the question of substance abuse.

At times the patient's dramatic or manipulative style may lead to behavior typically inappropriate to a professional relationship, such as when he or she notices your new watch or hairstyle, compliments you on your good taste in clothing, or asks personal questions about your social relationships or sexual preference. *Interviewing the Patient Who Exhibits Dramatic or Manipulative Behavior,* below, presents some guidelines for deflecting this type of behavior and getting beyond the dramatics into a more effective form of communication.

WHAT TO SAY
Interviewing the Patient Who Exhibits
Dramatic or Manipulative Behavior

- Listen and observe as the patient talks. Ask yourself, "What does the patient gain by this behavior?"
- Remain calm, gentle, and firm. Understand your boundaries.
- Feed back what you hear, using frequent summaries to regain or stay in control.
- Remain descriptive, not judgmental or evaluative; focus on the how, not the why. For example, "I've noticed that when I try to ask you about drug use you tend to change the subject," as opposed to "Why don't you answer my question?"
- If the patient asks you a personal or uncomfortable question, try reflecting back with a statement such as "Well, we're really not here to talk about my opinion. I'm interested in hearing more about you. How did you handle that?"
- Identify the patient's strengths and feed them back, profiling the "healthy person within," as well as the patient who sits in front of you. For example, "I can see that you enjoy being an attractive woman and you enjoy being taken care of by a man. How do you meet those needs in your life?"

◆ **PRACTICE POINT**
Taking a thorough clinical history in a respectful atmosphere while demonstrating that you are in charge is the best way to build a solid relationship and establish an appropriate treatment plan.

Long-suffering, Masochistic Style

Long-suffering, masochistic patients seem to be rejecting help as they present a history of continual suffering from disease, disappointment, and other adversity. They see their lives as never-ending stories of bad luck. Often they disregard their own needs in order to help other people. Despite apparent humility, these patients may tend to be exhibitionistic about their fate. With regard to medical care, they may feel that no treatment will help them; when one symptom or illness disappears, another mysteriously takes its place.

The patient who copes by using a long-suffering style will not "buy" reassurance and optimism. In the interview, you should avoid being overly optimistic or cheerful. You should also steer clear of focusing on the patient's strengths or accomplishments (which might be a good strategy with most other patients) or making insensitive and patronizing remarks like "I'm sure you'll be feeling better in no time." These patients cannot be talked out of the severe nature of their suffering. Although they may not regard talking to a trainee as therapeutic, they may like the idea of being able to help you by permitting you to conduct the medical interview.

 PRACTICE POINT
Accept the patient's pessimism with a descriptive statement such as "It sounds as though you don't think there is much hope of getting better."

Consider the following interchange with an 82-year-old woman who is experiencing failing abilities and is trying to care for her severely demented 89-year-old spouse:

Clinician	**How have things been going for you?**
Patient	Well, not much different. Same as usual. Same problems, same lack of solutions. I'm not saying that anyone would give me a different answer, but I still don't have to like it.
	Yeah, you feel that you've gotten that answer to a lot of problems.
	I feel that I've gotten that answer everywhere. Everything that I have problems with. Everything, that is, except Dr. Jackson, who wants to operate on my throat.
	Which you don't want.
	No. Pretty hopeless, isn't it?

Well, I think you're doing about as well as anyone could do.
Well, I don't know, maybe I am. Again I say it's not good enough, but I don't suppose there's any good enough in a situation like that.
How do you feel about the medication right now? Do you think it's helped your spirits at all?
I like to believe it does. I can't be real sure because I don't know how I'd be feeling without it, but I try to imagine it soothes me some.
Good.
I don't think it's doing me any harm.
Good. What about getting some extra help at home? Have you made any progress with that?
I don't know. The reason I have resisted is because I had a sister-in-law who could not live alone and she had an endless succession of people that I know stole from her and robbed her.
The best thing is to get either someone that you know well or a person who is recommended by someone you trust.
That's true, but I don't think that person exists.
I wish there were something I could do to help.
I don't expect you to have solutions. It's just how things are. Nothing can change.

This kind of interchange is enough to make any clinician feel pretty hopeless as well. Note the patient's repeated return to the theme of no solutions. The most optimistic she gets (and it is not much) is "I like to believe" that the antidepressant she has been taking is helpful, at least "I don't think it's doing me any harm." The interviewer finally gives up making suggestions and begins to share the patient's pessimism: "I wish there were something I could do to help." The patient in turn—paradoxically—offers reassurance ("I don't expect you to have solutions").

Guarded, Paranoid Style

Some patients are inclined to be suspicious of health care professionals and the medical care establishment. They may recite a long list of slights from others and openly point out how the illness was mishandled; or they blame others for the origin of their problem. During stress, the patient may become even more anxious, guarded, suspicious, and quarrelsome. In turn, you may find yourself feeling constantly on guard, as if to avoid being "caught" in a competitive relationship.

Patients with a guarded or paranoid style often express disgust about their previous interactions with health care professionals. They may express that their clinicians not only failed them but also were insensitive and even perhaps in collusion with a system "rotten to the core." You may be presumed guilty by association. The patient may say with great exasperation, "All I want to know is if I've had a heart attack. Why doesn't my doctor tell me yes or no? Why is he keeping it from me?" It is rarely useful to unravel such a question, as you are unlikely to have the needed information, and the patient may think that you are taking sides. A better strategy is to acknowledge and accept the patient's suspicions with a statement such as "It must be terribly frustrating, not knowing." Then proceed with the interview by reminding the patient that although you cannot help with that particular problem, "I am interested in hearing more about the symptoms that brought you here." *Interviewing the Patient Who Appears Guarded*, below, presents some additional points to consider when interviewing the patient who behaves in a guarded or paranoid manner.

WHAT TO SAY
Interviewing the Patient Who Appears Guarded

- Remain friendly and courteous.
- Clearly explain your strategy for diagnosis and treatment: "When we get your test results, we'll know what to do next."
- Identify your role and clarify its limitations: "I am a senior student and I will discuss your symptoms with Dr Smith."
- Openly acknowledge the patient's suspicious attitudes; do not ignore them: "This must be terribly frustrating for you."
- Clarify your understanding of the patient's beliefs, while indicating that you do not necessarily agree with them: "I'm not sure about that, but I would like to hear more about your symptoms."

 PRACTICE POINT

When the patient makes a provocative statement, make sure not to contradict, argue, or try to convince the patient otherwise.

Superior Style

Patients exhibiting a superior style behave self-confidently and may appear smug, vain, or even grandiose. They often come across as persons who feel they are entitled to the best of everything. They may demand

the most senior clinician or the most well-known specialist, and act con-
descending or arrogant toward trainees or younger professionals. They
may attempt to control the clinician—sometimes by making excessive
demands and threatening litigation. Instead of developing faith or trust in
their clinicians, their relationships are characterized by entitlement.
Often, such patients react to situations that occur in the office or hospital
with anger and hostility—anger that can impinge upon you as caregiver.

The superior style may reveal itself for the first time when the patient
experiences unusual stress. Consider this example of a young actor who
had never had difficulty interacting with his clinician until he developed
a "cold or flu or something, which normally I would just wait until it went
away except I'm involved in a show right now." The dialogue continues:

Patient   And it's the leading role in a rather important production and we open
           this Thursday (clears throat) and I went into this cold.
Clinician   You open this coming Thursday?
           And I went into a cold; it feels like it's been in my system for about
           2 weeks, but then on about Thursday it started clearing up. Then
           because of an audition Friday morning I got like 6 hours of sleep. Friday
           I started to feel coldish, Saturday I felt terrible, yesterday I felt terrible,
           so I feel I just need some kind of prescription ... to be able to deal
           with it.

So this patient who would "normally just wait" suddenly feels entitled
to treatment for a problem that is self-limited and that has no definitive
therapy. It is as though the patient is saying, "I know there is no cure for
a cold, but because I'm the lead in an important production you must
make an exception and cure me." This sounds paradoxical and illogical. In
such a situation, the clinician and patient response might be:

**Clinician   There's no cure for the common cold! Actors are no different
           from anyone else!**
Patient   If you won't help me I'll find someone who will.

But the situation will likely go better if you respond:

**Clinician   I can understand your concern, what with this production and
           all. As you know, there's no cure for the common cold. But why
           don't I take a look at you and maybe I can recommend some-
           thing to get the symptoms under control so you'll feel in better
           form.**
Patient   Okay. I sure hope there's something you can do.

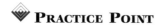 **PRACTICE POINT**

When dealing with entitlement behavior, acknowledge the patient's point of view and avoid the temptation to argue.

SOMATIZATION

The Nature of Somatization

Many patients have symptoms that are difficult to account for on the basis of "organic" disease. Some of these patients have syndromes that resolve over a relatively short period. Others have multiple and recurrent physical symptoms that span many years, many clinicians, and many diagnostic workups; yet the story as a whole never seems to make pathophysiologic sense. Sometimes the patient will tell you that "Doctors have never been able to find anything" or "They said it was all in my head." Others will bring you a series of medical diagnoses and treatments: gallbladder disease, uterine fibroids, osteoarthritis, degenerative disc disease, abdominal adhesions, and hypothyroidism. Although they ascribe their symptoms to these diagnosed disorders, these patients improve only partially and temporarily with appropriate treatment and soon develop new ailments.

Such patients suffer real pain and may develop real disability, even though their problems resist being placed into simple disease categories. Somatization is a process whereby people experience and express emotional discomfort or psychosocial stress in the language of physical symptoms. We consider somatization here for three reasons:

- Patients with functional somatic symptoms are frequently encountered in clinical practice, and they often consume large amounts of clinical time.
- Somatizing patients are often difficult to interview.
- The clinical interview and thorough review of the past medical history are critical to the diagnosis of somatoform disorders.

Differential Diagnosis of Somatization, page 262, presents a differential diagnosis for persistent somatization. In the somatoform disorders (see 3.b in the table), the process of somatization is a primary feature, and specific diagnostic criteria apply. A larger group of patients suffer functional somatic symptoms but do not meet specific criteria of the *Diagnostic and Statistical Manual of Mental Disorders, Text Revision,* Fourth Edition (DSM-TR-IV), for one of these conditions or for any other psychiatric disorder.

Somatizers use more medical services, require more sick leave and disability, and perceive themselves as less healthy than other office patients. Their interpersonal relationships, families, and ways of looking at the world are all affected by unending sickliness. Medical care itself may provide a "positive feedback loop" that validates the patient's sickliness, creates new anxiety ("If no one can find out what it is, it must be something strange and terrible"), and causes additional suffering.

DIFFERENTIAL DIAGNOSIS OF SOMATIZATION

1. Occult physical disease
   a. Syndromes of unknown etiology (e.g., fibromyalgia, chronic fatigue syndrome)
   b. Diseases with subtle, multisystem manifestations (e.g., systemic lupus erythematosus, multiple sclerosis, polymyalgia rheumatica)
2. Secondary somatization
   a. Secondary to known chronic disease
   b. Secondary to other psychiatric disorders
      Adjustment reactions
      Alcohol or other substance abuse
      Panic and other anxiety disorders
3. Primary somatization
   a. Transient functional somatic symptoms
   b. Somatoform disorders
      Hypochondriasis
      Conversion reaction
      Psychogenic pain disorder
      Undifferentiated somatoform disorder
4. Factitious disease (true malingering)

Somatization in the Clinical Interview

Somatization most commonly affects the clinical interview in one or both of two ways:

- **Patients may tend to amplify symptoms** of acute or chronic organic disease, or they may preferentially report physical symptoms of a condition, while deemphasizing emotional or psychosocial symptoms. This may occur in any illness, whether medical or psychiatric. One example of this process is "masked" depression, in which a depressed patient emphasizes such symptoms as fatigue, headache, insomnia, or weight gain while being unaware of, or disinclined to volunteer, depressed mood or hopelessness as symptoms. In such cases, the interview is directed toward identifying suppressed symptoms that complete the diagnostic pattern of depressive disorder, as well as assessing the physical symptoms.

- **Patients may report numerous psychophysiologic disturbances** (e.g., headache, backache, palpitations, breathlessness, or irregular bowel movements) mediated through autonomic or other known pathophysiologic mechanisms. Most people experience these sorts of problems at one time or another in their lives, and when symptoms persist, each can be diagnosed as part of a separate syndrome, such as irritable bowel syndrome, fibromyalgia, "tension" headaches, and premenstrual syndrome. However, if you obtain a history of multiple, recurrent, or disabling syndromes of this type, consider somatization as the likely cause. Don't lose sight of the forest because you are carefully studying every tree.

In clinical practice, you will commonly encounter amplified symptoms and psychophysiologic complaints, either separately or in combination. Virtually any symptom can be a manifestation of somatization; it need not be odd, complex, or inexplicable. When evaluating the role of somatization, focus on the pattern, logic, and context of symptoms, rather than on trying to decide whether one type of symptom (e.g., dizziness) is more likely than another type (e.g., dysuria) to represent somatization. Look for "positive" features in the clinical history suggesting somatization, rather than taking the "negative" approach of ruling out every conceivable physical disease. *Characteristics of Patients and Symptoms Suggestive of Somatization,* below, presents nine such positive characteristics. If two or three of these are present, consider the hypothesis that the patient's symptoms are at least partly attributable to somatization. You can test this hypothesis by directing your interview toward identifying additional features.

CHARACTERISTICS OF PATIENTS AND SYMPTOMS SUGGESTIVE OF SOMATIZATION

1. The symptom's description is vague, inconsistent, or bizarre.
2. The symptoms persist despite apparently adequate medical therapy.
3. The illness begins in the context of a psychologically meaningful setting (e.g., death of relative, conflict with spouse, or job promotion).

4. The patient denies any emotional distress or psychological role of the symptoms.
5. The patient has engaged in poly-doctoring, has had poly-surgery, or both.
6. There is evidence of an associated psychiatric disorder.
7. The patient has features suggesting a hysterical personality style.
8. Discussion reveals that the patient attributes an idiosyncratic meaning to his or her symptoms.
9. The patient has difficulty describing emotions or inner processes in words.

Adapted and abridged from Lipkin M Jr. Psychiatry and medicine. In: Kaplan H, Sadock B (Eds.). *Comprehensive Textbook of Psychiatry*, 5th ed. Baltimore, Williams & Wilkins, 1987.

 PRACTICE POINT

Given a vague symptom that persists despite therapy, explore the symptoms' cognitive or emotional meaning ("What do you think is causing this?") and search for evidence of such psychiatric disorders as major depression or panic disorder.

Interviewing the Somatizing Patient

What can you do in the interview to help the somatizing patient? Consistent application of good listening and responding skills is the basis of any effective encounter, laying the groundwork for effective therapy. Although difficult, it is necessary to build a trusting relationship and validate the patient's suffering. Somatizers often fragment their health care. Careful attention to the past history may require obtaining the names and addresses of numerous clinicians and sending for the patient's records. A patient who doesn't think it is relevant may not volunteer the names of a cardiologist and dermatologist when seeing you for a gastrointestinal complaint. Try to establish goals, indicating that if a syndrome has been present for a long time, a similarly long period of treatment may be required before it improves or resolves. Remember to devote some time, even if only a couple of minutes, to "healthy talk" in each interaction. This will be difficult at first because the patient may find any topic other than his or her symptoms irrelevant and perhaps suspicious. However, genuine empathic concern may break through the "body" barrier and allow the person who somatizes to be more open with you. Finally, schedule regular and frequent follow-up visits so that the patient does not need a new or worsening symptom as a "ticket of admission" to see you again.

Interviewing the Patient Who Somatizes, below, presents a few pointers for use in your encounters with somatizing patients.

WHAT TO SAY
Interviewing the Patient Who Somatizes

- In the initial assessment, obtain a complete patient profile, including functional status, occupational history, and family constellation, even though the patient may want to limit the discussion to symptoms.
- Pay particular attention to the sequence and details of the past medical history. "Tell me what happened first."
- Examine the patient to avoid missing disease and to validate the patient's concerns by showing that you take the symptoms seriously.
- If the patient presents multiple symptoms and concerns, agree on which of them need attention first. "Let's decide which problem to tackle first."
- Sometimes an explicit contract is helpful; you agree to address the patient's concerns systematically, and the patient agrees to accept reassurance if there is no cause for alarm: "I recommend checking out the abdominal pain first. If the tests are normal, can we stop testing?"
- Avoid "vague reference" (see page 173). Although you may not be sure of a symptom's underlying cause, you can still explain its operation and your plan for treatment in physiologic terms, such as "Your intestine feels painful when it is stretched or goes into spasm."
- Speak of the body, not of the mind. It is generally not useful to explain symptoms as originating in the mind because this approach makes the patient feel that the symptom is "all in your head."
- When talking about "stress" or "tension," relate those concepts to physiologic parameters (e.g., the autonomic nervous system), which cause the disagreeable sensation or symptom: "When you get anxious, your heart beats faster."

DIFFICULT FEELINGS IN THE MEDICAL INTERVIEW

The patient's feelings or emotions frequently influence the clinical interview and may interfere with communication. The same is true of the clinician's feelings. Strong emotions may produce behaviors that prevent you from obtaining accurate information, making good clinical judgments, educating patients, and establishing therapeutic relationships.

Experienced clinicians find that empathic responses not only help the patient feel understood, but also facilitate the interview by making it more efficient, accurate, and therapeutic. Other basic strategies to help deal with feelings that threaten to subvert the interview include:

- Elicit the patient's permission, perhaps with a question such as "Is it all right if we go on?" If the answer is yes, show your appreciation. If the answer is no, accept the patient's noncooperation and ask for the reasons in a nonthreatening way, recognizing the patient's right to refuse.
- Indicate your willingness to compromise within limits. For example, you could ask, "Would it help if I came back in an hour? Rescheduled the appointment? Talked louder? Talked slower?"
- Prepare the way for potentially threatening questions. For example, "You have had a lot of back pain, and from what you tell me, it has also made you quite depressed. ... Has it affected your marriage? Your sex life?"
- Try to remain "in sync" with the patient, particularly when you notice that he or she feels upset or misunderstood. For example, "Just now, as you were describing your pain, you got a very worried look on your face. Did I say something that upset you?"
- Remain calm.

◆ PRACTICE POINT
When the patient's or your own feelings get in the way, you need to identify and acknowledge them so that the interview can proceed successfully.

Anxiety

Every illness produces at least some anxiety, if not outright fear, in the patient. Common sources of anxiety are feelings of helplessness, fear of pain and disability, inability to accept warmth or tenderness, fear of expressing anger, and, of course, uncertainty about the future. When people are anxious, they tend to intensify their customary ways of coping with the world. For instance, a compulsive patient may become more particular and a paranoid patient may become more guarded. Signs of anxiety that may appear include facial flushing, sweating, rapid speech or silence, cold hands, fidgeting, or even trembling. The anxious patient may be difficult to interview until the anxiety has been acknowledged and discussed. In *Interviewing the Anxious Patient,* below, we describe a few ways that might help you begin to defuse your patient's anxiety.

WHAT TO SAY
Interviewing the Anxious Patient

- Be unhurried and calm in your manner.
- Sympathize, but remember that too much sympathy may magnify the patient's fears.
- Be specific as to what you expect of the patient—for example, in preparing for a physical examination: "Take off your top, put this gown on, and sit here on the table."
- Be specific about what is normal or not normal and explain your actions: "Now I'm checking the size of your thyroid and it feels normal" or "While you get dressed I'll take a few minutes to review your file."
- Tell the patient that anxiety is normal and appropriate: "Most people feel this way. It is okay to feel scared."

Consider this example. A 57-year-old woman saw her primary care provider for an annual examination. The thought of an examination, even on a day when she had no worrisome symptoms, made her nervous; she was so distraught that her stomach felt queasy, and her red lipstick was coated with antacid as she entered the office. It was clear (in retrospect) that just showing up for the examination was a major effort. Everything, fortunately, was in order. The clinician had only one prescription:

Clinician	**Everything is fine. I have only one recommendation, and that is that I'd like you to get a mammogram.**
Patient	Oh my God! You mean I've got cancer? Not my breast!
	No, no, of course not. No, I recommend a mammogram for all my patients over the age of 50. It's routine.

As though the clinician were not leveling with her, the woman continued:

Patient	I couldn't stand to lose a breast; chemotherapy is awful. I already have thinning hair, you know; chemotherapy makes that worse. No, I won't do that—I can't.

In retrospect, this patient's fragile adaptation to her clinical encounter was shattered by the suggestion of a routine screening test. She evidently thought that the recommendation was targeted, not routine, despite her clinician's protests to the contrary. If we look back at how the clinician introduced the idea, we notice a possible contradiction: "Everything is fine ... get a mammogram." This anxiety-ridden patient thinks, "If 'everything is fine,' why do I need a mammogram?" The clinician might have been able to achieve the aim of getting her to have a mammogram (which, by the way, she never agreed to) by saying:

Clinician **Everything is fine. Your exam is completely normal. Just like you come for a Pap test because you know that's routine in all women, we also routinely recommend a mammogram for all women your age. Have you ever had one done?**

In this instance, the clinician reassures the patient by specifying the nature of "fine" ("Your exam is completely normal"), framing the screening function of the mammogram in a concrete way (comparing it to the Pap test), and anticipating the woman's worry by explaining the reason for the test before she can spin a fantasy of calamity.

Anger

While a patient's anxiety may make us sympathetic, anger is usually more difficult to handle. Patients behave in a hostile manner for many reasons. These reasons often have nothing to do with the clinician personally but rather relate to the patient's own situation, such as inconsiderate care by previous health care professionals, life disappointments, or perceived injustice. What makes one patient depressed may make another patient angry, and the seemingly angry patient may, in fact, be depressed. Review the guidelines in *Interviewing the Angry Patient,* below, for coping with anger in the interview as you consider the following examples.

WHAT TO SAY
Interviewing the Angry Patient

■ Recognize and acknowledge anger with a statement such as "I can see (hear or feel) that you are angry and frustrated," or, because many people do not like to be accused of being angry, "Waiting so long makes most people angry."

- If you are not sure that what you are hearing is anger, ask, "Are you feeling angry?"
- Explore contributing factors and identify any underlying feelings, such as fear, hurt, disappointment, or powerlessness: "If that were me, I think I'd be feeling hurt and powerless. Do you ever feel that way?"
- Accept the patient's reason even if you do not personally agree with it: "I hear what you are saying."
- If the patient's anger is justifiably directed at you, acknowledge your error: "We all make mistakes; and I'd like to learn from this one and correct it."
- If the anger is not directed at you, help the patient recognize ways he or she can deal with the anger-provoking situations.

In the first example, the clinician responds to a patient angered by a thoughtless comment:

Patient   You're just as insensitive as the rest of 'em.

Clinician   I am so sorry. I guess that was a foolish question to ask. Now that I understand you a little better, do you think we could start over?

In another example, a patient was angry after being interviewed in front of a group of students and residents at a psychiatric case conference. She is talking to her clinician following the conference:

Patient   I now know what it's like to be poor. I never would have been at that conference if I had my own private doctor. I know what it's like to be a guinea pig. That doctor asked about my early childhood when what I needed was someone to find out what's been going on over the last 10 years and how tough life has been for me so that he could help me. I thought he would be able to give me something to help my nerves right now, not just talk about my grandmother.

Although this patient reminds us of the patient who asserts entitlement (see pages 259–260), she has good reason for being upset. Talking about what she considered ancient history confused and frustrated her. The conference ended apparently without a definite formulation or plan of action, and although the clinician was actually attempting to remedy the situation by having her present at the conference, the patient may not have known that. An explanation and an acknowledgment of her feelings are in order:

Clinician **It certainly must seem strange to talk about old things when you feel so bad now and want relief. I can understand your frustration. Actually, the reason I wanted to talk with you is to discuss what to do next to get you to feel better. Because Dr. Smith had some good ideas that I think we should try. In fact, he suggested some medication that he thinks will be helpful, and I think so, too.**

The other aspect of her anger was a sense of being on display or of being experimented with (perhaps two sides of the same coin). She may have been surprised by the conference format, requiring her to sit in front of a room full of people she had never met before. Someone should have prepared her for what was to occur; if no one did, the clinician can only apologize by saying:

Clinician **I am so sorry, I guess I didn't really explain very well what was supposed to happen to you. I'm sorry you felt uncomfortable. But I did learn a lot about you that I think will help me to take better care of you.**
Patient   Okay. What I really need is to feel better.

◆ **PRACTICE POINT**
Accept the patient's anger by continuing to listen, while explaining the situation in a neutral fashion, even though a logical explanation will not necessarily change the patient's feelings.

Depression

We use the word *depression* in a number of ways. Depression may be a manifestation of a psychiatric disorder, a response to recent loss (such as death of a spouse), an expression of a pessimistic approach to life, or a transient feeling state. Major depressive disorder may be the underlying problem in a substantial percentage of patients who complain of fatigue, weakness, lack of energy, insomnia, backache, or headache; but depression as a feeling or response to illness is also common. Depressive characteristics include feelings of worthlessness, hopelessness, apathy, and guilt, together with a profoundly empty and lonely feeling. These are manifest in the patient's manner, tone of voice, posture, and speech. The patient may think slowly and talk little, speak softly and have a "flat" affect, look down or away from you, and be tearful.

◆ **PRACTICE POINT**
Make statements such as "You look sad" or "You look as if all this has gotten you down," which give the patient an opportunity to talk about depressed feelings, thereby facilitating other more "medical" aspects of the history.

Some patients have endured such tragic events that you fear being overwhelmed with sorrow. In such instances, it is appropriate to say that you, too, find the situation sad. In this way you demonstrate your sympathy, compassion, or fellow feeling. You are also a professional, however, and your feelings should be used constructively to help the patient. Consider this example: The patient is a 57-year-old woman who had coronary bypass surgery at age 53, followed 2 years later by a modified radical mastectomy for aggressive carcinoma of the breast. She is now suffering from metastatic disease and is about to lose her health insurance coverage because her husband's business is failing and they can no longer afford the premiums.

Clinician	**A lot of bad things have happened to you. You must be a pretty strong person to have endured all this. How have you managed?**
Patient	Well, I have my faith … and my family has been just wonderful to me.

Notice how the interviewer acknowledges the feeling content but, instead of getting deep into the tragedy, allows the patient to express her strength and her coping style. This technique serves the dual purpose of keeping both parties from being overwhelmed.

Often the best follow-up questions are simple statements such as "Tell me more about these feelings" or "Tell me more about it," or the use of simple prompters and facilitators such as "Mm hmm" followed by silence to encourage the patient to speak. This technique may uncover information vital to the diagnostic process:

Clinician	**You look sad. Is it about this chest pain you're having or something else?**
Patient	I guess I am sad. My chest has been hurting all week. Well … see … I don't know if I can say it … I get all choked up … excuse me [trying to hold back tears]. My mother died on Monday. Every time I think about her I get this choked-up feeling in here and it starts to hurt like my angina down into my arm.

In this encounter, the interviewer discovers the crucial connection between an exacerbation of angina and the recent death of the patient's mother.

Depression and Suicide Risk

Although perhaps more appropriate to a consideration of depression as an illness, no discussion of depression is complete without considering how to assess the depth of depression and risk of suicide. Some useful questions include:

- Do you get pretty discouraged or down?
- What do you see for yourself in the future? How do you see the future?

And, if answers to the above questions indicate a risk of suicide, ask:

- Have you ever thought of hurting yourself?
- Have you thought about doing away with yourself? Of ending your life? Of suicide?
- Are you having any thoughts of hurting yourself? Of killing yourself?
- Did you ever think about how you would do it?

The patient may need a few extra seconds (or even longer) to answer these questions. Far from putting the idea of suicide into their heads, most patients experience relief at the opportunity to talk about their feelings of suicide. Here is an example of an assessment of a patient who is seeing an internist for follow-up of abdominal pain and asthma:

Clinician	**Last time I talked to you, you were feeling pretty bad.**
Patient	You know, sometimes I scare myself.
	You mean ... have you ever tried to kill yourself?
	Yeah.
	How did you do it? How did you try?
	Uh, I turned on the gas once.
	What happened?
	Somebody, they smelled the gas.
	When was that?
	That's not the first time I tried to kill myself. One time I climbed up on the bridge.
	Uh hmm. What stopped you?

I don't know.
I'm glad you stopped. How are you feeling right now?

The need to assess suicide risk arises often in the context of routine clinical care. Notice how this clinician does not shy away from asking specific questions about past and current suicide intent. The clinician also reaches out to the patient by sharing genuine happiness ("I'm glad you stopped") that the patient is alive.

Denial

Denial is a common response to illness. It is evident in statements like "This isn't really happening to me," "I can't believe it," and "That wasn't blood I saw in my bowel movement—at least, I don't think it was." In some patients, denial is strong enough to make them ignore or forget symptoms. Alternatively, they may minimize a worrisome symptom and report it as a trivial event: "I had a little pain in my chest, but it only lasted an hour." Only later do you find out that the chest pain was severe and associated with nausea, sweating, and a feeling of impending doom.

Whereas some patients play down symptoms, others deny the emotional impact of a diagnosis or prognosis. At times, it is hard to tell the difference between denial and optimism, such as in the patient with a potentially lethal disease who smiles and says, "I'm a fighter. I know I can beat it." When patients accept bad news (see Chapter 14) with apparent equanimity, it is unclear whether they are realistically handling it well or engaging in denial. Try to assess the patient's understanding of what he or she is feeling. Two useful techniques are:

- Accept denial as the patient's unique and current experience.
- Inform the patient gently and calmly that many people feel differently, including you. For example, you can say, "Most people feel very sad when they hear they have a serious illness," or "I guess I would be worried."

◆ PRACTICE POINT
Denial can lead to serious delays in seeking care, but it may also be a useful mechanism for coping with bad news, so you should handle the patient's denial with circumspection and respect.

Consider this example of a young woman who came for a "checkup." This was her first visit to a new clinician. On palpating the abdomen, the clinician found a large mass, which later proved to be an enormous uterine fibroid. The patient seemed unaware that it was present, even though it was the size of a 5-month pregnancy. When she was told that a hysterectomy might be necessary, she appeared unconcerned. The clinician needed to find out if this 30-year-old childless woman understood and accepted what a hysterectomy would mean to her, or, alternatively, if she had not internalized the implications of surgery:

Clinician	**You don't seem very concerned at the idea of a hysterectomy.**
Patient	Well, if I have to have it, that's it.
	Do you know what a hysterectomy is?
	Well, I guess that's when they take everything out.
	Well, actually, it means the removal of the uterus or womb— that's where this fibroid is. Now the tumor is an overgrowth in the muscle, but even though it's not cancer, it may be impossible to remove without removing the uterus. Now your ovaries, which are the glands next to the uterus that make female hormones like estrogen, you've heard of estrogen? [Patient nods.] Okay, the ovaries would not be removed. [Draws picture.] They would stay, so your hormones would still work right.
	But I still couldn't have babies.
	That's right, you couldn't have babies. What do you think about that?
	I don't know. I guess I never thought much about it, not being married and all, but I guess it hasn't really hit me yet. I'm more worried about the operation itself.

Notice how the interviewer gently probes the patient's knowledge and offers a clear explanation as to what will happen. The patient is not denying the outcome of the surgery but is, perhaps, delaying dealing with it pending resolution of her more immediate fears about the operation itself, and the clinician determines that her approach is a reasonable one.

THE CLINICIAN'S FEELINGS

The clinical encounter may be highly charged with emotion. For you as a clinician, just as for the patient, the interaction may bring out attitudes and behaviors that reflect previous experience and relationships. The sicker the patient, and the more helpless and dependent he or she is, the more likely it is that the patient's attitude toward you will reflect previously learned attitudes, styles, and coping behaviors. Sometimes these attitudes are manifest in ways that may appear totally irrational. For example, a patient who has had an angry, competitive relationship with his father may perceive a male clinician as a powerful authority and may become antagonistic, sarcastic, and competitive, even though the clinician has done nothing that would ordinarily elicit such a response. Similarly, female health care professionals may encounter seemingly irrational responses based on the patient's early experiences with their mothers. Although you may not be able to figure it out at the time, seemingly irrational behavior often has a reason and constitutes important data about your patient.

On the other hand, you also experience feelings about your patients, sometimes extremely strong or negative feelings. You may try to hide these emotions because you think they are inappropriate, or believe they will interfere with your objectivity in caring for the patient. Some patients are extremely likable, others less so, and some are positively unlikable. A few patients will so upset you that their presence on your office schedule threatens to ruin your day. Some will make you angry, and others will make you sad. You will find a few patients so humorous that you wonder whether your response to them is "professional." You may even feel

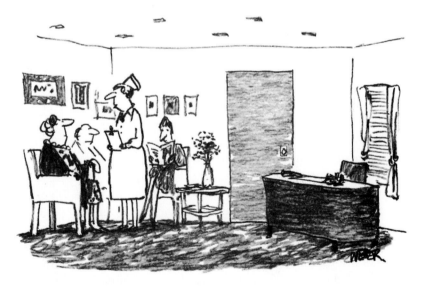

"The doctor will see you now, Mrs. Perkins. Please try not to upset him."

sexually attracted to certain patients and therefore become embarrassed or behave awkwardly.

There are two crucial points to remember about such feelings:

- First, the patient's behavior pattern probably engenders similar feelings in other people. Therefore, your negative response might be useful clinical information, helping to explain some of the patient's difficulties.
- Second, your response, particularly if it is strong or exaggerated, probably also represents an interaction with factors in your own life history and personality—so-called *counter-transference.*

The best approach to such feelings is first to identify and acknowledge them. Ask yourself, "How is this patient making me uncomfortable? And why?" The answers to "how" and "why" questions will allow you to identify behaviors in the patient that help your assessment. For example, do you dread seeing this patient because he or she makes too many demands? If all demanding patients seem to put you on edge, you should be self-reflective enough to understand that fear of being exploited or manipulated is a particular problem for you. You can't change your personality, but you can develop support systems that may help you in coping with demanding patients. Alternatively, perhaps you are uncomfortable with patients who are depressed or dying; you are afraid that there is nothing you can do for them. What can you do for yourself as you struggle with these difficult interactions? Here are a few suggestions:

- Recognize and acknowledge the feelings as *your* personal response to the patient, thereby bringing you into the equation and reminding you that these are *your* problems, not the patient's. You might cope with such patient-engendered emotion in the immediate situation by excusing yourself and stepping out of the room for a few moments to regain your composure (e.g., performing a short breathing exercise or meditation technique).
- Manage patients who tend to cause you emotional roadblocks by planning ahead and organizing physical, temporal, and personal factors in your office to optimize the situation. For example, if you tend to react excessively to a given patient's anger when he has to wait a long time to see you, you can schedule his appointment on a light day, or at the beginning of office hours. If a patient rattles you because she has numerous complaints when you are

concerned about maintaining adequate patient flow, schedule her appointment at the end of the day.

- Share your feelings with a supportive colleague who can help in these situations. Ideally, you should identify at least one colleague with whom you can informally (and mutually) discuss these issues and derive emotional support.
- Formalize this sharing activity by joining or establishing a group of clinicians that meets regularly. You can assist one another in understanding and coping with interactive problems that are encountered in practice.
- As you become comfortable with these feelings, share them with the patient and thus improve his or her self-understanding. The opportunity to create a real connection with your patient can be the basis for a professional intimacy as you learn more about each other over time.

◆ PRACTICE POINT

Health care professionals who get in touch with their feelings and discuss them with colleagues are more likely than others to "survive" difficult interactions.

SUMMARY—Difficult Patient-Clinician Interactions

Although we'd like all interviews with our patients to go well, sometimes our best efforts to apply basic skills go awry. When this happens, our ability to get accurate and precise data, as well as our relationship with the patient, may be impaired. We may ascribe too much importance to one symptom, too little to another, or entirely miss a vital point. In this chapter, we explored common sources of interviewing problems, including interactive styles, somatization, and difficult feelings. Although it is useful from a learning perspective to discuss each as a distinct category, problems rarely occur in pure form, and a number of common approaches are helpful to diagnose and treat the "sick" interview:

- View the problem as one involving the interaction itself rather than only the patient. All patients (and all clinicians) have personality styles and feelings; problems arise when either party exhibits a mismatched or exaggerated response.

- Try to diagnose the problem. (Is this seemingly angry patient really depressed? Are these requests reasonable? If not, why not?)
- Observe the basics of good interviewing technique (open-ended questions, time for the patient to respond, use of summaries and interchangeable responses).
- Accept and respect the patient's feelings and coping style.
- Focus on good interactions, which, repeated over time, lead to productive relationships.
- Establish an appropriate level of control over the relationship, which means setting goals, limits, and guidelines. Remember that the patient also wants to control his or her frightening feelings and will appreciate help in dealing with them.
- Develop strategies to enhance your ability to cope when you feel yourself reacting too emotionally to certain patients or situations. Such strategies will help you maintain your empathic focus on the patient.

CHAPTER 14

Telling Bad News

Something New and Dreadful

There was no deceiving himself: something new and dreadful was happening to him, something of such vast importance that nothing in his life could compare with it.

Leo Tolstoy, *The Death of Ivan Ilych*

RESPECT FOR PATIENTS' AUTONOMY

Telling bad news is among the most difficult interpersonal situations that clinicians encounter, but the idea that one should inform a patient that he or she has a potentially lethal disease is a relatively new one in medicine. As recently as the 1960s, most American physicians routinely misled cancer patients about their diagnosis and, especially, the prognosis of their condition. This paternalistic tradition was based on the belief that knowledge of a fatal illness is generally harmful to patients: they lose hope of being cured, the argument goes, and this causes more suffering and perhaps even shortens their lives because they lose the "will to live." The last 40 years have seen a remarkable reversal of these beliefs. We now know that the large majority of people in our society desire to know their prognosis and that such knowledge is far more helpful than harmful. Of equal importance is the development of greater respect for patient autonomy and self-determination as a fundamental principle of medical ethics. We now have a better appreciation of patients' rights, especially the right to choose (or refuse) treatment. This right demands that patients be given adequate information about their diagnosis and prognosis, as well as the risks and benefits of therapy. Today it is standard practice for patients to be told the "news" of their condition, whether it be good or bad.

During the same period, however, another change has taken place. We have come to neglect many of the more positive features of the traditional approach to caring for dying patients. In the past, when little could be done to change the course of fatal illness, clinicians emphasized care; if they couldn't cure, they could at least remain faithful, available, and supportive to dying patients and their families. Witness the traditional images of nighttime house calls and bedside vigils. Now that medicine has enormous power to intervene, we tend to focus almost exclusively on technical aspects of what we can do for a patient: Can the cancer be cured? Will chemotherapy induce a remission? When the answer to such questions is negative, we often conclude that our role is finished and say, "There is nothing I can do." We feel uncomfortable, so we minimize our interactions with the patient, rather than using the therapeutic power of the clinician-patient relationship to provide physical and emotional support.

BARRIERS TO COMMUNICATING BAD NEWS

Barriers to Telling Bad News, below, summarizes several psychological and professional barriers that clinicians encounter when faced with communicating bad news. These barriers are personal and cultural, and they must be overcome to communicate bad news with clarity and empathy.

BARRIERS TO TELLING BAD NEWS

- **Denying defeat:** There is always a chance.
- **Confusion instead of clarity:** Professional language disguises the truth.
- **Destroying hope:** The patient needs the will to live.
- **Keeping your distance:** Having feelings is unprofessional.
- **Disappearing:** There is nothing I can do.

The Clinician Delays: Denying Defeat

Given the wide array of available diagnostic tests and treatment options, it is natural that clinicians tend to wait until the last possible minute to tell bad news. In a sense, they convince themselves the news is not really that bad, at least as yet. After all, this argument goes, additional tests should be done. Perhaps the cancer has not metastasized; perhaps the heart failure is not as bad as we anticipate. Why discuss the prognosis before the picture is entirely clear? Why create useless anxiety? Alternatively, after unsuccessful cancer surgery a clinician might ask herself, "Why discuss our failure to remove the whole tumor? Let's wait until the patient is stronger and better able to take the news." This approach essentially denies the reality of terminal illness by continually postponing discussion until more information is obtained. This form of denial flounders on the shoals of respect for self-determination and the doctrine of informed consent: a patient cannot make informed choices about his or her care without knowing what the problem is and the risks and benefits of treatment options.

The Clinician Filters the Truth: Confusion Instead of Clarity

When clinicians do give bad news, they often do so obliquely or in a language that the patient doesn't understand, hiding behind "medicalese" rather than addressing the patient's human concerns in simple, clear language. Alternatively, they may use vague language that is literally true ("The tumor isn't responding as well as we would like it to") but does not convey the existential meaning of the situation. The following example of an interaction with the family of a dying patient illustrates this type of miscommunication:

Clinician   **Your mother's condition is deteriorating, and we don't expect her to do too well.**

Patient   [Family] Thank you, doctor; we know you are doing your best.
            Well, so far we've been able to keep her blood pressure up with pressors.
            [Family] That's good, isn't it? At least the blood pressure isn't a problem.
            [Clinician leaves] [Family to each other] Thank goodness, he didn't say she's dying.

The use of complex descriptions about what can be done to disguise honest discussion about what it means is probably the most common form of miscommunication in caring for dying patients. This type of interchange is illustrated in Leo Tolstoy's *The Death of Ivan Ilych* when Ivan Ilych realizes that "something new and dreadful was happening to him, something of such vast importance that nothing in his life could compare with it." His doctor blathers on about technical details, such as a possible "floating kidney." Later, Ivan Ilych goes to another doctor, who tells him that the problem is "a tiny little thing in the caecum," and then proceeds to describe what must be done: "Stimulate the energy of one organ, depress the activity of another." But neither doctor addresses the most important issue: "To Ivan Ilych only one question mattered: was his condition serious or not?"

The Clinician Wills to Live: Not Destroying Hope

In the past, clinicians justified their reluctance to "tell it like it is" with the thought that the truth would harm the patient by destroying hope and causing loss of the will to live. It seemed reasonable then that truthfulness was at odds with the Hippocratic dictum, "Help, or at least do no harm." We now know this belief about not destroying hope to be generally false, yet it is still difficult, when faced with a real patient in a real situation, not to think that perhaps the truth should be watered down or delayed in *this* particular case. There is a sense in which the better the relationship we have with a patient, the more difficult it might be to avoid the loss-of-hope fallacy. If a patient is important to us, it is easy to imagine many ways in which bad news might cause harm. Alternatively, clinicians who see themselves as detached technicians might have an easier time of it—if you can't imagine the patient as a real person with a real story, psychological harm isn't of much concern.

The Clinician Is Detached: Maintaining Distance

Health care professionals may not want to confront their own feelings about dying. They may also be frightened by the patient's, or a family member's, potentially strong emotional response to the news. Clinicians who are extraordinarily skillful at detached, technical aspects of medicine may at the same time be insecure in dealing with sensitive interpersonal relationships. This leads dying patients to feel emotionally abandoned.

The Clinician Vanishes: Disappearing

When patients become terminally ill, their clinicians seem to vanish—no more rounds, no more office visits, no more interaction. There are a number of reasons for this disappearing act. First, if a clinician views office visits in a purely technical light, he or she might feel there is no justification for frequent visits—after all, the patient is no longer on active treatment.

Likewise, the hospital clinician may be overwhelmed with work and feel he or she has no time to spend just "socializing" in a dying patient's room. Second, terminally ill patients usually have difficulty getting around; because house calls are rare nowadays, these patients may find it physically difficult to see their clinicians. Finally, many clinicians find it emotionally difficult to care for dying patients; oriented toward aggressive therapy and attempts to cure, they are extremely uncomfortable with the maxim, "Don't just do something; sit there."

EMPATHY AND INTERACTION IN TELLING BAD NEWS

Setting the Stage

The first step in effectively communicating bad news (see *How to Communicate Bad News*, below) is to prepare yourself for the encounter and to select an appropriate setting. In the hospital, this preparation means choosing a relatively quiet time to sit by the patient's bed, a time when you don't have to jump up and finish rounds or answer pages. Some patients prefer the presence of a spouse or other family members; others prefer to receive the news on their own. The old practice of informing the family first and then deciding whether the patient should be told is disrespectful, paternalistic, and a breach of clinician-patient confidentiality. When a patient is elderly or extremely ill, it often seems natural to speak with a family member first about diagnosis or prognosis. In some cases, this approach may be appropriate if consistent with the patient's known wishes, but you should make it clear that the patient also has a right to know. We make this generalization for American culture, in which self-determination is a paramount moral and legal value. In other cultures, dying persons may expect their families to play a larger (or even exclusive) role in managing their care.

WHAT TO SAY
How to Communicate Bad News

Set the Stage and Be There

- Choose a quiet setting: "Can we meet in the patient lounge area at the end of the hall?"
- Give the news in person, not by phone: "I'd like to meet with you to go over your test results."

■ Allocate adequate time for discussion: "Let's schedule at least 30 minutes, more if we need it."

Tell the News

■ Use simple, clear language: "I'm afraid I have bad news."
■ Avoid minimizing the problem: "We have the results of the biopsy, and I have to tell you that it is cancer."
■ Assess the patient's emotional state: "Do you want to continue now?" "Do you want to talk about your feelings?"
■ Express sorrow for the patient's situation: "I am so sorry to have to tell you this."

Continue the Interview

■ Assess how the patient feels after receiving the news: "What is it like for you after hearing this?"
■ Reassure the patient of your continued availability: "I am going to work with you on a plan to deal with this."
■ Communicate a plan for care if not cure: "I will be there for you."

◆ PRACTICE POINT

Tell the news to the patient first, preferably with one or more family members present, unless the patient indicates in advance that you should discuss diagnosis and prognosis with someone else.

Being There

Giving bad news over the telephone is almost always a bad decision. Consider the following example:

Clinician [By telephone] **The bad news is that you have a brain tumor. The good news is that we think it's a meningioma, which means it'll be easy for us to get to.**

Patient [Long pause.] What, what are you saying? I don't know what you mean.

I mean it's probably a benign tumor on the outside of your brain, so we can remove it by surgery.

Uh, I don't know what to say. ... Can I come in and talk with you about this?

> **Okay, yes, we can do that. Call Judy. Let's make an appointment for next Tuesday.**

This clinician's insensitive "good news/bad news" opening demonstrates insensitivity to the human dimension of his message. He seems to believe that having a meningioma is a wonderful opportunity for the patient and nothing to be upset about. When the patient requests a meeting, this physician blithely suggests a future date and asks the patient herself to set it up ("Call Judy"). He has neither allowed adequate time for discussion of the news today—after all, the patient can't suspend her feelings until next week—nor assessed the patient's emotional state to determine what needs to be done immediately.

How could this situation have been handled better? First, the clinician or his staff could have called to arrange a prompt appointment to discuss the test results. Second, he could have approached the topic in a direct and emotionally appropriate manner without minimizing the issue or hiding behind euphemisms. For example, "I would like to meet with you this afternoon to review your test results. Are you able to do that?"

◈ PRACTICE POINT

Never give bad news by telephone. Be available to the patient immediately, as well as in the future.

Telling the News

The patient will already know by your behaviors (e.g., an intake of breath, an uncharacteristic hesitation) that something is wrong; in fact, your selection of a quiet place or invitation to a family member will broadcast that you are about to say something difficult. It is best to avoid the natural temptation to tiptoe up to the main point by beginning with small talk or side issues. You can better help the patient by spending the entire time explaining the situation, answering the patient's questions, and providing emotional support. There is also a risk that, if you begin slowly, you will end up by minimizing the problem, stopping at half-truths, or leaving important facts unexplained. Here is an example of a clinician beginning to tell bad news in a clear, straightforward way.

Clinician   **Good morning, Mr. Lee. How are you feeling today?**
Patient   Better than I did a week ago.

> **I'm glad of that. We have some very serious matters to discuss regarding your health. Do you feel ready for this discussion?**
> Well, I want to know.
> **It's hard to ever be ready for bad news. This is not easy. I need to let you know that we got the results of your test back. ... As we had feared, the lump is a malignant tumor, cancer.**

In this case the clinician moves almost directly from "We have some very serious matters to discuss" to "It's hard to ever be ready for bad news." Her one intervening question is, "Do you feel ready for this discussion?" An important aspect of this type of encounter is assessing the patient's emotional state both directly by specific questions and indirectly through paralanguage and nonverbal cues (see Chapter 2, Respect, Genuineness, and Empathy). The clinician should acknowledge the difficulty of the situation and adjust the pace and form of the presentation based on an assessment of the patient's emotional needs. It is appropriate to express sorrow for the patient's pain. This may involve not only verbal expressions of concern, but also nonverbal evidence of solidarity, such as maintaining good eye contact, reaching out and touching the patient's hand or sleeve, or even shedding tears.

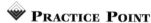 **PRACTICE POINT**
Preface your remarks with a clear statement such as "I'm afraid I have bad news."

Continuing the Discussion

As the discussion progresses, it is important for the clinician to monitor the patient's understanding of the information and his or her emotional response to it. Patients who have just received bad news are unlikely to remember complex information about diagnostic strategies or treatment options; often, however, one or more specific tasks may need to be done quickly, such as further diagnostic studies to delineate the extent of disease, or urgent radiation therapy in the case of threatened spinal cord compression. In such cases, it may be necessary to discuss technical issues during the same conversation in which you reveal the bad news. To help facilitate the patient's retention of information, follow the guidelines suggested in Chapter 18, Education and Negotiation (page 362). Other useful suggestions include:

- If the patient agrees, encourage at least one other family member to participate in the discussion.
- Illustrate your major points with pictures, charts, or drawings.
- At various points during the interview, check back with the patient (and family member, if present) to assess understanding and invite questions.
- Make an audiotape of the discussion for the patient to review at home.
- If available, lend the patient a DVD or videotape that describes the condition and diagnostic and treatment options.
- At the end of the encounter, summarize and recheck the patient's understanding.

◆ PRACTICE POINT

When telling bad news, it is best to stick to the major points, reiterate them, offer to answer questions, and arrange for your continued availability, including a prompt follow-up appointment.

Emotional Responses

Calm and "Coping"

Patients' emotional responses to bad news vary greatly. Some may seem calm and cool, focusing entirely on technical details. This reaction (or lack of reaction) tends to relieve the anxious clinician, who might conclude that his or her patient is coping exceptionally well with the situation. However, extreme calmness or detachment suggests that the patient either hasn't really understood the news, or hasn't emotionally connected with it. It might be useful for the clinician to draw attention to this lack of response: "I notice you are taking this situation very calmly, but in my experience many people react differently."

Angry and Challenging

Other patients display anger and hostility. One of the authors cared for a middle-aged man who had, in a period of weeks, developed facial flushing, shortness of breath when lying down, and other symptoms of superior vena cava syndrome, which resulted from a tumor that compromised venous return to the heart from the upper part of his body. Because it took 2 weeks to accomplish the diagnostic studies and arrange a mediastinoscopy, which ultimately revealed non-Hodgkin's lymphoma, the patient responded to the news with angry accusations about what he perceived to be a delay in diagnosis. Why hadn't we acted more quickly? Why wasn't the hospital more efficient? In such cases it is always best to acknowledge the anger without minimizing it or trying to explain it away—for example, "I know this is devastating news, and I understand why you are upset. But I do want to help."

Some patients will combine anger with denial, aggressively challenging the diagnosis while at the same time demanding a second opinion. Again, the clinician should acknowledge the shocking nature of the news and support the patient or family member in obtaining another opinion (e.g., "I think that's a good idea, do you have someone in mind?") if he or she so desires.

Despondent and Hopeless

The response that clinicians fear most is for the patient to collapse in tears. Consider this interchange with a patient who has just learned he has pancreatic cancer:

Patient   Oh, my God! Oh, my God! [He and his daughter hug. She is sobbing.] Oh God, oh God, oh God, oh God. [Patient also begins to cry.] [After moving a box of tissue to a table beside the patient, the clinician remains quiet for about 60 seconds.]

Clinician **I'm sorry to have had to tell you this ... I know it's devastating news. [Another 15-second pause]**

[Daughter, looking up] What do we do now?

[Patient, with his head down, almost garbled] There's nothing to do, nothing ... nothing.

I can't imagine how terrible and hopeless you must feel, Mr. Brandy. You must be overwhelmed right now ... [He leans forward, reaches out and puts his hand on the patient's forearm.] But I need you to understand this—there is a lot that we can do to relieve your pain, and get you up and around, and get you feeling better. And I'm going to stick with you; we're all going to stick with you.

[Patient] But I'm going to die!

Yes, you will. But you're a long way from dead yet.

This complex interaction illustrates what many would consider a "worst case" scenario. Yet the clinician not only uses his skill to keep the situation afloat, but he is also able to begin the process of palliative care by assuring that he will relieve the patient's symptoms and will not abandon him. First, by remaining silent, he allows the patient and his daughter to express their grief, while communicating his empathic presence (e.g., offering the box of tissues). Second, he avoids false reassurance ("Now, now, this is no time to lose hope") and the tendency to deflect the conversation to safer topics, such as additional tests or treatment options. Instead, the clinician voices his own sadness and provides an empathic (interchangeable) response by correctly labeling the news as "devastating." Likewise, he is honest in admitting that he "can't imagine how ... you must feel."

At the same time, the clinician initiates palliative care by reinforcing the therapeutic bond (e.g., touching his vulnerable patient) and by stating clearly and firmly the two most important messages the patient needs to hear at this point: "I may not be able to cure you, but I can certainly help to relieve your suffering; and no matter what happens, I will not abandon you." This example leads us into a brief consideration of interviewing in palliative care.

 PRACTICE POINT
Acknowledge and accept the patient's emotional response to hearing bad news. Avoid giving false reassurance.

INTERVIEWING IN PALLIATIVE CARE

In many cases, bad news ushers in a period of intensive therapy that leads to remission or cure. In others, disease-altering therapy is either ineffective at the outset, or the disease later recurs following an initially good response. Thereafter, treatment is directed exclusively toward relieving symptoms and improving the patient's quality of life. Quality of life includes physical, emotional, and spiritual dimensions.

 PRACTICE POINT
The relief of suffering is *always* a primary duty for clinicians. In terminal illness the clinician focuses on relieving the patient's suffering directly, even when it is not possible to alter the disease process.

As the role of palliation increases toward the end of life, clinicians encounter the same barriers that made it difficult for them to communicate bad news in the first place. They tend to avoid opportunities for clinician-patient communication and to focus on physical aspects of care (as opposed to emotional, social, or spiritual aspects) more tenaciously than ever. Yet, if anything, the role of the interview in data gathering, trust building, and general patient care becomes even greater during terminal illness. *How to Initiate a Conversation about End-of-Life Care*, below, presents a number of questions that you might use in interviewing palliative care patients in order to learn about (and to indicate your interest in) their existential concerns.

WHAT TO SAY
How to Initiate a Conversation about End-of-Life Care

- "What concerns you most about your illness?"
- "How is treatment going for you (and your family)?"
- "As you think about your illness, what is the best thing that might happen?"
- "What is the worst thing that might happen?"
- "What has been most difficult about this illness for you?"
- "What are your hopes (expectations, fears) for the future?"
- "As you think about the future, what is most important to you?"

Adapted from Lo B, Quill T, Tulsky J, 1999. Discussing palliative care with patients. *Ann Intern Med* 1999; 130:744–749, at 745, with permission.

Understanding the Patient's Goals

It is important to formulate and communicate a plan for continued care, even when remission or cure is no longer possible. At this point open-ended conversation with the patient (and often the family as well) allows you to ascertain the patient's personal goals, as well as his or her medical needs. In end-of-life situations these goals may evolve over days or weeks and may include statements such as:

- "I hope that I'll be able to see my grandson's third birthday."
- "If only Joyce and her mother would learn to get along better."
- "I'd like to get out and visit the lake again."
- "When the kids come, I want to be awake enough to enjoy it."

In terminally ill patients such goals provide an ongoing stimulus for hope. By working toward their fulfillment, the clinician can nourish her patient's realistic hope, even when there is no chance of cure or life extension. However, to do so you must encourage patient trust and self-disclosure.

◈ Practice Point

Patients continue to find meaning in their lives by setting goals for themselves and hoping to achieve them, even though no life-extending treatment is possible.

Alleviation of Pain and Other Symptoms

Patient report is the "gold standard" for assessing the severity of pain and other symptoms commonly experienced by palliative care patients. Accurate assessment of physical (e.g., pain, nausea, fatigue, breathlessness), cognitive, (e.g., irritability, poor concentration) and emotional (e.g. anxiety, depressed mood) symptoms depends on open communication between clinician and patient, rather than results of laboratory tests or imaging studies. Consider the following case of a 47-year-old woman with end-stage ovarian cancer. The patient is in a home hospice program, and her clinician is making a house call.

Clinician	**How are you feeling today?**
Patient	I'm okay. I've been staying out of bed in the morning. I go downstairs when Joyce comes; she helps me. And I've been trying to eat.
	How about in the afternoon?
	Well, I usually go up to bed. I can watch my programs in bed. And sometimes one of the ladies from church comes over. We have this group; we're working on a quilt.
	How about your pain?
	It's better. I'd say it's okay. I don't take the extra pain pills.
	You mean, you don't need the breakthrough morphine because you're satisfied with the pain relief you're getting from the MS Contin?
	Yea, I don't like to take extra pills, they make me groggy.
	Okay, but I want to hear about how much pain you're having. Tell me, why do you go up to bed?
	I guess it's my side. It gets so uncomfortable late in the morning. It … it just feels better if I prop myself up in bed.
	So the pain in your side increases enough to make you want to stay in bed?
	I guess you could call it pain; you know, that deep gnawing feeling I get. Not the sharp pain.

But you don't take the breakthrough morphine pills?
Like I say, I'm afraid they would make me sleep all afternoon.
On a scale of 10, like we usually do, where would you put this deep gnawing feeling?
Oh … oh, I'd say 8.

In this example the patient initially reports that she is doing "okay." However, the clinician notes that her formerly active and independent patient is spending her afternoons in bed. Moreover, when asked specifically about pain, the patient's response is vague, except to say that she doesn't like to—and evidently doesn't—take the morphine tablets that she is supposed to use as needed for breakthrough pain. Why not? Because she is not having pain? Because she tried them and found they made her groggy? Or for some other reason? The clinician proceeds to assess the pain, which the patient admits is severe enough to send her to bed, although it is a "deep gnawing feeling" rather than, strictly speaking, pain. In fact, the "deep gnawing feeling" is moderately severe (8 out of 10).

There is a lot of work yet to be done here. The clinician must attempt to identify more specifically the barrier preventing her patient from taking the morphine tablets. It may be fear of addiction, or a belief that suffering serves as restitution for her sins, or a genuine concern that additional morphine would sedate her too much. In each case there may be an appropriate intervention by the clinician or another team member (e.g., chaplain) to resolve the barrier.

◈ PRACTICE POINT
Assessing a symptom through patient report is the gold standard. However, patient report includes not only statements about character and severity, but also how the symptom affects the patient's functional status and plans.

Existential or Spiritual Suffering

During the last phase of illness, even clinicians who appropriately increase their sensitivity to, and expert treatment of, the patient's physical and emotional problems, sometimes fail to take the next step and address the patient's existential or spiritual suffering. *How to Explore Spiritual Issues in End-of-Life Care,* page 293, suggests some further questions that help explore the more specifically spiritual concerns of the dying patient.

WHAT TO SAY

How to Explore Spiritual Issues in End-of-Life Care

To Open the Topic

■ "Is faith or spirituality important to you during this illness?"

■ "Has faith (spirituality, religion) been important to you at other times during your life?"

■ "Do you have someone to talk to about religious (spiritual) matters?"

■ "Would you like to explore religious matters with someone?"

To Initiate Further Discussion

■ "What do you still want to accomplish during your life?"

■ "What might be left undone if you were to die today?"

■ "What is your understanding about what happens after you die?"

■ "Given that your time is limited, what legacy do you want to leave your family?"

■ "What do you want your children and grandchildren to remember about you?"

Adapted from Lo B, Quill T, Tulsky J, 1999. Discussing palliative care with patients. *Ann Intern Med* 1999; 130:744–749, at p. 746, with permission.

Non-abandonment

Probably the worst news that a patient can experience is for his clinician to say, "There is nothing more I can do," or, alternatively, for the clinician simply to withdraw and disappear. The patient with progressive life-threatening illness needs to hear (and hear often) that his clinicians remain concerned about his welfare and will not abandon him, with such statements as:

- "No matter what happens, I'll do my best to see this through with you.... I won't abandon you."
- "I want you to know I'll continue to be available. You can always call me if you have questions or problems ... I'll get back to you."
- "My goal is for you to be as comfortable and functional as possible. We have good medications to help us do that. You and I will work on this together."

Because dying patients tend to have diverse and often pressing needs, ideally they should be cared for by a multidisciplinary team of clinicians who meet regularly to coordinate patient care. In this way, each individual clinician can commit to addressing specific needs related to his or her expertise, while at the same time reinforcing the efforts of other team members in other areas.

INTERVIEWING AND ADVANCE DIRECTIVES

An advance directive is a written statement ("living will") or an explicit arrangement with another person (health care proxy or durable power of attorney) that permits a patient's wishes regarding treatment to be honored, if and when the patient loses health care decision-making capacity. The Patient Self-Determination Act is a federal law requiring that hospitals and certain other health care facilities inform patients about advance directives. The goal of this law is to give patients the opportunity to formulate their own treatment goals and to express them, or to appoint a surrogate decision maker prior to the eventuality of their losing decision-making capacity. However, a seriously ill patient just admitted to the hospital is generally not physically or psychologically prepared for a thorough discussion about health care choices near the end of life. Likewise, clinicians treating critically ill patients are not likely to set a high priority on explaining advance directives and their meaning.

◆ PRACTICE POINT
The best time to interview patients regarding advance directives is during their ongoing outpatient care, particularly in the primary care setting.

How can you put the concept of an advance directive into action? First, you should ideally inquire about whether a patient has a living will or has designated a health care proxy in your initial medical interview of every adult patient. If you use a structured questionnaire to obtain preliminary data, such a question may be included on the questionnaire. When you ask about the patient's health beliefs and values as part of the patient profile, you may also include a query about the existence and character of an advance directive.

Advance directives should be explored further in the ambulatory setting with patients who suffer from serious chronic or progressive illnesses. Such patients should receive information about written advance directives and health care proxies, keyed to the appropriate legal requirements in your state.

◈ **PRACTICE POINT**
You should inquire about an advance directive as part of the base-line assessment of every new adult patient.

Discussing Advance Directives

When initiating a discussion of advance directives, set the stage by clearly stating the issue, rather than making assumptions about the patient's prior knowledge or asking pointed questions about potential treatment choices. Let's examine three examples of clinicians asking patients about end-of-life decisions:

- "Now we need to talk about living wills. You ought to consider signing a living will, because, if you become incompetent later in this illness, we need to know what you would want us to do if, let's say, we had to put you on a breathing machine."
- "As I said, there is nothing more we can do to stop the disease from progressing, so we are going to be faced with some tough questions sooner or later. For example, if your heart stops, would you like us to do what we can to try to start it up again?"
- "Now we need to talk about what kinds of treatment decisions you would like somebody to make for you if you lose your ability to make your own decisions. What I'm thinking about is something we call a living will or a health care proxy. You've probably heard about living wills. They are written statements that tell us what you would like us to do or not to do if, let's say, your illness reaches the point where we have to put you on a breathing machine and there is no hope that you will recover. A health care proxy is just a person you choose to speak for you and to make all your medical decisions for you if you become so ill you can't make your own choices. Lots of people have both living wills and health care proxies. Would you like to discuss more about this now?"

In the first case, the clinician assumed that the patient would know what "a living will" and "incompetent" mean, and thus failed to explain the terms or put them in perspective. The second clinician jumped immediately to a specific question about cardiopulmonary resuscitation, after beginning on a negative note: "there is nothing more we can do." The third clinician, however, was careful not only to set the stage for discussing the issue, but also to allow the patient to decide whether the discussion should continue at that point. She was explicit about the meaning of living wills and health care proxies and indicated they were not incompatible. Also, she did not frame her reference to "breathing machine" as a leading question. The exchange might continue in this way:

Patient   I don't know, doctor, I've heard about living wills, but I'm not sure I know enough about them.

Clinician   **Well, I can give you a brochure that I think will answer a lot of your questions about living wills, and also it tells how to designate someone you trust to make decisions for you. I can also give you the form for designating a proxy, so you can see what it looks like.**

OK, but … I don't know, talking about this makes me feel like it's all over, you know, like there's no hope.

I can understand why you would feel that, but it really means nothing of the sort. There's a lot we can do for you and a lot you can do for yourself. And you and I will work together on this. I'll respect your decisions every step of the way. That's really why I bring the issue up now–to make sure that we can continue respecting your choices and values if something happens and you can't tell us at the time. I guess you could call it a type of preventive medicine.

A major point in this dialogue is the clinician's attempt to defuse the patient's understandable anxiety when confronted with the issue of advance directives. In this case, she makes sure that the patient understands that he is not "signing over" his participation in decision making, but is rather extending his participation beyond the point it would normally end. Unlike the clinician in the second example, she is also alleviating the patient's feeling that "living will equals nothing-more-we-can-do."

◆ **PRACTICE POINT**
When discussing advance directives with patients, approach the topic as a normal part of patient care and clearly explain the concept in laypersons' terms.

CULTURAL CONSIDERATIONS

In Chapter 12 we explored cultural competence in the patient interview. In this section we consider cultural differences in the way people handle (or hear) bad news about their own health or the health of loved ones. Each patient is a unique person with his or her own history and life trajectory. Never assume that a Hispanic patient will behave according to some generalized Hispanic pattern, an African-American patient will approach life-threatening news in a traditional African-American manner, or a middle-class white person will behave in a "typical" fashion. The key is to develop awareness of your patient's unique life narrative in the context of their cultural heritage.

◆ PRACTICE POINT
Avoid cultural stereotypes when telling bad news and providing end-of-life care.

Cultural competence will assist you by helping you to recognize your own cultural blind spot. Remember that most of what we have said thus far about talking with the dying patient is, in fact, heavily grounded in the cultural values of self-determination, independence, and privacy. When we employ such practices as truthfulness, informed consent, and confidentiality, we demonstrate respect by acknowledging the patient's autonomy. In other cultures, autonomy may be balanced by or even secondary to more communal values, especially when confronting sensitive situations such as terminal illness. For example, the dying patient's family may be expected to play a prominent decision-making role, and to shoulder major responsibility for providing nurture and hope. Remember, too, that patients will almost always try to handle their serious illnesses in ways that seem best, given their own life narratives. Their approaches or strategies will reflect cultural values *in some way,* although you cannot predict *precisely what values,* or even precisely what culture, without listening carefully to your patient.

Family Decision Makers

One of us was taking care of a 56-year-old Chinese woman with ovarian cancer. A few weeks earlier she had been working at her usual job as a hospital nurse and was feeling perfectly normal. Suddenly, she developed abdominal pain and swelling. After the diagnosis was made, we sat down to tell her the bad news, only to discover that the patient, who had appeared to be completely acculturated after living and working in the United States for many years, expressed discomfort with talking about personal medical matters. She avoided eye contact. She asked no questions. Her only comment was that she continued to believe benign fibroid tumors were responsible for her symptoms. It was evident that our attempting to share the name of her diagnosis—even tentatively—caused extreme anxiety. The conversation went on:

Clinician   **I can see that you don't feel like talking right now. You're tired. I know you had trouble sleeping last night.**

Patient   It's okay, though, doc. I think I'll sleep, just as long as I get that Restoril along with the morphine.

Yea, I'll make sure of that. Uh, is there anyone else I should talk to?

[Pause] Ling. You should talk to Ling first—I think she's coming in later after work. She'll know what to do.

Well, I could have them page me. Uh, shall I try to come here and talk with her in your room?

No, it's okay. I'm tired.

This patient was a medically sophisticated nurse. Notice that she uses the correct names of her medications. Notice also that she is no shrinking violet. She specifies exactly what she wants—for Ling to handle the medical information: "She'll know what to do." In fact, Ling was an older sibling who was far less educated and more traditional than the patient was. Ling had emigrated from China with their mother only 2 or 3 years earlier. During subsequent care, Ling assumed a maternal role, arranging for our patient's medical care and handling her affairs. She indicated that her sister should not be told the prognosis because she would lose hope and "dwell on negative things."

◆ PRACTICE POINT

While respecting and supporting the patient's autonomy, it is also important to appreciate the role of family decision makers.

Cultural Circumlocutions

In some traditional Native American communities, such as the Navajo, people believe that any conversation dealing explicitly with death or dying may expose them to grave harm. They believe that such behavior might hasten death, possibly by attracting malevolent spirits or by increasing the person's vulnerability to spirits already causing the illness. Either way, their belief is that saying the words will make it so. Navajos also avoid talking about the dead or visiting places where someone has recently died. In some Mediterranean cultures, individuals may have similar concerns regarding the Evil Eye. For example, if you speak about death and dying, the words may attract the Evil Eye, which could then lead to disaster. In these communities the question is not so much "To whom do you reveal the bad news?" but "In what ways might you speak about end-of-life issues at all?" This cultural feature is particularly difficult when it comes to the question of withholding or withdrawing life-sustaining therapy. To provide culturally appropriate care, some clinicians have found it effective to initiate discussion about end-of-life decisions by couching the whole scenario as a story or a hypothetical event affecting other people.

Clinician **I've heard it said that some people, when it comes to using a machine to breathe for them–this is if they ever get so sick that they can't breathe on their own–what I've heard is that these people don't like to be hooked up to the breathing machine. What do you think about that?**

To many Americans this type of statement sounds like beating around the bush. However, to some Native American families it might serve as a point of entry into a complex discussion, much of which the clinician would consider tangential if she understood the language. In such communities, however, both group consensus and avoidance of direct speech about death constitute important values.

SUMMARY – Telling Bad News

We began this chapter by exploring several barriers to communicating bad news to patients. In summary:

- Clinicians tend to deny to themselves that the situation is as bad as it is and, therefore, delay telling the news.
- They often use vague or complicated language.
- They may believe that patients will lose hope once they know their prognosis.
- Clinicians may also become emotionally distant and disappear.

To provide good care for terminally ill patients, these barriers must be overcome. When telling bad news, the clinician should:

- Set the stage by providing a comfortable environment and allowing sufficient time.
- Begin with a direct statement such as "I'm afraid I have bad news to tell you."

- Provide verbal and nonverbal expressions of sorrow and support.
- As the interview progresses, monitor the patient's emotional response, realizing that it is difficult for persons to take in and process so much significant information at one time.

Good continuing care for the critically ill and dying patient demands that the clinician be both emotionally and physically accessible. At the same time, he or she should recognize that the suffering of dying patients is multidimensional. Appropriate palliative care involves giving patients the opportunity to express and discuss emotional, existential, or spiritual suffering, as well as physical functioning.

Advance directives help ensure that patients' wishes are respected even if they lose decision-making capacity. A question about a living will or health care proxy should be part of every initial medical interview. Advance directives should be explored further with patients who suffer from serious chronic, progressive, or terminal illness. The subject requires a direct and clear explanation, followed by willingness to answer questions and provide emotional support.

Finally, dying and death are sensitive topics. Telling bad news must always be considered from a cultural perspective. Because respect for autonomy is paramount in contemporary Western culture, our default position emphasizes forthrightness and truthfulness. However, you should recognize that in our multicultural society, patients and families bring other values to the table as well, requiring us to individualize our approach. Cultural sensitivity *does not* mean that we should create stereotypes of cultural practices; it *does* mean that we should pay careful attention to the needs and desires of our individual patients.

CHAPTER 15

Talking with Patients about Complementary and Alternative Medicine

A Great Many Remedies

If a great many remedies are suggested for some disease, it means the disease is incurable.
Anton Chekhov, *The Cherry Orchard*

INTEGRATING COMPLEMENTARY AND ALTERNATIVE MEDICINE

Complementary and alternative medicine (CAM) is among the most rapidly expanding areas of clinical practice. A large percentage of your patients will have tried some form of unconventional therapy for their health problems, and many will be using CAM concurrently with the clinical treatment that they obtain from you. Yet these patients are often reluctant to tell you about their experiences with other practitioners. In this chapter we will discuss the context and importance of talking with patients about their use of CAM. Although "CAM" is a convenient acronym, we actually prefer the term *integrative medicine* because it suggests a kind of "big tent" in which patients and practitioners work toward comprehensive care that is integrated into the patients' belief system and also into a broad humanistic perspective on healing.

CONSIDER THE CONTEXT

Many mainstream clinicians are surprised that CAM is so popular. The remarkable scientific and technologic developments of the last century have given medicine the ability to prevent, cure, or ameliorate much human illness. Scientific methodology has permitted us to create high standards of evidence for evaluating treatment effectiveness. In this context, some argue, alternative and traditional therapies don't make the grade. They haven't been shown to be effective, nor do they "fit" the rest of what we know about pathophysiology. Therefore, CAM ought to wither away, rather than becoming a growth industry. Mainstream clinicians also complain that most CAM therapists and modalities are unlicensed and unregulated, so that quality control or evidence-based guidelines are difficult or impossible.

Despite these objections, we live in an era in which a wide diversity of therapies and healing systems are flourishing, and for good reasons. Between 30% and 40% of adults use at least one form of unconventional therapy each year. These therapies are most frequently used for chronic bothersome symptoms and non–life-threatening conditions; but they are also often employed in conjunction with standard medical treatment for serious and progressive diseases such as cancer. Interestingly, over 80% of those who use alternative therapy for a health condition also employ standard medical treatment for the same problem, although about 50% to 75% of these persons do not inform their medical doctor about the unconventional therapy.

DEFINITION AND DESCRIPTION

Table 15–1 presents a helpful taxonomy of integrative or complementary and alternative therapies. It is important to understand that integrative medicine as we use the term ranges widely, from body-based systems of healing such as homeopathy and chiropractic, to spiritual systems

TABLE 15–1

A TAXONONOMY OF TYPES OF COMPLEMENTARY AND ALTERNATIVE MEDICINE	
Varieties of Healing Practices	*Examples*
Professionalized or Distinct Medical Systems	Chiropractic
	Acupuncture
• Organized into medical movements with distinct theories, practices, and institutions	Ayurvedic medicine
	Homeopathy
Religious Healing	Pentecostal churches
• Religious practices that facilitate physical healing	Christian Science
	Catholic charismatic movement

Varieties of Healing Practices	Examples
Natural Health Reform • Alternative dietary and lifestyle practices	Megavitamins Macrobiotics Organic foods Vegan diet Herbal medicine
Ethno-Medicine • Practices rooted in the medical or religious traditions of various cultures.	Puerto Rican spiritualism Haitian vodun Hmong healing practices African-American rootwork Mexican-American *curanderismo*
Mind Cures • Belief that mental forces are the preeminent arbiters of health	Mind-over-matter therapies Mind-body medicine Christian Science
Non-normative Scientific • Mainstream medical techniques used for unapproved purposes or in unapproved ways.	Chelation therapy Hyperbaric oxygen Immune modulation
Folk Healing Practices • Traditional healing practices of a limited and unorganized nature occurring in specific groups or communities.	Copper bracelets for arthritis Chicken soup for common cold "Feed a cold, starve a fever" Red string for a nosebleed
New Age Healing • A connection between the spiritual and physical realms involving esoteric energies	Crystals and magnets Astral energy Reiki, qigong

Adapted from Kaptchuk TJ, Eisenberg DM. Varieties of Healing. 2: A Taxonomy of Unconventional Healing Practices. *Ann Intern Med.* 2001; 135: 196-204.

such as Christian Science; and from ancient cultural traditions such as Ayurvedic medicine to contemporary New Age therapies. Some of these forms of therapy exist as complete explanatory systems of illness and healing; others are fragmentary. Some are amenable to scientific testing; others are not. Some view themselves as synergistic with mainstream medicine; others oppose at least certain aspects of mainstream medicine.

There is no bright dividing line between standard medicine and CAM. Rather, the line tends to be fuzzy and practices may overlap. For example, acupuncture, a technique from traditional Chinese medicine, has entered the mainstream as an important modality for pain control. Likewise, such herbal remedies as St. John's wort and feverfew are now widely recommended by mainstream clinicians. Also, whether vitamin therapy is a form of CAM or standard practice depends largely on who prescribes it and what he or she claims it will accomplish. The same can be said for various nutritional plans, exercise programs, and relaxation techniques.

For our purposes, however, there is no need to give a strict definition of CAM because we are interested simply in the patient's behavior and beliefs regarding therapy, *any therapy,* whether it is considered integrative, complementary, alternative, or mainstream, and how to talk with patients about their concerns and beliefs.

◆ PRACTICE POINT

In the medical interview it is important to learn what types of therapy your patient believes might be of help; what other practitioners he or she has consulted; and what treatment modalities were used.

WHO USES CAM?

Factors Associated with Patient Use of CAM, below, summarizes the characteristics of patients who tend to use CAM and the types of condition for which they use it. As you can see, well-educated people who are motivated to make their own decisions, who express a belief in natural or holistic healing, and who suffer from chronic and recurrent problems are likely to seek additional help from CAM.

FACTORS ASSOCIATED WITH PATIENT USE OF CAM

Characteristics of the Patient

- Higher socioeconomic group
- Desire to avoid toxicity or invasiveness of conventional therapy
- Preference for high personal involvement in decision making
- Dissatisfaction with attitudes and practitioners of conventional medicine
- A particular healing system as a part of a patient's cultural heritage
- Belief in the importance of a holistic health philosophy
- A transformational experience that changes one's view of life and illness

Characteristics of the Condition or Situation

- Failure of conventional therapy
- Failure of diagnosis
- Serious or chronic illness with poor prognosis
- Acute or chronic conditions for which conventional treatment is lacking or ineffective
- Certain specific medical problems: anxiety, back pain, chronic pain, urinary tract problems

Dissatisfaction with conventional medicine is also frequently a factor in patients subsequently choosing CAM. This may be a result of incorrect diagnosis, ineffective conventional treatment, or poor interactive skills on the part of the mainstream practitioner—clinicians who don't take the time to listen, who convey negative attitudes, who don't give understandable explanations, or who simply don't "connect" with the patient. When patients have had these types of experiences with several different clinicians, they may eventually give up on conventional medicine. Among the subgroup of persons who rely primarily on CAM rather than mainstream health care, most express distrust of and serious dissatisfaction with conventional clinicians.

◆ PRACTICE POINT

Patients often seek help from CAM because they value the concepts of balance, wholeness, and harmony in their lives. Other patients choose CAM because of personal or vicarious experience with insensitive mainstream clinicians who fail to listen or to provide coherent explanations.

For the most part, the rising popularity of CAM is not based on deeply held beliefs. On the contrary, today's integrative medicine movement is pragmatic. Although clinicians often find it surprising, patients are usually the best judges of what works for them. People seek out acupuncture, chiropractic, homeopathy, megavitamins, and other therapies simply because they are looking for something that works. A given person might try homeopathy one month and megavitamins the next, even though the conceptual systems underlying these therapies are irreconcilable.

However, some patients do choose treatment based on their deep cultural or religious background. This is often the case, for example, with traditional East Asian or Indian emigrants and Christian Scientists. It is risky, though, to jump to conclusions based on a person's religion or ethnic group. For example, one of us once encouraged an elderly Chinese woman to consider traditional Chinese approaches for treating her depression. Another internist had prescribed Prozac, but she couldn't take it because the drug gave her the "jitters." She also believed that psychiatrists were "for the birds." Several features—her age, her traditional lifestyle (not working outside the home), and her negative attitude toward psychiatry—suggested that traditional Chinese medicine might be just the "right cup of tea" for her. However, she was offended by a referral to a Chinese Holistic Health Center near her home. She proceeded to give a stern lecture about her belief that Western medicine was better. "You can't get rid of me that easy," she said, "I need your help." This response could have been avoided if we had explored her beliefs and expectations regarding her illness before jumping to a plausible, but unwarranted, conclusion.

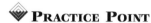 **PRACTICE POINT**

Do not assume that a patient will believe in the efficacy of an alternative healing system just because it is characteristic of the patient's culture or ethnic group. Alternatively, remember that such systems and practices may be important resources to assist you in treating selected patients.

LEARNING ABOUT CAM IN THE CLINICAL INTERVIEW

How do you find out where your patient stands on CAM? *Talking with Patients about CAM,* below, presents some guidelines for inquiring about your patient's use of other forms of health care.

WHAT TO SAY
Talking with Patients about CAM

- Ask as part of your standard medical interview, "What else are you doing to take care of your health?"
- Give permission for patients to raise the topic: "Have you seen anyone else about this problem?"
- Listen for "nondisclosing" clues: "You've read a lot about this; have you seen other types of practitioners?"
- Check with patients regularly regarding their explanatory models: "What do you think is causing this problem?"

- Seek more information from patients and other sources: "Do you have any articles you can share with me so I can learn more about this?"
- Become familiar with local patterns of use.
- Be frank about what you do not know: "I'm not familiar with this form of treatment."

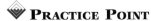

Introduce the Topic

The first step is to introduce the topic of CAM as part of your standard medical interview, either in the context of health maintenance and preventive medicine, or when evaluating a specific problem. After the patient tells you about any medical treatment he or she has had, you might ask, "And what else are you doing to take care of your health?" or "What else have you tried so far?" These are rather nonspecific queries, and patients will often use the opportunity to tell you about dietary or exercise programs. In some cases these programs will be related to alternative therapies; in others, they won't be.

Give Permission to Talk

Your acceptance of these particular "what elses," as indicated by your active listening and facilitative responding, may encourage the patient to tell you more. Useful follow-up questions are "What about other types of practitioners or other types of health care?" or "Have you seen anyone else about this problem?" This approach gives patients permission to talk about their alternative therapies if they wish to do so. In some cases they will not, possibly because they are embarrassed or uncertain about your reaction.

◆ PRACTICE POINT

Patients may believe that mainstream clinicians will disapprove of their use of CAM modalities. To dispel this concern, inquire about the patient's use of CAM modalities in an open and interested way.

Difficult Conditions

Be particularly alert to possible CAM use when patients suffer from chronic symptoms or conditions for which mainstream clinicians often provide unsatisfactory treatment. These conditions include chronic headaches, back and neck pain, fatigue, dizziness, and obesity, among many others. In such cases you might include an inquiry about CAM as part of your routine history.

Nondisclosing Clues

A nondisclosing clue is a verbal or nonverbal indication that the patient has something to say that he or she is *not* telling you. Listen carefully for nondisclosing clues, which may appear in any part of your interview.

Here is an excerpt from an initial encounter between a general internist and a young woman with a 9-month history of fatigue, poor concentration, and repeated respiratory infections. For most of that time, she had been able to maintain her busy schedule as a corporate attorney, but in recent weeks the condition "laid me low" and forced her to severely limit her workload. She has already described the narrative of her illness, including the fact that she has sought help from two doctors: an endocrinologist, who "put me through a lot of blood tests and told me there is nothing wrong," and an urgent care doctor, who "keeps giving me antibiotics."

Clinician	**And what else have you been doing for your health?**
Patient	I can tell you I've read every book I can get my hands on about it.
	You mean about your health problem?
	Yeah, chronic fatigue … or there's other names for it, too. Most of them say it's a problem with the immune system.
	So you've been told that you have chronic fatigue syndrome?
	No, actually, the doctors told me that I was depressed, or one of them did, Dr. X. He tried to give me Prozac, which was ridiculous. Dr. Y at the urgent care, she doesn't say anything, just that I should slow down.
	Gee, not having any answers must drive you up the wall. Feeling so terrible all the time and just not knowing.
	There has to be something. I'm not imagining this.
	And what about other practitioners? I mean, other types of health care?
	Well, I went to this chronic fatigue specialist, I think he started out as a chiropractor and nutritionist, but now he specializes in chronic fatigue. And he put me on this regimen to build up my immune system, you know, vitamins, and some other stuff, herbs, like St. John's wort. It's pretty complicated.
	And how's it going?
	Uh, it's only been a month or so, but I think there's improvement, I mean it's hard to tell.

Note how the patient initially responds by telling the doctor how many books she has read about her condition. No doubt she has also surfed the Internet for additional information. What is her conclusion? "Most of them say it's a problem with the immune system." It seems unlikely that a patient with her education and personality would have been satisfied with two doctors who are neither helping to relieve her symptoms nor providing her with a good explanation of her problem. These features—her job, her personality, and the fact that she has read so much—are *nondisclosing clues* that she might well have sought CAM treatment. The clinician continues with an empathic response tailored to the patient's need to get to the bottom of things, "Gee, not having any answers must drive you up the wall." Perhaps this additive response helps her develop sufficient trust to mention the chronic fatigue specialist that she is currently seeing. The clinician evidently accepts the additional data, although the tone and nonverbal features of his response ("And how's it going?") could make a big difference in how the interview proceeds.

At this point the internist is left with more questions than answers. Why is the patient seeking his help? At first she said her symptoms had worsened in the last month, but now she says, "I think there's improvement" from her new regimen of vitamins and herbs. The internist can pursue one of several paths. He could gently confront his patient with this discrepancy and ask for clarification, "I'm a bit confused here. You said earlier that things are steadily getting worse, but now it sounds as if the vitamins might actually be helping." Another possibility would be to avoid an explicit confrontation, but, after completing the history, go back to the basics of who, what, when, where, and why. "What leads you to come to me now? What would you like me to do for you?"

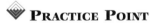 **PRACTICE POINT**
Keep alert for nondisclosing clues that suggest the patient employs CAM modalities.

The Patient's Explanatory Model

Before pursuing the issue either way, it would be useful to learn a bit more about this patient's *explanatory model.* She has already explained that her previous doctor thought she was depressed and that "most of them" (authors of books about chronic fatigue) think it is an immunologic problem. But she has not spelled out her own belief. This may be difficult to pin down for two reasons: she may not yet be willing to trust this new clinician with her private thoughts on the matter, or those thoughts may not be entirely clear or consistent, even to the patient herself.

Let's consider another example. A middle-aged man with hypertension comes to see a new clinician for an initial evaluation and checkup. He explains that in the past he had taken a prescription for his blood pressure, but it had run out and he had not refilled it.

Patient	I don't believe in eating chemicals.
Clinician	**You mean you don't like to take medicines? Not even for your high blood pressure?**
	Well … I used to take a lot of different things, but they never seemed to help. My doctor kept changing them, you know, adding new ones. The pressure never budged, and then I found out it was only high when he checked it, or his girl checked it. So I said, why do I need all this aggravation?
	So you don't take any medications now?
	Naw. No chemicals.
	So not even aspirin or something for headache?
	Naw. I don't get headaches since I started this stuff called feverfew; it's an herb.
	Feverfew? Isn't that …
	It's natural, perfectly organic.
	Do you take any other organic pills or herbs?
	Yea, my wife gets a lot of stuff from the health food store. We go to Vitamin Central.
	Do you know what all of it is?
	Yeah, well, there's vitamin E and zinc and … I'm telling you, doc, the stuff is all natural.

In this case the patient obviously believes that "natural" or "organic" substances are not "chemicals." Chemicals can hurt him, but natural substances such as vitamins and herbs will not hurt him. This belief probably played a role in his decision to discontinue his antihypertensive medication. It may have also been responsible, at least in part, for his dismal medical experience—"a lot of different things" that "never seemed to help." Finally, it highlights the question of why the patient is now seeking a new clinician. Sure enough, the man had selected this particular clinician from a panel of available internists because the insurance company's book indicated that the doctor was board certified in preventive medicine, as well as internal medicine. The patient indicated that to him preventive medicine signified vitamins, herbs, and other forms of "natural" therapy.

What are the clinician's options at this point? Note how he demonstrates basic skills of interviewing by showing respect for the patient's approach, despite his concern about the high blood pressure. It appears that to gain this patient's trust, the clinician must either avoid prescribing medications at all or teach him that in some cases "chemicals" are beneficial. Such teaching will require a better understanding of why he thinks drugs are unnatural and harmful in the first place. Simply telling him the facts (e.g., "herbs contain chemicals, too, you know") is unlikely to help. It will be more useful to explore the basis of his belief (see Chapter 12, Cultural Competence in the Interview) and then to negotiate a mutually acceptable plan (see Chapter 18, Education and Negotiation).

◈ PRACTICE POINT

When noncompliance with mainstream treatments is based on strong beliefs (e.g., the negative effects of chemicals, the importance of balance or "nature," the fear of impurity), simple causal explanations or expressions of anger or disappointment are not likely to change the beliefs and behavior. You need to explore the source of the belief and its centrality to the patient's life.

Seek More Information from Patients and Other Sources

The hypertensive patient we just met takes feverfew for his headaches, along with unspecified doses of vitamin E and zinc. The previous patient with chronic fatigue is on a complex regimen of vitamins and herbs, including St. John's wort. What do you know about these vitamins, minerals, and herbs? What are they supposed to do? What are their potential adverse effects or toxicities? Should you obtain more detail about the specific course of treatment the chiropractor or chronic fatigue specialist has prescribed? Does it include spinal adjustment? Or colonic cleansing? Or mental visualization?

- *Learn from the patient.* Ask for more information from the patient, especially if the CAM modality is ongoing, or if it involves chemicals that may interact with the treatment you prescribe or may have toxicities of their own. The patient may be able to give you a brochure or handout describing the treatment and its rationale. CAM practitioners often provide such materials to their patients (a practice that mainstream practitioners would do well to imitate). Finally, you might write down a few questions for the patient to ask the CAM therapist.

- *Learn from other sources.* Try to find out possible risks and benefits of your patient's CAM therapy by checking journals, books, and Web sites, as well as by asking appropriate CAM practitioners for information.

Find Out about Local Patterns of Use

CAM use by your patients will vary widely depending on the nature of your practice and the characteristics of the community in which you practice—for example, older patients vs. younger patients, inner city vs. suburban, culturally homogeneous vs. culturally diverse, or East Coast vs. West Coast. Good patient care demands that you develop at least a general awareness of other health care resources available in the community, among which are CAM services or practitioners. Thus, if your practice includes a concentration of immigrant Indian families, you should be sensitive to their possible use of Ayurvedic medicine and how it might interact with therapy you prescribe. Similarly, if you serve Hispanic patients in the Southwest, respectful high-quality care demands that you be alert to situations in which they might seek help from a *curandero,* or traditional spiritual healer.

It's Okay to Say You Don't Know

If patients trust you with information about their CAM use, they might ask what you think about it. Do you approve or not? Or they might bring in magazine articles, Internet printouts, or brochures about the "latest fantastic cure for insomnia" or "we guarantee a 20-lb. weight loss in 20 days, or your money back." If your patient has cancer and is considering forgoing indicated primary chemotherapy in favor of macrobiotics, it would be important to reply, "This form of treatment doesn't seem logical or make physiological sense." But often the relative risks and benefits will be less obvious. It is reasonable to tell the patient that you do not know. In this context you should:

- Indicate the rationale for medical treatment.
- Indicate the expected benefits and risks of medical treatment.
- Help the patient to formulate his or her questions about the CAM therapy being considered.
- Encourage the patient to request satisfactory answers to these questions from the CAM practitioner.

- Make it clear that you are willing to continue seeing the patient and discussing the matter.
- Agree to disagree, if necessary, while maintaining respect and open communication.

❖ PRACTICE POINT
When you don't know the answer to a patient's question, it is best to admit that you don't know.

INTEGRATIVE PRACTICE

Once you are aware that your patient is employing CAM, there are important questions to consider:

- Do the CAM therapies interfere with medical care that you believe is appropriate, or do they have toxicities that may harm the patient?
- If not, am I able to work within the patient's belief system to provide high-quality integrative medical care?

Consider the following example. At a subsequent visit to your office, the patient with chronic fatigue brings copies of laboratory work performed by her holistic practitioner. She shows you the results of a hair analysis in which the magnesium content is low and a positive blood test for reactivity to *Candida* (a type of yeast commonly found in the environment). She goes on:

Patient   He said that the magnesium was because of my diet and he recommended some changes there, but he wanted you to prescribe an antibiotic for the *Candida* allergy. He said the first thing to do is to clear it up, and it might take a long time. Sometimes people have to take antibiotics for months.

Clinician   But you don't actually have an infection.
He said there's no obvious infection, yes, but I'm extra-sensitive to it ... like I react to the spores in the air, which activates my immune system all the time.

The CAM practitioner has given this patient an explanation of what she needs—but, unfortunately, from you. The chronic fatigue specialist says he is treating her "holistically" for an overactive immune system and you have to do your part by prescribing an antibiotic to suppress the offending agent. The problem, however, is that there is no scientific basis—no studies, no evidence, no rationale—for the concept of Candida allergy as a cause of chronic fatigue, and you wish to avoid using an expensive and potentially harmful antifungal agent. Although you also want to avoid criticizing the other practitioner, the chronic fatigue specialist has put you on the spot by using a medical test inappropriately and suggesting a course of mainstream medical treatment. How can you decline while remaining empathic and respectful of the patient? Our clinician might respond:

Clinician **I think I understand what your chronic fatigue doctor explained to you, and I know it sounds reasonable. But the thing is, I don't think you actually have a yeast infection. Infection means that the germs get into your tissues and your body tries to fight them off. You see, these yeasts are everywhere, on the skin and so forth, and everybody has a certain amount of sensitivity to them. So lots of people have positive tests whether or not they have chronic fatigue. But that's not what's causing your illness. And, unfortunately, the antibiotics for *Candida* have a lot more side effects than the antibiotics we use every day for sinus infections or strep throats.**

He might go on to explain the adverse effects and other risks of antifungal agents. There are two crucial factors in this interchange. The first is the clinician's tone and manner—his nonverbal and paralanguage communication, as well as the actual words. He wants to maintain trust and support the patient, while at the same time explaining why he disagrees. Unfortunately, he has no "magic bullet" alternative to prescribe, so it is especially important that he convey his ongoing concern for her. Second, he must give her the opportunity to ask questions and to discuss the point until she understands his explanation.

◆ **PRACTICE POINT**

Patients often use CAM therapies for symptoms and conditions for which mainstream medicine offers limited benefit. If the patient believes CAM is helpful, it is inappropriate to dismiss or denigrate it. However, if you believe the CAM practice is risky, or if it interferes with treatment that you prescribe, then carefully explain the situation, while affirming your support and the patient's right to choose.

Unlike the previous case, you will usually not be asked to participate in your patient's CAM therapy. Instead, you will have to judge whether the CAM therapy is consistent with the treatment you propose, and if not, what you should do about it. Here is an example of an elderly woman, blind from glaucoma, who was undergoing chelation therapy, as well as standard medical treatment, for cerebrovascular and heart disease. Chelation involves IV administration of ethylenediaminetetraacetic acid (EDTA), an agent that binds calcium or other cations in the blood, thus removing them from the body when EDTA is excreted in the urine. Chelation is effective in treating lead poisoning, for example, by removing excess lead from storage in the body, but there is no credible evidence that chelation removes calcium from arterial plaques. Moreover, it requires repeated IV treatments that may be dangerous and are definitely expensive. Chelation for atherosclerosis is considered unacceptable by mainstream clinicians. In this example, the patient has already explained to her new clinician that she has been suffering for several months from "creeping numbness" in her legs. Her previous clinician conveyed the impression that this symptom was not serious. The new clinician has helped the patient become comfortable enough to explain her interpretation of the problem and what should be done about it.

Clinician	**You had this creeping numbness, and they didn't seem to know what to do about it?**
Patient	Well, no, and then after the stroke, my back actually … I told you about what the doctor said. He said it wasn't important, that it had already happened.
	That your back had already collapsed?
	Well, I didn't understand, I thought that it meant my backbones would fall down. I was talking to Dr. Smith about it, but he wouldn't do a thing. I mean, it didn't seem to bother him at all. And then my bitter fear for my legs. Then, it actually came to the point where my legs were just like a couple of logs. I would try to sleep at night and turn over and I would drag my legs.
	Is that what made you afraid?
	I was afraid. Well, I explained to Dr. Smith, "Look, Dr. Smith, there are people that lose the use of their legs and they go and use a wheelchair, but you got to have eyes to guide the wheelchair and I don't have that, so what am I going to do?" But it was like talking to the wall. Once he got very angry. "Do you think that if there would be something that would help you, I wouldn't do it for you?" Well, as if it was a sin for me

to be concerned about myself. So anyway, well, the situation was really awful, I was really fretting my mind all the time. I just lost the use of my eyes, next I lost the use of my legs, then what to do?

The patient had osteoporosis and vertebral compression fractures. Evidently she had tried first to attribute her leg numbness to the "collapsed" back, but her clinician vetoed that explanation and never provided an alternative. Moreover, he seemed to ignore both her symptom and her growing anxiety.

Clinician	**So what did you think, though? I mean, where did the numbness come from?**
Patient	Well, then I decided to go to Dr. Brown and he said "I'll chelate you and you'll have no more strokes." So that's when I made up my mind to go to the chelation and I did, and it's better.
	Do you mean Dr. Brown said the numbness was related to the stroke?
	Well, that's the only thing that made sense. Blockage of the arteries. That's what I thought. So chelation must help.
	You were afraid to tell me about this, too, weren't you?
	Well, you should have seen Dr. Smith. He got mad. I felt so sick that time, he got so mad … actually I don't know what was the matter with him. Like he was ready to get a nervous breakdown or something. [Long pause] The thing is, it's so cruel. It's so cruel. Maybe the chelation does do some good, and if it does then why deprive a patient, just because of politics, that's not right. You come to Dr. Brown's office and it's always filled with chelating people, you know. So, once I heard this woman telling, not to me, to others, about a friend she knew. How his legs were so bad they turned black and his doctor advised him to have them amputated. Well, that's a horrible prospect! But somebody told him about chelation, so he went and did it, and slowly the color came back in his legs. He started to be okay and he went back to work. This is hard to believe. And when he went to his doctor to show him, the doctor's response was, "If it was up to me I would still amputate." It's hard to believe such extreme cruelty.
	And your legs are better now?
	Yes, well, the numbness is still there, I can notice it, but it's not as bad, really, and I'm not afraid of it.

Notice in this scenario that the patient assumes that her numbness is due to "blockages" and infers that chelation will help. Her experience at

Dr. Brown's chelation center is quite positive; unlike Dr. Smith, Dr. Brown seems to know what he is doing. Moreover, she heard a miraculous testimonial about chelation's effectiveness. Had the new clinician not made her comfortable and shown interest in her beliefs, he would not have learned that she attributes her symptom to calcium deposits ("Where did the numbness come from?") and had sought out chelation. Nor would she be able to discuss her fears ("You were afraid to tell me about this, too, weren't you?").

The clinician is faced with a patient who has spent much time and money on a form of treatment that mainstream clinicians consider worthless. Earlier clinicians had let her down, both by saying there was nothing to be done despite her "bitter fear for my legs" and by becoming angry when she raised the issue of CAM. The main point from this clinician's perspective is that she feels better, her symptoms are largely resolved, and no academic discussion of quackery will alter that fact.

What does a respectful, empathic clinician do next? Consider the questions posed at the beginning of this section.

- Do the CAM therapies interfere with medical care that you believe is appropriate, or do they have toxicities that may harm the patient? In this case the answer is "yes." Chelation is expensive and potentially toxic (risks), but it provides the patient with no benefit. In fact, the patient's numbness is likely neurological, rather than vascular, in origin.
- Am I able to work within the patient's belief system to provide high-quality integrative medical care? The patient seems willing to accept standard medical treatment, provided the clinician pays attention to her symptoms. Or, perhaps more importantly, pays attention to her. She may well be amenable to decreasing or discontinuing her reliance on CAM if she becomes aware of a desirable alternative. The next step would be to arrive at a mutually acceptable course of action through the process of negotiation, which we discuss in Chapter 18, Education and Negotiation.

SUMMARY — Talking with Patients about Complementary and Alternative Medicine

CAM is a rapidly growing component of the health care system. In primary care practice, it is likely that nearly half of your patients have used or are using CAM, although most of them will not initially tell you about it. Highly educated, self-directed persons who are concerned about the invasiveness and toxicity of conventional medicine are likely to seek out CAM, as will those who are dissatisfied with conventional practitioners, particularly if they have chronic, ill-defined, or poorly treatable conditions. A common theme in these patients' stories is that allopathic clinicians simply don't take the time to listen to them.

You should introduce a discussion of CAM by including relevant questions in your standard interview, as well as by giving the patient permission to broach the topic, listening carefully for nondisclosing clues. To enlarge and clarify the discussion, ask about the patient's explanatory model and request specific information about the type of CAM therapy used. Differentiate clearly between what you know and what you do not know about a given therapy and support the patient in efforts to obtain answers to important questions about benefit and risk. Also ask yourself:

- Is the alternative therapy really dangerous?
- Does it prohibit necessary medical care?
- Can you work within the patient's belief system to provide good care?

If the answer to the last question is "yes," the next steps include negotiation and education.

CHAPTER 16

Ethics and the Law

Respecting Patient Rights

The patient has a right to considerate and respect-ful care ... to obtain relevant, current and under-standable information ... to every consideration of privacy.
American Hospital Association Patient Bill of Rights

UNDERSTANDING AUTONOMY AND BENEFICENCE

We live in a pluralistic society in which persons of many communities with different ethical perspectives live side by side. Despite this diversity, there is surprisingly wide agreement about principles of health care ethics, especially the importance of *caring* (beneficence), which serves as the moral basis for health care professions, and *respect for self-determination* (autonomy), which serves as a fundamental moral standard of our society. The claim that individuals have rights with regard to health care (e.g., the right to privacy, the right to refuse treatment, the right to die) is ground-ed in respect for autonomy. Alternatively, the claim that the state or soci-ety should provide benefits to us (e.g., the right to health care) is based on the principle of beneficence.

When applied to clinical situations, **autonomy** and **beneficence** often conflict. Clinicians frequently encounter situations in which respecting the patient's autonomous decision appears to work against the patient's best interests. Patients sometimes choose courses of action that are clearly detriments, at least from the clinician's perspective. In general, both ethics and the law place greater weight on adults' autonomous choices about health care than on clinicians' moral commitment to help

319

patients who seem to be making bad choices. The latter practice is called **paternalism** (i.e., acting as if the clinician were a parent who does what he or she thinks is best for the child, no matter what the child wants).

PATIENT RIGHTS

Professionalism in health care begins with respecting patient rights. This respect involves a relationship characterized by truthful disclosure, informed consent, and confidentiality, as well as a commitment to doing your best to help your patient. The commitment to beneficence entails a number of additional ethical rules—for example, patient advocacy and avoidance of conflicts of interest. Although these are fundamentally ethical and professional considerations, the importance of health care in our society is such that the states and the federal government have developed a body of law to ensure patient rights while also promoting public welfare. This chapter explores these concepts in the context of good clinician-patient communication.

INFORMED CONSENT

When patients cooperate with you during the interview, physical examination, or routine testing, their behavior implies consent. Throughout this text we develop the concept of **transparency** with reference to the process of the patient-clinician encounter. In essence, the clinician should provide sufficient information to make the meaning of the process, diagnosis, or procedure *transparent* to the patient. This process includes allowing the patient to ask as many questions as needed and answering them to the patient's satisfaction. Transparency also applies to the more formal process of **informed consent.**

When clinical procedures and treatments are invasive or risky, ethics and the law set a higher standard of responsibility in disclosing information about risks, benefits, and alternatives, as well as in ensuring that the patient actually has the capacity to make health care decisions. This process is codified in the legal doctrine of informed consent. Clinical students often perform procedures for which patients must provide informed consent, including documentation by signing a consent form. How do you go about obtaining informed consent? How do you know the patient has the mental and emotional capacity to provide consent? How much information do you need to provide? The following section suggests answers to these questions.

INFORMED CONSENT REQUIRES CONVERSATION

Your clinic or hospital has consent forms with standardized language that meets legal requirements. Although consent forms may serve as an outline to guide discussion, remember that the patient's act of signing this form does not in itself constitute informed consent. Although it does serve as prima facie evidence of consent, the signed form may be challenged in court if there is opposing evidence that the patient was poorly informed, incompetent, or coerced.

To fulfill legal requirements for informed consent, four conditions must be met:

- The patient must demonstrate health care decision-making capacity (see page 324).
- The consent must be voluntary (i.e., no evidence of coercion or undue influence).
- The patient must receive adequate information about the nature of the procedure, its benefits and risks, and alternative courses of action.
- The patient must demonstrate that he or she understands this information.

◆ PRACTICE POINT
Informed consent is a process involving conversation and understanding; it is not just a piece of paper.

HOW MUCH INFORMATION IS ENOUGH?

Informed consent requires skillful clinician-patient interaction. The goal of the disclosure part of the interaction is to provide all the information that a "reasonable person" would want to know about a procedure or treatment before deciding whether to accept or reject it. The courts in many states have set the "reasonable person" as a standard for disclosure because it focuses on the needs of the patient, rather than simply on the custom or convenience of health professionals. However, what a "reasonable person" would want to know is subject to interpretation and, therefore, somewhat subjective. For example, you might safely conclude that a person would want to know about the common complications of a procedure and about serious complications that are less common or even rare. But how rare is rare? One in 10,000 cases? One in a million? An advantage of the transparency model is that, once given basic information about rationale and outcome, the patient is encouraged to ask questions, thus indicating his or her personal threshold for the disclosure required to make the decision.

◆ PRACTICE POINT

You have sufficiently informed a patient about a treatment or procedure when you have disclosed the information about rationale, benefits, risks, and alternatives that a reasonable person would want to know, and when the patient has had the opportunity to have his or her questions answered and demonstrates understanding of the answers.

The therapeutic core qualities of empathy, genuineness, and respect (see Chapter 2) build trust and facilitate the consent process. Clinical students should pay particular attention to the need for genuineness. Perhaps you are about to perform your first lumbar puncture or your second paracentesis (the first was unsuccessful). Should you reveal your inexperience? What do you say when the patient asks what percentage of your previous patients developed post–lumbar puncture headaches? You should not evade these questions, give misleading information, or pretend to be experienced. This is an awkward and sensitive situation, but it must be dealt with head-on. Here is an example:

Clinician   **I am a medical student. I've seen this procedure done several times, and I've been taught how to do it, but this will be my first attempt to perform it on my own. But you should understand that the resident physician, Dr. X, will be there beside me, directing me in every step.**

Your resident or preceptor should reassure the patient and explain his or her role, including readiness to step in if it becomes necessary. The patient, of course, has the right to refuse to let you do the procedure and to request someone more experienced.

◆ PRACTICE POINT

A reasonable person would want to know the skill level and experience of the clinician performing a procedure. Hence, informed consent requires that you disclose the fact that you are a learner under supervision.

BARRIERS TO INFORMED CONSENT

You should be aware of real, and sometimes insurmountable, barriers to informed consent (see *Barriers to Informed Consent,* below). Two of these are especially relevant to clinical trainees. First, some patients believe that decision making ought to be in the hands of clinicians, and they therefore opt out of the decision-making process and defer to others' judgments. In these cases clinicians should understand that taking responsibility for a decision is a completely separate issue from desiring information. Such patients may want to be thoroughly informed about what is going on. You should not confuse ready acceptance of a procedure with lack of interest in its rationale or outcome. Students may contribute a great deal in these situations because they can spend time listening to their patients' concerns and answering their questions.

BARRIERS TO INFORMED CONSENT

Patient Characteristics

- Patient does not "hear" the disclosure because of denial, conflict, or ambivalence.
- Patient does not understand the lines of authority and which clinician is responsible.
- Patient desires information but believes that the actual decision should be made by the clinician.

Clinician Characteristics

- Clinician does not understand the rationale or requirements for patient involvement in decision making.
- Clinician does not communicate well.
- Clinician does not allot adequate time to disclose information thoroughly and answer questions.

Nature of Clinical Decisions

- Treatment decisions evolve over time, rather than being quick and clear.
- Numerous decisions must often be made.
- Decision-making process often involves input from a number of different people.

Second, the health care environment often confuses patients because there is so much new information and so many decisions to be made; the decisions occur at different times, and frequently a variety of people are responsible. Thus, it may be difficult for a patient to generate the attention and focus needed to make a particular decision on a given occasion. Again, the student can play an important role by taking the time to explain these features and answer questions.

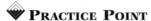 **PRACTICE POINT**

Even if a patient says, "I'll do whatever you think is best," you should continue to inform him or her about what is going on and why.

DECISION-MAKING CAPACITY

In health care we assume that an adult person has the capacity to make his or her own decisions unless we have evidence to the contrary. In other words, our default position is that adult patients can (and should) make decisions for themselves, even when they are sick or elderly. Clinicians sometimes use the terms *competence* and *decision-making capacity* interchangeably. This is inaccurate and confusing, because the terms refer to two very different concepts that only partially overlap:

- *Competence and incompetence are legal terms.* Only a court can determine incompetence. A judge may ascertain that a patient is either globally incompetent or incompetent in a specific arena, such as managing finances. If a person is incompetent, the court appoints a guardian to serve as his or her decision maker. Thus, when you take care of a legally incompetent patient, you conduct the informed consent process with the patient's legal guardian.
- In the clinical context, *decision-making capacity is a more limited concept that refers to a person's ability at a given time to make decisions about his or her health care.* In many cases decision-making capacity waxes and wanes over the course of a serious illness, or even over the course of a single day (e.g., some patients, referred to as "sundowners," are clear-minded in the daytime but become delirious at night). Normally, the treating clinicians determine whether a patient lacks decision-making capacity; if so, they turn to that patient's health care proxy (see Chapter 14, Telling Bad News, page 294) or to another surrogate, such as a family member, to engage in decision-making.

STANDARDS FOR JUDGING CAPACITY

Sometimes it is obvious that a sick person lacks capacity. Examples include patients who are:

- Comatose or semicomatose
- Delirious or confused due to acute illness
- Severely demented
- Severely developmentally delayed
- Actively psychotic, with delusions, hallucinations, and disorganized thinking
- Infants and young children

Remember, however, that dementia, psychosis, and developmental disorders vary widely in severity; a given patient may be affected sufficiently mildly that the condition does *not* interfere with his or her decision-making capacity.

As noted, our default position is to assume that the patient has capacity, unless there is convincing evidence to the contrary. Some clinicians think that a patient's refusal of medically indicated care in itself constitutes such evidence. In other words, if a patient's decision is the "right" one from our point of view, we presume rationality; if the decision is "wrong," we suspect impaired reasoning. For example, an elderly man with diabetes makes all of his own decisions in the hospital until he decides to forgo surgery for his gangrenous foot, at which point the clinicians decide that he lacks capacity because "he doesn't know what's good for him." By this standard, every person who chooses to refuse aggressive treatment might have his or her wishes overruled by well-meaning but paternalistic clinicians.

◆ PRACTICE POINT

A patient's refusal of the medically recommended treatment option is not in itself evidence that the patient lacks capacity; alternatively, the patient's willing acceptance of a recommended option does not necessarily mean that the patient has capacity.

Clinical assessment of capacity should be focused on *process* (how the patient arrives at a decision) rather than on *outcome* (whether clinicians think it is the "right" decision). This standard demands that we look at the decision-making process as it relates to the issue at hand, rather than making judgments based on other data about the patient, such as her his-

tory of forgetfulness, or the fact that he is sometimes incontinent or confused. Authorities suggest four criteria for assessing capacity. The patient
must be able to:

- Communicate a choice
- Understand information about a treatment decision
- Appreciate the medical situation and its consequences
- Use logical processes to evaluate information and compare options

Assessing Patient Decision-Making Capacity in the Interview, below, presents a series of questions that will help you to convert these general considerations into data that are useful in determining capacity. We want, in

---

WHAT TO SAY
Assessing Patient Decision-Making Capacity in the Interview

Component of Health Care Decision-Making Capacity	Example Questions to Evaluate Patient's Capacity
Awareness of Illness and Ability to Describe	Can you tell me why you are in the hospital? Do you know the name of your illness? Tell me what happened to you.
Comprehension of Treatment and Benefits	What will happen to you if you don't get treated? Do you understand what treatment is recommended? What does that involve? What will it do for you? Are there any other treatment options? Which treatment do you prefer? Tell me how the treatment you prefer is better than the others for you.
Comprehension of Risks	What are the possible harmful or unpleasant effects of the recommended treatment? What are the possible harmful effects of the treatment you prefer?
Decision-Making Process	What concerns or worries do you have about the treatment? Do the benefits of the treatment you prefer outweigh your reservations? Why? Tell me more about that.

(continued on following page)

Component of Health Care Decision-Making Capacity	Example Questions to Evaluate Patient's Capacity
Personal Belief System (Especially if Patient Refuses Treatment That Is Likely to Be Highly Beneficial from a Medical Perspective)	If you do not receive this treatment, there is a very good chance that you will die soon, or become permanently disabled. Do you believe that? How does this enter into your decision? How would you explain your decision to a close friend or family member? Are you a religious (or spiritual) person? If so, how do you understand your decision in relation to your religious faith (or spirituality)?

Adapted in part from Searight HR. Assessing patient competence for medical decision making. *American Family Physician* 1992;45: 751–759 (Table 2).

particular, to emphasize two features of this process. First, it is important that the patient demonstrate adequate understanding of the risks and alternatives, as well as the benefits of the proposed treatment. For example, the clinician might say, "I just explained the benefits and possible complications of the procedure, but I want to make sure you understand what I said. Could you tell me in your own words?" Second, it is crucial to distinguish between *logical thinking process* and *correct or reasonable conclusion*. A patient's fundamental beliefs or values might be different from yours. Using those beliefs as premises, he or she could logically—and reasonably—reach a conclusion you believe is wrong. For example, Christian Scientists believe that illness is illusory and represents an error in perception that can be corrected by study and prayer. A Christian Scientist might reasonably decline medical treatment because acceptance of treatment implies lack of faith, and lack of faith is spiritually damaging. Clinical expertise extends only to assessing the patient's best interest from a medical perspective; patients have a more global view of their welfare, based on religious, cultural, or other values.

◆ PRACTICE POINT

Decisions about medical care are essentially value decisions, determined by religious, cultural, and personal beliefs, as well as by biomedical factors.

Children and Adolescents

Infants and young children are excluded from making their own decisions. Almost everyone would agree that a 6-year-old child cannot make a voluntary, informed decision about the risks and benefits of surgery, but what about a 13-year-old boy or a 16-year-old girl? Neither one has reached the age of majority, so from a legal perspective they have no right to make their own medical decisions, unless they fall into certain categories recognized by the state. These categories include:

- *Emancipated minor*—a minor who is married, or who has left the family home and independently supports himself or herself
- *Special groups*—minors who seek health care for contraception or sexually transmitted diseases; or who are pregnant and seek treatment related to pregnancy

Morally and legally, we treat adolescents who belong to the first group as if they were adults with decision-making capacity. Those belonging to the second group are entitled to similar autonomy and respect, including confidentiality from their parents, but *only* within the specific range of health services specified by law (i.e., reproductive medicine and sexually transmitted disease). However, children and adolescents should be involved in their own care as much as possible, consistent with their level of maturity. Our default position, especially when treating adolescents, is to demonstrate respect for their autonomy and to make it clear to parents that our interactions with their teenage daughters and sons are, for the most part, confidential (see Chapter 10, Pediatric and Adolescent Interviewing, page 206), although we, of course, encourage teenagers to share the relevant personal information with their parents.

Psychiatric Evaluation of Decision-Making Capacity

When we believe a patient may lack capacity because of a thought disorder or other serious psychiatric problem, it is important to seek expert psychiatric or psychological consultation to assist in the determination. The following are a few guidelines derived from the clinical interview:

- *Extreme ambivalence* may lead a patient to switch his or her decision abruptly several times during a short period. The patient says yes, then no, then yes, then no, perhaps with increasing agitation.

This behavior is a "red flag" indicating that further psychiatric or neurological evaluation is required.

- *Impairments of attention span, judgment, memory, and intelligence* may interfere with the ability to understand information and to appreciate consequences of the medical situation. When these are subtle, or the patient compensates for them by using intact social skills, it may be necessary to obtain more expert evaluation.
- *Presence of psychiatric symptoms* or an identified psychiatric disorder does not in itself mean the patient lacks capacity. In particular, the common syndrome of clinical depression (if not severe) does not necessarily impair decision-making ability for health care.
- *Assessing the capacity to reason logically* is subtle, and some courts have considered logical handling of data to be too strong a criterion to require as evidence of competency. Psychiatric consultation may be helpful in this assessment. In any case, knowledge of the patient's beliefs and value system is required to understand what makes him or her tick.

CONFIDENTIALITY

Confidentiality is an ancient concept in medicine. The Hippocratic oath states, "What I may see or hear in the course of the treatment or even outside of the treatment in regard to the life of men ... I will keep to myself holding such things shameful to be spoken about." Twenty-five hundred years later, the American Medical Association (AMA) expresses a similar duty in its Principles of Medical Ethics: "A physician shall ... safeguard patient confidences within the constraints of the law." Confidentiality is also an important duty for all other health professions, as expressed in their traditions and ethical codes. Confidentiality honors both the principle of autonomy (i.e., respect for privacy) and the principle of beneficence (i.e., leads to better outcomes in terms of trust, openness of communication, and willingness to seek help).

Legal Limits and Exceptions to Confidentiality

However, confidentiality is a limited or qualified duty, rather than an absolute duty. The AMA Principles of Medical Ethics specify confidentiality only "within the constraints of law." For example, unlike attorney-client or confessor-penitent confidences, information revealed by patients to clinicians is not protected from discovery in a court of law. *Exceptions to Clinician-Patient Confidentiality*, below, presents a list of legal exceptions to the rule of confidentiality. Most of these result from legislative action, in the form of statutes, or administrative action, in the form of regulations. In general, the objective is to protect either the patient (e.g., child abuse), other persons (e.g., communicable disease), or both (e.g., gun or knife wounds). Other exceptions to confidentiality are included under the concept of *dangerousness*, which demands that the clinician assess the risk that the patient is likely to harm himself or others, a determination usually based on verbal evidence obtained during a clinical interview (e.g., the patient with a mental disorder who indicates that he intends to kill his girlfriend because she is a CIA agent, or a patient with an uncontrolled seizure disorder requesting clearance for a driver's license).

EXCEPTIONS TO CLINICIAN-PATIENT CONFIDENTIALITY

Required by Statute or Regulation*

- Specified communicable diseases
- Gunshot wounds
- Certain types of knife wounds and burns
- Child abuse or neglect
- Dog bites
- Court subpoenas

Dangerousness: Threats of Harm to Patient or Others

- Threats to harm or kill others
- Suicidality
- Development of health conditions that cause serious risk to others if patient continues to perform a regulated activity (e.g., driving a bus, flying a plane)

Related to Employment, Licensing, Insurance, and Administration

- Requests by third-party payer
- Specific types of health information reported to a clinician employed by company
- Licensing requirements (e.g., drivers, pilots)

*These are examples; specific requirements differ by jurisdiction. Get to know the law in your state.

Ceding the Right of Privacy

A patient, of course, may always cede the right of privacy and permit his or her personal health information to be shared with others. For example, patients may request that their medical records be sent to other clinicians, insurance companies, or governmental agencies for cases such as disability determination. *However, this process may present an ethical problem in situations where patients are likely to allow disclosure of their personal information without knowing that they are doing so.* Nowadays, patients frequently have only limited awareness of the extent to which their information may be shared with third-party insurers, employers, and others. These disclosures may be authorized by patients who have signed standard releases at the beginning of their association with a clinic or an individual encounter.

Moreover, there are many situations in which clinicians have obligations to a third party in addition to the patient (or even instead of the patient). Though the patient may have signed a release form prior to seeing such a clinician, he or she may not be fully aware that this clinical interaction is different from an ordinary one in which confidentiality is expected. Here are two examples:

- Clinicians employed by a company, or under contract with a company, to assess and treat occupational injuries or to determine work fitness.
- Independent medical or psychological examiners paid by government agencies to assess functional status and disability.

In such cases the clinician should begin by clearly stating his or her role, including the fact that the company or agency will receive a full report of the examination.

HIPAA Privacy Regulations

In Chapter 9, Communication in the Office Setting, we discussed how the Health Insurance Portability and Accountability Act (HIPAA) has recently introduced new legal "muscle" to strengthen confidentiality of personal health information. HIPAA privacy regulations protect medical records and other individually identifiable health information, whether on paper, in computers, or communicated orally. *Representative Elements of the HIPAA Privacy Rule,* page 332, presents the major elements of HIPAA as they relate to confidentiality. Note that HIPAA:

- Enables patients to find out how their personal health information may be used by clinicians, including how it may be shared with others, thereby preventing situations arising from conflicts such as those described in the previous section
- Limits release of information to the minimum reasonably needed for the purpose of the disclosure
- Generally gives patients the right to examine and obtain a copy of their own health records and request corrections

REPRESENTATIVE ELEMENTS OF THE HIPAA PRIVACY RULE

Access to Medical Records. Patients have the right to see and obtain copies of their medical records and request corrections if they identify errors.

Confidential Communications. Patients can request that their health care facilities and professionals take reasonable steps to ensure that their communications with the patient are confidential.

Limits on Use of Personal Medical Information. Health professionals have limits on how they may use individually identifiable health information.

Written Privacy Procedures. All covered entities must have written privacy procedures, including who has access to protected information, how it will be used, and when it may be disclosed.

Notice of Privacy Practices. Health care facilities, physicians, and other health professionals must notify patients how they use personal medical information.

Employee Training and Privacy Officer. Covered entities must train their employees in their privacy procedures and must designate an individual to be responsible for ensuring that the procedures are followed.

Prohibition on Marketing. There are limits on the use of patient information for marketing purposes.

Complaints. Patients may file a formal complaint regarding the privacy practices of a health care facility or professional.

Stronger State Laws. The federal privacy standards do not affect any state laws that provide stronger privacy protections. Rather, the federal law sets a national "floor" of privacy standards to protect all Americans.

To accomplish this enhancement of confidentiality (and empowerment), HIPAA creates new duties for health care facilities and professionals, as also indicated in *Representative Elements of the HIPAA Privacy Rule.*

TRUTHFULNESS

In Chapter 9 we discussed truthfulness in ambulatory care situations, especially with reference to disability determination, insurance forms, work excuses, and other third party interactions (see page 190). We also explored the ethical, cultural, and therapeutic dimensions of truthfulness in telling bad news (Chapter 14, page 281). Finally, our consideration of informed consent earlier in this chapter presupposes truthful disclosure about diagnoses and the benefits and burdens of therapy. In this section we highlight several common—but misleading—objections clinicians sometimes raise to telling it like it is.

"We Never Really Know the Truth"

Some clinicians avoid being truthful by claiming that clinicians never really know the whole truth. Medical knowledge, they say, is probabilistic. Judgments based on probability and clinical judgment may be wrong, so why confuse the patient by being too direct and explicit? To respond to this objection, we must distinguish between truthfulness, a moral quality that we should all strive for; and Truth (with an uppercase T), which is indeed frequently unknown. Truthful interactions include admitting one's uncertainty and, in the case of students, explaining one's limited role or responsibility. They also include inviting the patient's questions and answering them in understandable terms. This type of disclosure is required for informed consent.

For example, in the following exchange a young man has been referred to an ophthalmologist because of persistent redness and irritation of both eyes. The clinician ascertains that the patient has iritis, an inflammation of the iris that is often associated with such systemic diseases as Reiter's syndrome, sarcoidosis, and Lyme disease. The clinician has explained the eye problem and its treatment but is concerned that there might be an underlying inflammatory disease.

Clinician	**And here is a prescription for some blood tests, too. Just to make sure everything is all right.**
Patient	Blood tests? I thought you said this was just an eye irritation.
	It is, but these are just tests we routinely do in cases like this.
	But do you think it might be something serious?
	No, but you can never be too careful.

This patient may or may not accept this vague reassurance emotionally, but he certainly has not had his questions answered in a truthful way. The ophthalmologist literally does not know the truth about whether there is a systemic problem, and he wants to avoid frightening the patient. He may also dread the number of questions he might have to answer if he were more forthright with this well-educated young man. The clinician's attitude can be summed up as "get the tests now and we'll talk later."

Here is how the clinician might present the same information in a more truthful manner:

Clinician **And here is a prescription for some blood tests, too. Based on what you've said and my examination, I think your iritis is a simple inflammation of your eyes and nothing else. But sometimes iritis can be the first sign of more generalized illness, especially some types of arthritis or infection. So it is best to do these blood tests to make sure there isn't anything additional we have to treat you for.**

Patient   That sounds scary. Could this be serious?

I have no reason to think it is. Most cases of iritis are localized conditions that get better quickly with the drops. And remember I asked you all those questions about fatigue and joint pains and muscle pains? It sounds like you're in good shape. But there is always a chance we could pick up an early sign if by any chance you were going to develop one of those other conditions. So I think it's a good idea to get the blood tests.

In this case the clinician is being truthful, while at the same time acknowledging his uncertainty. He stresses the high probability that no systemic problem will be found (true) but also acknowledges the low, but real, probability he might be wrong. The patient may or may not be satisfied at this point. He may ask for more information about the possible systemic diseases, or press the clinician for more specific probability estimates. The clinician should answer these to the best of his ability.

 PRACTICE POINT
A clinician's willingness to explain the situation in a clear, straightforward way usually enhances the patient's trust in the clinician and tends to defuse anxiety.

"Don't Tell Me; I Don't Want to Know."

Some clinicians generalize from the fact that sick persons often use denial as a defense mechanism to claim that patients in general do not want to know the truth. This is simply not the case. Studies have repeatedly shown that most people want to know the truth about what is happening to them. Even though patients often defer to their clinicians in making decisions ("I'll do whatever you think best, doc"), this does not mean they want to be ignorant of the facts. Surveys also show that patients value being informed about their condition more highly than they value making their own decisions about treatment.

◆ PRACTICE POINT
Patients who show little interest in actively participating in health care decisions may still want to be thoroughly informed about their condition.

Occasionally patients tell their clinician, "If it's cancer, I don't want to know. Don't tell me." Such statements signal a need for the clinician to listen attentively and explore the issues with the patient by asking:

- Do you really mean you do not want to learn about your problem?
- Do you think that understanding your situation would allow you to live more fully and help you cope with whatever happens?

In a small percentage of cases, denial (and perhaps magical thinking) is so strong that the patient decides to waive his or her right to know. Other patients may waive their right to know because of cultural barriers. In all such cases, someone must be identified to represent the patient, and that person must be fully informed. As part of the waiver process, you and your patient should ascertain just who the surrogate will be.

"Laypeople Just Can't Understand."

Clinicians sometimes claim that patients cannot understand medical facts. Medicine is so complex that laypeople have no way of knowing all the subtleties involved in a complicated case. Even if this were true, it is irrelevant. The patient needs to know what a reasonable person would want to know about the condition, not what a trained scientist would want to know. Explaining medical facts is an important clinical skill.

◆ PRACTICE POINT
If you cannot explain a process to a patient in accessible language, you probably do not thoroughly understand what you are talking about.

"He Is Too Fragile to Bear the Truth."

Some clinicians claim that the truth will cause harm. This notion exemplifies the paternalistic attitude that clinicians know what is best for their patients and ought to pursue it independent of their patients' wishes. Even if accurate information were sometimes harmful, respect for autonomy would usually tip the balance in favor of truthfulness. However, knowing the truth is rarely damaging; rather, it generally has a positive effect on patients.

This generalization has an exception known as *therapeutic privilege* (i.e., treatment may be undertaken without adequately informing the patient). For example, severely disturbed patients may respond to bad news with decompensation of their psychiatric condition. In such cases, a clinician might contemplate waiving the truth on the basis of predictable harm. However, these situations require careful consideration and usually psychiatric evaluation. The mere fact that a patient is chronically anxious, or has hysterical outbursts, or is clinically depressed does not limit his or her right to know the truth. The clinician should be particularly cautious of accepting family judgments: "Don't tell Aunt Clara. She won't be able to handle it. She's likely to go off the deep end." Such statements should serve as "red flags" that sensitive inquiry is necessary, but we should not use them as waivers of responsibility to our patients.

SUMMARY—Ethics and the Law

Respect for the principles of autonomy and beneficence is the foundation of ethical clinical practice. We make this respect operational in the medical interview and in our continuing conversations with the patient. Health care law promotes patient autonomy by requiring informed consent and by setting privacy standards, and it promotes the public welfare by setting certain limits on confidentiality. In this chapter we discussed the following:

- Informed consent is a process that is based on respect for patient rights. It requires disclosure of all the information about a procedure or treatment that a reasonable person would want to know before making a decision. Disclosure is embedded in a conversation in which the patient has adequate time and encouragement to have all his or her questions answered.

- Many barriers to informed consent exist, but most of them can be minimized by openness and good communication skills.
- Assessment of decision-making capacity is a key component to carrying out the process of informed consent. Capacity relates to the patient's ability to make judgments about risks, benefits, and consequences of a given intervention at the present time. Lack of capacity for health care decisions does not necessarily imply legal incompetence.
- Confidentiality is an important ethical rule in health care, but it is limited by law in cases where personal health information has important public health implications, or where the information indicates dangerousness. Patients may cede their right to privacy and sometimes do so without being fully aware of what they are doing. HIPAA privacy regulations create a higher standard for confidentiality of health information and new requirements for health care professionals in protecting privacy.
- Truthfulness is a prerequisite for ethical practice in our culture. Although truthfulness may be limited in certain situations, either by patient request or therapeutic privilege, these cases should be uncommon and clearly justified by appropriate criteria.

CHAPTER 17

Malpractice and the Clinical Interview

The Sum of All the General Rage

He piled upon the whale's white hump the sum of all the general rage and hate felt by his whole race from Adam down.

Herman Melville, *Moby Dick*

GOOD COMMUNICATION IS THE BEST DEFENSIVE MEDICINE

A decade or two ago, the issue of malpractice prevention would not have been addressed in a textbook on clinical interviewing skills. Clinicians then thought (as many still do) that there are only two ways of trying to avoid negligence suits. The first, of course, is minimizing clinical mistakes, although we all know that a lawsuit may follow an adverse outcome even if no mistakes are made. The second approach is practicing "defensive medicine"—that is, making some of your medical decisions on the basis of perceived liability risk rather than on the basis of good clinical judgment. Usually this approach involves excessive diagnostic testing. For example, an emergency medicine physician might routinely order computed tomography (CT) scans on patients with head injuries, even if the clinical circumstances do not warrant the scan. Similarly, an internist or neurologist might order a magnetic resonance imaging (MRI) scan on all patients with headache, knowing, of course, that very few such scans are clinically indicated.

Studies of malpractice claims, however, have repeatedly demonstrated two remarkable findings:

- **Defensive medicine *does not* prevent malpractice suits.** If a patient has a bad medical outcome, the fact that the clinician ordered inappropriate tests does not reduce the risk of a lawsuit. The best policy, in fact, is to follow clinical guidelines—what is known as the standard of care.

- **Good clinician communication *does* prevent malpractice suits.** A patient who feels that the clinician listens to and understands him or her is not likely to sue that person, even if a bad outcome occurs.

In other words, good communication is the *real* defensive medicine. Because this finding is so consistent across studies and striking, malpractice insurance carriers now sponsor seminars on communication skills. Clinicians who complete these seminars often receive discounts on their malpractice insurance premiums (a sure sign that this training works). An empathic, compassionate approach with good interactive technique leads to better diagnosis and therapy and also enhances patient satisfaction. Satisfied patients generally do not sue.

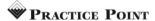 **Practice Point**

If an adverse outcome occurs, the strongest predictor of a malpractice action is a preexisting poor clinician-patient relationship.

These findings have implications for clinical interviewing. In this chapter we focus on specific aspects of the clinician-patient encounter relevant to malpractice prevention: earning trust through the mastery of basic skills, building a negligence-free relationship, transparency, communicating with other members of the health care team, and keeping good records.

EARNING TRUST THROUGH MASTERY OF BASIC SKILLS

Some clinicians, especially older ones, believe that patients do not trust health care professionals the way they used to. These clinicians express nostalgia for a time when patients were silent, faithful, appreciative, undemanding, and trusting. Although such a time probably never existed, it is true that we live in a culture in which people have particularly high expectations of health care and assert themselves when they feel betrayed, injured, or abandoned. Nowadays you have to *earn* a patient's trust and satisfaction. The mantle of professionalism no longer gives you immunity from being questioned, contradicted, or sued.

Let us be clear about the role and meaning of *competence*. Because the health professions are technical fields, there is a widespread belief in our culture that technical competence is what makes a good clinician. But the concept of "technical competence" is usually considered applicable only to skills related to the machines and procedures of advanced technology. The other technical aspects of clinical practice—for example, the clinical skills this book discusses—are either not considered fundamental to good practice or are redefined as nontechnical personal qualities that are nice but not essential. This line of reasoning concludes that "good bedside manner" is desirable but secondary. After all, you often hear people ask, "Would you rather have a pleasant, communicative surgeon, or a competent one?"

When it comes to medical negligence issues, however, technical competencies in *both* spheres—your scope of clinical practice and your interactive skills—are paramount. We assume that you will make every attempt to avoid errors of scientific knowledge and judgment. Our concern here is with the *other* sphere of technical competence.

◆ PRACTICE POINT

The evidence indicates that "interactively competent" clinicians engender trust and satisfaction in their patients, and they experience fewer negligence suits.

In a well-known study that compared primary care physicians who do not get sued to those who do, the investigators found that the two groups demonstrated similar performance in strictly informational aspects of the encounter—that is, asking relevant questions ("What can you tell me about the chest pain?") or providing information ("This medication may make you constipated"). However, the clinicians who had not been sued engaged more often in the behaviors listed in *Interview Behaviors of Clinicians Who Don't Get Sued,* below. Facilitative responses give patients

---

WHAT TO SAY
Interview Behaviors of Clinicians Who Don't Get Sued

- Facilitative responses—paraphrases, mirrors, and statements such as "Tell me more about that"; "Uh huh"; "Anything else?"
- Inquiries about what the patient thinks or understands about the problem: "What do you think is causing this?"

- Interpretive statements: "Let me explain what this means."
- Orienting statements—instructions about the flow of the visit: "First I'll examine you and then we'll discuss the possible causes."
- Orienting statements—transitions: "Now I'd like to find out about how your health has been in the past."
- Humor and laughter: "You are such a good sport. You must be the world's expert on using crutches."

Source: Levinson W, Roter DL, Mullooly JP, Dull VT, Frankel RM. Physician-patient communication. The relationship with malpractice claims among primary care physicians and surgeons. *JAMA* 1997; 277:553–559 at p. 557.

permission to talk and to tell their story in their own way (see page 54). These responses demonstrate that the clinician cares about what the patient has to say and, by implication, cares about the patient. Likewise, inquiries about the patient's beliefs suggest that the clinician is taking the patient-as-person seriously. Orienting statements demonstrate respect and help establish realistic expectations of the visit and, by extension, of the therapeutic enterprise.

For example, here is a segment from the interview of a 70-year-old man who is seeing a new clinician for the first time. Note all the statements that orient the patient to the visit:

Clinician **Okay.... Well, I think I have some idea now of your major concerns. What I'd like to do next is have you step over here [indicates examination table] and I'll take a look at you from head to toe. While we're doing that, you can give me some more details.**

Patient There was something else I wanted to apprise you of ... but I can't think of it.

Not to worry, it may come to you and when I'm done with the exam I'll give you time to collect your thoughts and see if you have any questions. How does that sound?

It sounds good.

[The clinician conducts and finishes the physical examination.] Okay.... That's all we'll do today. Let me step out for a few minutes while you get dressed. That will give me a chance to review the files you brought in. Then I'll come back and we'll make a plan.

In this example, the patient knows what is happening and that he is the clinician's focus even when the clinician leaves the room.

BUILDING BLOCKS OF A NEGLIGENCE-FREE RELATIONSHIP

In a general sense, this whole book is about avoiding malpractice litigation. The interview is a tool for malpractice prevention in at least four ways:

- Trust-building tool: empathy, respect and genuineness bring you closer to the patient.
- Diagnostic tool: the more you listen, the more you learn.
- Relationship-building tool: good conversations make good relationships.
- Therapeutic tool: good clinicians make good healers.

Remember that these functions overlap considerably; for example, it would be difficult, if not impossible, to master the interview as a diagnostic tool or an instrument of healing without first inspiring the patient's trust.

Let us now focus the discussion on additional behaviors that help prevent litigation. *Building a Negligence-Free Encounter,* below, summarizes these negligence-deflecting behaviors, which we will now review in detail.

WHAT TO SAY
Building a Negligence-Free Encounter

- Listen to what the patient says and doesn't say: "You are very quiet. Did something I said upset you?"
- Avoid trivializing or demeaning the patient: **not** "You worry too much."
- Acknowledge the patient's level of concern: "I can see you're very worried about this weakness."
- Strive for transparency in your reasoning and recommendations: "Here's what I'm thinking."
- Be clear about what you know and what you don't know: "What I know is that you are anemic. What I don't know is why."
- Never make promises you can't keep: "I can't promise that you'll get better, but about half the people with this problem do."
- Be available to the patient: "I want you to call me on Friday to tell me how you are doing." OR "My partner is on-call this weekend. I'll tell him what's going on."

Listen to What the Patient Says and Doesn't Say

Consider these comments by dissatisfied patients:

- "My last doctor never listened to me. There wasn't time.... I was always in and out of his office, like an assembly line."
- "The thing about Doctor Jones, he's got his own spiel.... You have to do it his way or else."
- "I just couldn't get a word in edgewise."
- "Doctor Adams just didn't understand me."

These statements share a high level of frustration and in some cases anger. The patients feel that they were not getting their message across; thus, they couldn't "connect" with their clinicians. No wonder they sought new clinicians. If one of them had a bad outcome or missed diagnosis, he or she might believe that Dr. Adams or Dr. Jones was negligent. What behaviors prevent this kind of frustration?

- **Allow enough time.** The first patient experienced a treadmill-like environment. He didn't feel he had time to explain anything, which at first frustrated him and later, perhaps, prevented him from trying to do so. Although the actual time you spend with a patient may be limited, there is no excuse for not listening actively and completely during the time you have. If you do so, the patient is likely to experience the encounter as lasting longer (*perceived time*) and to feel understood.
- **Keep quiet.** In the second and third cases, the clinicians evidently had their own agenda, rather than the patient's agenda, in mind. They may have been friendly or reassuring, but they took over the conversation. Remember to allow patients the time to state *their* concerns, even those concerns that don't surface in the first few seconds of the interview.
- **Keep listening not only to what is said, but also to what isn't said.** When the patient says, "Dr. Adams just didn't understand me," we learn only the outcome, not the specific problem. Dr. Adams may have thought she was doing a good job taking care of the patient's verbal complaints, but the patient didn't feel safe enough to express her real concern. The nonverbal cues, the hand-on-the-doorknob phenomenon, the seeming magnification of mild or simple health problems—all these slipped past Dr. Adams, who was focused solely on addressing the explicit concerns.

Avoid Trivializing or Demeaning: Acknowledge the Patient's Level of Concern

Next, consider these tortured outbursts:

- "Who does he think he is? He just walks in with this high and mighty air about him, like he's God or something. He doesn't even sit down. He just says, 'Well, the good news is your tests are normal. So it's not your heart. It must be in your head.' Like I'm making it all up."
- "So she told me to take Celebrex for 2 more weeks. I've been taking Celebrex a month now and I'm in pain. I can't get out of bed in the morning. And she tells me it can't be that bad, I should have more patience."

The first clinician demeaned the patient's assessment of her illness, turning her into a "psycho" or "crock," because to most people symptoms that are "in your head" are less real than symptoms that are "in your body." The clinician thinks the patient should be happy because she doesn't have cancer or hypothyroidism, but he ignores the fact that she is suffering from symptoms that she doesn't understand.

The second clinician trivialized the patient's experience. The patient has disabling symptoms that the medication does not relieve. After a month there is little reason to believe the same drug will lead to a major improvement. Nonetheless, the clinician says, "It can't be that bad." Of course, it can—it *is* that bad! Why wasn't this clinician listening? Maybe she had a preconceived notion that the patient was dramatizing his symptoms. Maybe she couldn't think of any better treatment. Maybe she was just having a bad day. In any case, she lost her patient's confidence.

◈ PRACTICE POINT
To avoid demeaning or trivializing, address your patient's level of concern with interchangeable, empathic responses.

A patient's concern is real, even if *you* believe it is unwarranted. Moreover, in some cases it will turn out that *you are wrong*—the first patient might have occult cancer, and the second might have an unusual form of arthritis that you failed to diagnose. If so, you might end up with a lawsuit as well as a dissatisfied patient.

Strive for Transparency

By *transparency* we mean that the patient should be able to visualize or understand your reasoning, to see through what you are saying to what you are thinking. Consider this explanation given by a cardiologist:

Clinician   **OK, Mr. Marsden, what we have here is a lesion in the left anterior descending artery, looks like about a 90% occlusion, and then there's a 100% occlusion of the first perforator. We need to send you to the hospital as soon as possible.**

Several behaviors facilitate transparency. First, *don't use jargon.* Clinicians often speak opaquely. Because so much of our time and energy are invested in the culture of medicine, medical terms trip lightly off our lips. Words like "occlusion" seem perfectly clear and natural to us, and certainly more precise than "blockage." We may not take the time and trouble to translate.

Second, *explain how and why you came to the conclusion.* Another aspect of clinical transparency is to explain your conclusions or recommendations. Mr. Marsden's cardiologist couches his explanation in medical jargon—it sounds ominous, but the patient has no way of judging specifically what it means for him. The recommendation is blunt: "You need to go to the hospital as soon as possible." Why? What's the danger if I don't go? How long will I be there? Are there any alternatives? The clinician needs to explain more and in a way that Mr. Marsden understands. We will discuss this question of transparency in more detail, but remember that we should always be eliciting informed consent when we expect patients to follow our instructions.

Finally, remember that conversations with patients are always, in a sense, cross-cultural and, as such, may result in misunderstanding. Sick people live in the culture of illness, vulnerability, and fear. Clinicians live in the culture of health, technique, and knowledge. Thus, even an encounter between a middle-class African-American clinician and a middle-class African-American patient is a cross-cultural experience. The language and culture discrepancies often manifest themselves as misunderstandings about what was said or not said during an encounter. Sometimes a clinician who thinks that she has completely explained the benefits, risks, and alternatives to a procedure or treatment will discover later that the patient had absolutely no idea what she was talking about.

Be Clear about What You Know and What You Don't Know

Consider the following excerpt:

Patient   So she kept telling me it was my heart. ... She had me on the patch and three or four different pills—headaches, weakness, you wouldn't believe it. So I said they just seem to make me sicker, and what about the burning and the sour taste? But, no, she said it was definitely my heart, but I probably couldn't have more heart surgery, since I already had a quadruple bypass.

This patient was experiencing several chest symptoms. Because of his past history of severe coronary artery disease, the cardiologist was treating him medically for angina, despite features also consistent with gastroesophageal reflux (for example, he often developed the pain when lying down). Without a referral, he went to a gastroenterologist suggested by a friend and was discovered to have severe inflammation of his lower esophagus, secondary to chronic reflux. Why didn't the cardiologist at least consider this possibility, especially when the anti-angina treatment wasn't working? We don't have enough information to answer that question, but the case highlights two issues about diagnosis and disclosure. First, if you believe there are possible competing diagnoses, let the patient know. For example, "Given everything we know about your condition, I'm pretty sure this is angina. Let's increase your medication and see. If by any chance it doesn't get better, then we need to go back to the drawing board and think about whether there is some other problem like excess stomach acid." Second, if you *don't* believe there are possible competing diagnoses, ask yourself why. Are you missing something? Have you closed your eyes prematurely to additional data? Are you sure you understand the whole picture? Naturally, in many cases you will have a high degree of certainty, but you should always keep your eyes open for conflicting or unexpected features and share these with the patient. ("Here's what I'm thinking. ...")

Admit Your Errors

When it comes to medical mistakes, honesty is almost always the best policy. It is also an extraordinarily difficult policy. Most of us are tempted to avoid the pain and embarrassment of admitting a clinical error by arguing that the error was trivial or the patient is better off not knowing. We also firmly believe (and sometimes are willing to admit) that fear of malpractice litigation influences our decision.

◈ **PRACTICE POINT**
Patients have a moral right to know if they are the victims of medical error. This moral right is now the law in some states.

Never Make Promises You Can't Keep

Listen to this patient, who has suffered for years from debilitating back pain:

Patient   The doctor said if I had the operation everything would be okay, my back would be fine, no more pain, no more painkillers. So I had the operation and it's been hell ever since—why it's worse than it was before.

Clinicians commonly hear stories like this. Nonclinicians do, too—at cocktail parties, in the elevator, at the supermarket, on the bus. Wherever you go, you encounter people who are dissatisfied with their health care, often because of what they consider a broken promise. A failed surgery is one example. Whether or not the surgeon actually said "Everything will be okay" is a moot point; the patient feels betrayed.

Medicine is fraught with uncertainty. We want to help our patients, and sometimes in the process of providing encouragement, we say the equivalent of "Everything's going to be all right," even if the diagnosis or prognosis is unclear. In the case of back surgery, patients must be selected carefully, and even then the outcome (relief of pain and disability) varies greatly. If this middle-aged man's orthopedic surgeon actually said "No more pain, no more painkillers," he was taking a risk that turned out to be unwarranted. However, patients often can't relate to statistics; they are looking for definitive answers. Thus, some patients will interpret a clinician's vague assurance as a clear-cut promise, and others will listen to a jargon-filled explanation, which they can't understand, and decide that it means whatever they want it to mean. When the prediction proves false, these individuals will be convinced that their clinician misled them.

Avoiding promises you can't keep is part of informed consent (discussed in Chapter 16, Ethics and the Law) and requires that you present the benefits (including the probability of success) and risks (including the probability of adverse outcomes), along with alternatives and your assessment of them. This conversation needs to be in clear, under-standable language. The patient whose back surgery was unsuccessful might have been satisfied had his surgeon presented the procedure in this way:

Clinician **Now that I've explained what the surgery is and what we're try-ing to accomplish with it, I want to emphasize an important point. The back problem that you have is very complicated. We don't fully understand the relationship between slipped discs–which you definitely have–and the severe back pain, which you also definitely have. Sometimes people continue to have back pain even after surgery. So I want to tell you that we can't promise anything. That's important to realize–it's tough, but it's true. All I can say is that in my professional judgment, sur-gery is the best choice we have right now. I think it will give you the best chance of relief, but remember it's still a "chance" of relief, not a sure thing.**

Be Available

The following patient's experience is, unfortunately, not uncommon:

Patient   I'd call his office time and again and they'd say 'We'll give him the mes-sage, Joyce,' and then I'd wait, but he'd never call back. Finally, things really reached a head. I couldn't take the pain any more, I was desper-ate, and then I got short of breath ... but I simply couldn't get through to him. He never called back. Finally, this other doctor called and he didn't seem to know what he was talking about."

If you are a trainee just entering clinical practice, your responsibility for patient care is limited and you are unlikely to face the on-call situation described by this patient. However, professional availability is an attribute that begins at the beginning—in your clinical interview and the initial clinician-patient encounter. The patient needs to be taken seriously and to sense that you are *available* to her as a person, that you will respond to her anxieties and concerns, and that you will *not* hold yourself distant and aloof. Similarly, if you are helping to care for a patient in your role as a trainee, your availability should be sustained over time, whether during a hospitalization, a clerkship, or a preceptorship. In this case, you have a responsibility to explain the characteristics and limits of your availability:

"I'll come to see you every day, Mr. Jones, but I'm a student and I won't be here on night call."

Most patients understand that their clinicians can't be on call 24 hours a day, 7 days a week. The issue here has to do with your overall pattern of responsiveness to the needs of patients. Many malpractice claims arise out of unanswered phone calls, or from inappropriate recommendations made by an on-call clinician whom the patient doesn't know and who is unfamiliar with the case. This is a complex topic, but here are a few basic guidelines on availability:

- Return patient calls promptly.
- If another clinician screens calls and responds to some of them, explain the system to your patients and reassure them that you are available if needed.
- If you encourage patients to call at a certain time of day, make sure your patients are aware of that time.
- Clarify what patients should expect on nights and weekends.
- If you are going to be away, make appropriate arrangements for coverage and inform patients who seem likely to have problems during your absence.

TRANSPARENCY IN EVERYDAY CLINICAL INTERACTIONS

In our everyday interactions with patients, we assume that they understand what we are saying and agreeing to what we are doing. When patients answer our questions during the interview, submit to a physical examination, take prescription drugs, or allow themselves to be stuck by needles or penetrated by x-rays, their actions constitute implied understanding and consent. When more invasive procedures and more specialized therapies pose sufficient potential risk to patients, we obtain explicit consent before performing them. The more we allow patients to see through what we are saying to what we are thinking in everyday matters, the more natural this process becomes when it has to be explicit—a natural extension of what we do every day. This consent must be an informed judgment based on adequate information about benefits, risks, and alternatives. In Chapter 16 we explore the moral and legal doctrine of informed consent and the controversies about how truly "informed" consent can be in medical practice, especially when it involves desperately ill patients and complex treatments. We focus here on the interactive process that allows patients to be informed and to participate in making the decisions about the management of their health problems.

Here is an example of a clinician aiming for transparency regarding the treatment of a patient's hypertension. Note how the clinician attempts to make his thought process clear so that the patient can "check" it and ask questions if he doesn't understand.

Clinician **I know you're concerned about your blood pressure, so let me tell you what I'm thinking. We know that we can reduce the risk to your health by treating your blood pressure, and we know that there are a number of very safe and effective medicines that have been used for many years. In your case the blood pressure isn't too high, we'd call it "mild," and you don't have any other serious health conditions, so we'll begin with a "mild" pill that you can take just once a day and that usually doesn't have many side effects. So here's what I'd like to recommend for you [names the medication and possible side effects]. So what do you think?**

The important issue here is that consent is obtained in the context of a conversation during which the clinician gives clear explanations and assesses the patient's understanding. Although we often think of informed consent only in the context of risky procedures, consent is a part of the most ordinary patient interactions. Such a conversation may lead to negotiation and compromise if the patient objects to proposed procedures or treatments; in addition, the conversation usually has the potential to be reopened at a later time. Transparency in everyday clinical interactions builds trust and facilitates the consent process—an important component of malpractice suit prevention.

COMMUNICATION WITHIN THE HEALTH CARE TEAM

Medical treatment is often extremely complicated. In the case of cancer, for example, treatment may require the interaction of primary care doctors, oncologists, surgeons, radiation therapists, and other clinicians. Cardiovascular, respiratory, neurological, and psychiatric disorders each involve a different array of specialists. Nowadays, even patients who have relatively minor health problems may engage the services of a team of professionals—for example, a family physician, a gynecologist, a dentist, a chiropractor, and a massage therapist. Communication among these

professionals is important. When the illness is severe, or different therapies may interact to cause risk of harm, communication is even more
important. If a clinician is unaware of important clinical information
because he or she has not communicated with a consultant or other member of the health care team, it may constitute negligence. Likewise, poor
communication among team members often leads to mixed messages for
the patient. Even if all parties share the same facts, different ways of presenting those facts may confuse the patient and make it appear that the
clinicians disagree. Guidelines for communication among professionals
were presented in Chapter 8, pages 155–156.

◆ PRACTICE POINT
**Good communication among clinicians and other medical profes-
sionals reduces the risk of adverse outcomes and litigation.**

KEEPING GOOD RECORDS: DOCUMENTATION, DOCUMENTATION, DOCUMENTATION

The Clinical Record

Written communication is often as important as the clinician-patient
interaction itself in preventing malpractice suits. When patients experience bad outcomes, they or their families may question the clinician's
diagnosis or treatment, even when they are otherwise satisfied with the
care they received. In other cases, they might be unable to remember critical aspects of the story, like a recommendation you made or a treatment
you prescribed at a certain point in time. They might believe incorrectly,
for example, that you failed to follow appropriate diagnostic or therapeutic guidelines.

The clinical record helps you remember *what* actually happened and
when it happened; this information is likely to be useful in explaining and
discussing the situation with the patient. Moreover, the record serves as
crucial documentation that can be used to ascertain the quality and appro-
priateness of your patient care; thus, your chart entries are of great importance. Table 17–1 presents a convenient mnemonic—the five Cs—to
remind you that clinical progress notes should be contemporaneous,
clear, comprehensible, concise, and complete. The third column of this
table presents some useful guidelines for achieving each "C" in your own
practice. Here are a few additional pointers specifically aimed at liability
prevention:

TABLE 17-1

THE UNIMPEACHABLE CLINICAL RECORD		
The Record Entries Should Be	**Which Means**	**To Accomplish This, You Should**
Contemporaneous	Written or dictated during or shortly after the patient visit	Set aside time to create your notes between patients. Organize a private "space" for writing or dictation.
Clear	Legible, uncluttered	Think before you write. Use a standard format or form. Dictate when possible.
Comprehensible	Logical and accurate representations of your clinical thinking and judgment	Think twice before you write. Read over before you finish and sign. Use a standard, step-by-step approach in your thinking.
Concise	To the point, with no excess verbiage	Keep your goal in mind. Remember the reader.
Complete	Inclusive of all the essential issues and aspects of the clinical situation	Ask yourself, "Who is this patient? What is the problem? What can be done? Have I explained it?"

- Always write (or dictate) your notes promptly, so that you don't forget any details of the interaction before documenting its content.
- If you do not receive a consultant's report in a reasonable period of time, ask for it.
- Although it is important to be concise, be sure to include all relevant information regarding differential diagnosis, reasons for diagnostic tests, and reasons for treatments you prescribe. (This is another aspect of transparency.)
- If a patient declines a test or treatment that you recommend, document not only the refusal, but also your explanation to the patient and possible remedial measures ("Will bring this up again at next visit" or "Patient asked to think about it and will give me a call").

- Use nonjudgmental language when a patient does not follow your recommendation (e.g., the word "declines" is preferable to "refuses" or "fails").
- If a declined test or treatment is particularly important, revisit the options with the patient within an appropriate period.

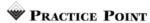 **PRACTICE POINT**

Approach the written record as a document that the patient may read at some time in the future.

What a Difference Some Notes Make

"Delay of diagnosis" is frequently the claim on malpractice suits. This situation occurs when a patient seeks help for a condition that eventually proves to be a serious illness (usually cancer), but for one reason or another the diagnostic process takes a long time. For example, a woman might present to her gynecologist with a lump in her breast. The gynecologist orders a mammogram, which appears to show that the lump is a manifestation of fibrocystic disease rather than malignancy. What to do next? The gynecologist might recommend a repeat mammogram in 2 or 3 months. Let's say the patient returns in 3 months, has a mammogram and ultrasound as recommended, and the lump proves to be cancer. She then undergoes definitive treatment, but the cancer is very aggressive and in a year or so she develops metastases. Some such patients might question the gynecologist's original diagnostic plan. What if she had had the ultrasound and a biopsy when she first went to see him? If the cancer had been discovered earlier, perhaps she could have been cured. In her pain and anxiety, the patient may blame the gynecologist for the bad outcome, claiming that the diagnosis was inappropriately delayed.

The crucial factor here is whether the clinician followed accepted clinical guidelines in waiting 3 months before repeating the test or ordering other tests. If he did, there is no basis for a suit—he was practicing state-of-the-art medicine, which in this case is evidence based. On the other hand, if the standard clinical guidelines recommended an immediate ultrasound, then he may well have been responsible for a delay in diagnosis. Whether the delay actually contributed to the patient's bad outcome is a moot point. The cancer may have been so aggressive that earlier diagnosis would not have prevented its spread. However, the combination of a clinical mistake (failure to follow standard practice) and a bad outcome is usually considered by juries to be prima facie evidence that the mistake resulted in the outcome.

What would have happened if the gynecologist's recommendations were correct, but the patient had not returned in 3 months? Let's say she waited 6 or 8 months, then went back to the gynecologist because the breast lump had gotten bigger. A similar scenario followed—she proved to have cancer, which by that time had spread to her lymph nodes and bones. If this patient subsequently decided to sue her gynecologist, a great deal would depend on (1) written documentation in the chart of the original conversation and recommendation and (2) evidence in the written record of measures that the gynecologist might have taken to remind her of the need for a follow-up mammogram. The office note should specify what was said and how it relates to the standard practice or clinical guideline. It should also indicate the manner of follow-up, such as a prescription for a repeat mammogram in 2 or 3 months and a follow-up office appointment. For something so important, there should also be evidence of a "tickler file" or some other method of initiating contact with the patient if she misses the follow-up appointment. For example, the office might send a standard reminder letter to patients who miss repeat mammograms or Pap smears, or an office staff member might even leave a telephone message inviting the patient to call for another appointment. If the clinician forgets to write down the plan or to document its importance, a lawsuit becomes an issue of the clinician's word against the patient's. And the patient is, after all, the person who suffers the misfortune. The clinician's word—no matter how sincere—may not convince a jury of the patient's peers.

◈ PRACTICE POINT

When a diagnostic plan is both reasonable and clearly documented, there is no basis for a "delay of diagnosis" suit.

On the Record

No matter how careful you are, you will sometimes make mistakes while writing in the clinical record. Your mind might wander, and soon you find yourself jotting down the wrong material—an incorrect observation or plan, for example, or perhaps a correct observation, but placed in the wrong patient's chart. More frequently, if you dictate your notes, you will identify errors of transcription. Sometimes, too, you might change your mind in the process of recording a note. Suddenly, the clinical data "click" into a different pattern. Aha! You want to pursue a new course of action, but you have already written a summary outlining your original plan. What should you do?

It is tempting to pursue either the *snuff-it-out* or the *throw-it-out* approach. *Snuff-it-out* means that you take a pen and carefully scribble over your sentences so that they disappear in a pool of blue or black lines, or at least can no longer be understood. By all means, suppress the temptation to snuff it out. Defacing the medical record raises serious doubts about your truthfulness when the record is used as evidence in malpractice litigation. The *throw-it-out* approach is also inappropriate, perhaps even worse, because it may require you to rewrite not only the present clinical entry, but also other entries on the page you toss out. Here are some guidelines for correcting errors in the health care record:

- Strike through the incorrect passage with a single line, so that the original writing can still be read and understood.
- Make your corrections.
- If the correction is a word, a date, or a short phrase, enter it above or in the margin of the incorrect entry.
- If the correction is longer, enter it in the text below the incorrect material as a continuation of the note.
- Initial and date your corrections. (This date should be the same date as the original entry.)
- Explain clearly why you are correcting the entry.

◆ PRACTICE POINT
The clinical record is also a legal document that must not be defaced or destroyed.

SUMMARY — Malpractice and the Clinical Interview
The best way to prevent malpractice suits is to practice with a high degree of technical competence: competence in the skills of clinical interviewing and clinician-patient interaction, as well as competence in your sphere of professional practice. By becoming an empathic, respectful practitioner who listens well and responds appropriately, you will generate trust and satisfaction among your patients. To avoid malpractice claims, pay particular attention to these guidelines:

- Listen to what the patient does and does not say.
- Avoid trivializing or demeaning the patient.

- Acknowledge the patient's level of concern.
- Strive for transparency in your reasoning and recommendations.
- Be clear about what you know and what you do not know.
- Never make promises you can't keep.
- Be available to the patient.

In addition, pay careful attention to obtaining consent. Employ a transparency standard for evaluating the information you provide and your patient's response. Likewise, look closely at your communication with other health professionals involved in a patient's care. Make sure they know what you are doing and you know what they are doing. Do not expect information simply to fall into place; seek it—by letter, phone, E-mail, or fax. Finally, remember that documentation is essential. Make your progress notes contemporaneous, clear, comprehensible, concise, and complete. Also document your attempts to follow up on missed appointments or tests. When you make a mistake writing in the patient's record, correct the mistake carefully and transparently so that others can understand what you are doing and when you are doing it.

CHAPTER 18

Education and Negotiation

Not through Argument but by Contagion

The faith that heals, heals not through argument but by contagion. But to heal, faith must have substance. A speculative balance of probability is not enough. The faith that heals must have deep roots in the personality of the healer.

W. R. Houston, *The Doctor Himself as a Therapeutic Agent*

INFLUENCING PATIENTS

Among the outcomes of the clinician–patient encounter, we pay particular attention in this text to data collection and hypothesis generation and testing—the diagnostic function of clinical interviewing. However, we also set the stage for relationship building. Therapeutic relationships are built on a series of encounters; each clinician-patient interaction has the potential to influence the way the patient behaves, thinks, and feels.

These three types of influence are interdependent and in practice often occur together. You influence *behavior* by asking patients to undertake diagnostic studies, take medication, return for follow-up visits, stop smoking, start exercising, and so on. When patients change their behaviors in these ways, we say that they are compliant, adherent, actively involved in their health care, or "good patients." Second, you influence how patients *feel*. If the encounter is positive, patients may feel less lonely, less anxious, less depressed, or more able to cope with their problems; if the encounter is negative, the patient may feel anxiety, anger, and greater feelings of confusion or powerlessness. Your patient may walk away either relieved or sorely distressed. Finally, you influence the way patients *think*. Through education and negotiation, patients may change their concepts of what illness is and what should be done about it. They may learn to understand themselves differently. In these ways, each encounter may either add to or subtract from the burden of suffering. This influence is what Michael Balint had in mind when he taught "the doctor is the drug."

In other words, your treatment of the patient is not just the intervention you prescribe. The drug is only a small part of the influence you have on the patient and the healing process. Even as you complete your initial interview and physical examination, you bring other influences to bear in managing the patient. You may simply be ordering further diagnostic studies while explaining your preliminary findings and expecting the patient to return. Even so, you want to maximize the probability that the patient actually obtains the studies, follows your advice, and returns to your office. Clearly, the best diagnoses and plans in the world are useless without patients' cooperation. You also want to do what you can to make the patient feel better starting today, rather than next week or next month. Insofar as possible, you want to reduce anxiety and relieve suffering.

◈ PRACTICE POINT

A skillful interview grounded in respect, empathy, and genuineness is the first step in enhancing your patient's active participation in health care and reducing the suffering caused by anxiety and uncertainty.

How do you maximize the chance that your influence will be positive and beneficial? In this book, we are concerned with the technical skills of medical interviewing. Using these skills has multiple effects. Good technique maximizes objectivity and precision, and it facilitates good clinical decision making. At the same time, good technique influences the patient to follow your advice and to leave your office with a sense of well-being and relief. Sick persons seeking medical help are frequently in a crisis situation, a time when seemingly small interventions may have significant outcomes. *Any clinician-patient interaction is likely to influence the suffering of a sick person.*

Most treatment requires active patient cooperation. Unless the patient is comatose, it is difficult to imagine a situation in which the behavioral component of therapy is not significant. Although "compliance" is a common term in medical parlance, it has two drawbacks. First, the word suggests that the clinician's orders are uniquely right and that a patient who fails to be 100% compliant will have a less-than-successful outcome. Second, it suggests a passive, plastic patient rather than an active, participating one. To some extent, the word "adherence" escapes the second connotation, but still implies the first. The patient must adhere, albeit actively, to the clinician's correct regimen. Rather than using either of these terms, we prefer to talk about clinician-patient cooperation in reaching the desired goal and to consider how the clinician influences the patient's behavior. In cooperation, as opposed to compliance or adherence, both parties contribute to finding and implementing the best solution. This chapter describes how clinicians influence patients in the course of everyday clinical interactions. We show how these interactions are learning experiences that can be used to encourage personal responsibility and behavioral change. In Chapter 9, we presented simple steps to enhance patient understanding in the office. In this chapter we discuss in more detail what works in conveying information, not only with regard to instructing patients but also with regard to establishing appropriate expectations about the illness and its treatment. Then we consider the art of negotiation and its component skills and behaviors, concluding the chapter with an extended example of clinician-patient negotiation.

EDUCATION

Conveying the Information

Why don't patients follow their clinician's instructions? A number of factors explain this apparent lack of cooperation, or so-called noncompliant behavior:

- **Personality**—Factors in the patient's personality structure interfere with cooperation.
- **Psychodynamics**—Defense mechanisms, such as denial, prevent cooperation.
- **Interpersonal dynamics**—Emotional issues arising from the clinician-patient interaction prevent cooperation.
- **Economics**—The patient cannot afford the prescribed treatment.
- **Culture and beliefs**—The patient's beliefs about the illness interfere with cooperation.
- **Cognitive factors**—The patient simply doesn't understand what is to be done and why.

Although each of these factors plays a part at least some of the time, studies indicate that the cognitive factor is critical and often present even when other factors also play a role. Patients frequently do not remember much of what the clinician says. Simply put, people can't do what a clinician recommends if they can't remember it. Investigators agree that patients, on average, initially remember 50% to 60% of the information that clinicians give them, and subsequently retain about 45% to 55% of what they can initially recall. Interestingly, neither intelligence nor age of the patient seems to be a decisive factor in how much is remembered. Even writing down the information, which would seem to be a fail-safe method, does not always lead to better cooperation or increase the amount of information remembered. Notably, patients who have a moderate level of anxiety about their problems are more likely to remember than if they have either very high (paralyzing and distracting) or very low (nonmotivating) anxiety levels.

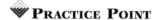 **PRACTICE POINT**

The first step in ensuring patient involvement is to make sure that the patient understands what you are saying and remembers it.

How do you do that? Consider the following example:

Clinician **So we're going to treat your hypertension with this diuretic and ...**

Patient   My hyper-tension? But I don't feel tense ...

We'll see how things go and we'll keep adding drugs until we get things in control.

I don't know, with my job and all, I can't afford not to be sharp.

It is easy to see the clinician's errors. Not only the words but also the style of this segment of the interaction suggest a range of problematic behaviors and missed opportunities. We are left wondering whether the clinician, who must have taken the patient's blood pressure (perhaps several times) during the interaction, has been silent all this time, thereby raising the patient's anxiety by saying nothing about blood pressure until the very end, then using the word "hypertension," which seems common enough but can be misunderstood by even a well-educated patient. The clinician is rushing to a discussion of treatment before even explaining the diagnosis. She is also vague about what the patient can expect, thereby increasing uncertainty and anxiety. Note, too, that the use of the word "drug" in relation to the word "hyper-*tension*" appears to leave this patient, a high-powered attorney, completely confused. He associates "drug" with "sedative" or "tranquilizer," and expresses his fear of becoming less "sharp" in his work.

Consider how the clinician might have facilitated better understanding by adopting the measures listed in *Conveying the Information,* below. The following transcript suggests how the same clinician might, on a better day, share her findings with the patient:

Clinician **Well, as I mentioned during my exam, when I take your blood pressure it is repeatedly above normal.**

Patient Yeah, you said that and it's making me kinda worried.

Well, we consider normal anything under 140 over 90 [writing this out and showing it to the patient], and yours is 160 over 105.

Uh huh, umm.

Another word for high blood pressure is "hypertension," even though it has nothing necessarily to do with tension or feeling tense. It just means that your body has reset your blood pressure at a higher level, like a thermostat. What I'd like to do next is explain to you what this means.

WHAT TO SAY

Conveying the Information

- Use words and phrases the patient is likely to understand: "Hypertension is the medical term for high blood pressure."
- Be concrete and specific about the nature of the problem, the treatment, and expected outcome: "Your blood pressure problem is not serious but you do need to take a pill every day to treat it. I will explain how this medicine will make you feel and what good it will do."
- In particular, give the name, purpose, mechanism (in lay terms), schedule, and duration of any prescribed medication: "The name of the medicine is atenolol and you will take one every morning. I will want you to keep taking it, provided that you feel well on it, even after your blood pressure comes down."

In this example the clinician has given a few explanations that will influence the patient through better transfer of information. The patient may well be more satisfied than in our first example and go home less anxious and confused about his condition. In addition, the clinician anticipated one of the common errors in patient understanding ("it has nothing to do with tension"), not only laying the groundwork for the proposed plan of treatment, but also making it easier for the patient to reveal other possible misconceptions he might have.

Checking for Understanding and Enhancing Memory

Once you have conveyed information to your patient it is necessary to ensure that your patient understands what you have said. Words and diagnoses that are routine for you are not so for your patient. A good case in point is the previous example, in which the patient hears that his blood pressure is related to "tension" even though the clinician said no such thing. Observing your patients' facial expressions and body language and allowing them to ask questions will avoid misunderstanding. Such misunderstanding may lead to failure to follow your recommendations. *Checking for Understanding,* below, describes how to check that your patient understands what you are saying. And, of course, once the patient understands, it is essential that he or she actually remembers the information or instructions. *Enhancing Memory,* below, describes various methods to enhance patients' memory.

WHAT TO SAY

Checking for Understanding

- Inquire about how much the patient understands: "Do you understand what I mean by high blood pressure?"
- Ask the patient to repeat explanations and instructions: "Can you repeat back to me how you are going to take this medication so I can be sure you understand?"
- Give corrective and supportive feedback: "Very good, you got most of it right. Just remember to take your pill with food."
- Encourage questions: "Is there anything that you have questions about?"

WHAT TO SAY

Enhancing Memory

- Write down instructions for the patient: "Let me write this out for you."
- Provide instructional material, such as brochures and printed handouts: "Here's a pamphlet that will help. I want you to take this with you."

■ Refer the patient to specific Web sites for further information: "I know you like checking on the Internet. Here's the name of a good site."

NEGOTIATION

Although patients cannot follow your advice unless they understand and remember it, they may reject your advice because they disagree with it. Your knowledge of the patient's personal and cultural beliefs about illness and healing will help you to view the situation from the patient's perspective. You then have several options. You can modify your therapeutic plan to accommodate the patient's health beliefs, attempt to modify the patient's beliefs through education and persuasion, or negotiate a therapeutic alliance, which involves some give and take on both sides. Negotiation—using discussion and compromise to arrive at a settlement of some issue—is a method of conflict resolution that respects the values of all parties. In practice, negotiation is a way of optimizing patient cooperation and is a sign of respect for the patient's autonomy. Your goals are to influence behavior, decrease anxiety, and increase the patient's sense of mastery over the problem. How can you accomplish these ends in the clinical interview?

In a successful clinical encounter, you reach agreement with the patient in four different areas:

- Agreement on what the clinical information is
- Agreement on the nature of the problem
- Agreement about what can or should be done
- Consent for procedures or treatments

The characteristics of your patient, your own traits, and the qualities of the relationship may facilitate or hinder reaching agreement. It is important to understand the patient's comprehension, decision-making processes, beliefs, and environment in order to have the greatest positive influence on the patient's behavior. These components restate in different terms the familiar themes of respect, empathy, communication skills, and acknowledgment of the patient's beliefs and expectations.

◈ PRACTICE POINT
You are able to influence patients when you respect them, communicate well, and understand their point of view.

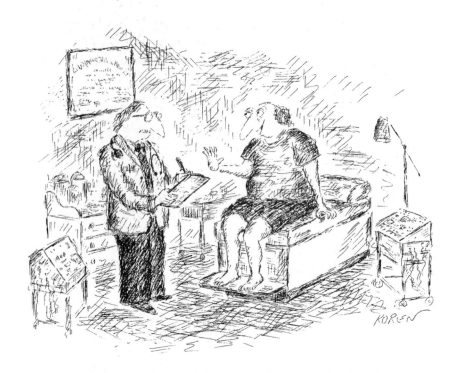

"Please, Doc—nothing too aggressive. I'm kind
of attached to my symptoms."

In day-to-day practice, education and negotiation occur together and
may take only a few moments. For example, here is a middle-aged patient
with bronchitis returning to see the clinician because of increased coughing:

Patient   It's going on 8 days now, doc. I was better 2 days ago, but then the
          coughing started up again yesterday. I'm not bringing up that thick, yel-
          low stuff any more—it's dry, hacky—but I'm still coughing a lot. What
          about an antibiotic?

Clinician **Well, here's what I think is happening. It sounds to me as if
          you've turned the corner, the infection has cleared up, but your
          throat is still raw and irritated. Things are healing.**
          Well, I do feel better … it's just this cough.
          **Do you think you can hang in there another 24 hours? Just use
          the cough medicine. Then if you're not clearly improving we'll
          go with an antibiotic.**
          That sounds good. Should I call you around this time tomorrow?

In this case the patient has already told the clinician that his wheezing is gone and his cough is no longer productive. Overall, he feels better, the fever is down, and on physical examination his chest sounds clear. Yet the patient quite reasonably interprets his dramatic (but dry) cough as a sign of worsening infection and believes that he needs an antibiotic. The clinician first reframes the situation—the dry cough represents healing rather than continued infection. The patient can accept this interpretation because it accords with other data ("Well, I do *feel* better"). The clinician then presents a counterproposal—let's see how it goes for the next 24 hours. The patient, who is now less frightened, accepts the plan, at least in part because he recognizes the clinician's logic and concern.

The next example is from an interview with a 71-year-old patient who has chronic obstructive pulmonary disease (COPD) and bronchospasm. Although she has wheezing throughout both lungs because COPD is chronic, she does not experience herself as being ill.

Patient	I smoked my last cigarette that day I had those tests.
Clinician	**I'm really glad you're not smoking. And I know how hard it is for you.**
	I'm determined this time. I don't want to be sick.
	I really would like you to be on an inhaler … it's not good for you to be wheezing all the time.
	But don't I sound better to you? I haven't smoked at all, I think I'm better, I'm not a medicine person.
	Well, not smoking will definitely be better for you. It will be a big help. Still, your lung condition has been going on a long time. There's a lot of inflammation and spasm in your breathing tubes. You know how short of breath you get.
	But I believe that everything will heal naturally if I just give it a chance. I mean, by not smoking.
	Well, here's what we can do. Let's agree to wait and see how it goes, provided you call me if you have any trouble breathing, any cough or wheezing. How's that? [The patient nods.] How about we recheck things in 3 months?
	Okay, that's good. You'll see, my lungs will be clear as a bell.
	Okay, 3 months. And keep up the good work.

This patient is convinced that her health will improve if she stays away from cigarettes. She is experiencing a sense of mastery ("I'm determined this time") that leads her to interpret the situation in a favorable light ("But don't I sound better to you?"). The clinician knows that her patient has reversible bronchospasm and, in fact, would have less wheezing and better exercise tolerance if she were to use an inhaler regularly. She explains this to the patient in simple, understandable terms, while reiterating the long-term benefits of not smoking. However, the clinician also realizes that the patient's sense of empowerment is a critical factor in her self-image. Thus, the clinician proposes an alternative program that combines monitoring (return visit) and potential crisis intervention ("call me if you have any trouble") with respect for the patient's values and strong motivation.

We illustrate these concepts with a more extended case example, which demonstrates the interactive nature of clinical problem solving. The case illustrates negotiation both in the "give-and-take bargaining" and the "maneuver to find a path" senses of the word. The patient is a 25-year-old woman who came to her family physician's office with the complaint of a severe and persistent vaginal itch. She expressed her distress and summarized her problem in an opening statement that we encountered previously in Chapter 3, page 63.

Patient   Well, I have a terrible vaginal itch, and I don't know whether it's from vaginitis or whether it's the urinary tract infection, you know ... ah, my regular doctor treated me for vaginitis first.

Clinician That was Doctor X?
Uh huh, then I, um, got a urinary tract infection, then the vaginitis came back, but during the whole ordeal I've never got no relief.

We learn several important facts about this patient from her opening statement: she is suffering ("terrible," "ordeal," "no relief"); she is medically sophisticated ("vaginitis," "urinary tract infection"); and she is not necessarily well educated ("never got no").

The clinician performs an examination and checks a specimen of vaginal secretion under the microscope, finding that the infection is clearly caused by *Trichomonas vaginalis* and can be easily and effectively treated with a single dose of medication. At this point, both patient and clinician agree on the nature of the problem: it is a *Trichomonas* infection. To the patient, the end of her suffering is in sight. The clinician begins to write out a prescription. But on seeing the name of the drug, the patient makes an unexpected comment:

Patient   Flagyl. You don't have any ... there's nothing else you can take besides Flagyl, huh?

Until this point, it seems as though the clinician has made not only an accurate diagnosis but also a correct decision about therapy, with which the patient will be happy. But the patient, instead of being grateful for the expertise, is not satisfied. The negotiation begins:

Clinician   **It's the best for it.**
Patient   Okay, but I might … well, I'll try it.

It is easy to imagine a scenario here in which the clinician simply says "fine," and the patient is left to her own doubts about the drug, perhaps taking it, perhaps not. But the clinician, listening to her hesitation, replies:

Clinician   **What's the problem?**
Patient   I think I was allergic to that.
            Why do you think that?
            Because I remember taking Flagyl before, and it did something … I think I broke out in hives or something.
            Really?
            But I'll try it. If I break out I'll let you know, but I think I did.
            That's a worry … let me look at the record. It says here that you were sensitive to ampicillin and sulfa … now could it have been …? Oh, it does say Flagyl.
            I think it was just hives. Maybe I've outgrown it.
            I don't want you to take it if you had hives from it.
            Well, maybe I'll have … I'll have outgrown it 'cause I think it's been a while back.
            [Still looking through the chart.] Yeah, it does say Flagyl.

The patient actually begins with an interpretation ("allergic") of some past event associated with the drug. The two then exchange information, together trying to verify or refute that interpretation. The patient provides supporting evidence with the descriptive term "hives," while the clinician searches for other evidence by going through the patient's chart. (The patient is new to this clinician, but had previously been seen in the same clinic.) This is more than a simple discussion of evidence, however, as we can see both patient ("I'll try it") and clinician ("I don't want you to take it") apparently on the verge of decisions, albeit opposite ones. Perhaps, seeing the physician's concern and given her willingness to risk hives, the patient offers a new interpretation to the data ("Maybe I'll have outgrown it"). The clinician then offers:

Clinician   **What we could do is, we could treat your husband and we could treat you with something else, but …**

Patient   Well, if that's the best, I want that.

... most of the "something elses" aren't as effective.

Well, I'll take Flagyl. It can only break me out in hives a day like ... it'll probably go away in the morning.

I would be kind of worried about that before prescribing it for you because you could get an even more serious reaction to it.

Data have been exchanged ("I was allergic"), verified ("hives," written record), and now reinterpreted ("I've outgrown it"). The patient, echoing the clinician's "It's the best," rejects the notion of "something else" by reversing the implication of concession in her earlier statement on taking Flagyl ("Well, I'll try it"). In the context of the clinician's earlier statement, "something else" would have to be judged decidedly inferior. We are tiptoeing on a threshold-of-risk boundary: take Flagyl and get rid of the itch but risk an allergic reaction, or take something else and avoid the reaction but risk not curing the itch. Much of what the patient says in subsequent statements suggests that she places a higher value on getting rid of the itch than on avoiding an allergic reaction. She acknowledges that there is a risk involved but discounts it ("just hives"); the clinician, on the other hand, emphasizes that the risk is more than what the patient says ("You could get an even more serious reaction").

The decision has become problematic, and we begin to see patient and clinician engage in a dialogue regarding risks and benefits. Lacking the data necessary to value or weigh the risks, the clinician returns to a discussion of the evidence, by turning again to the written record to find the supporting data for the diagnosis of allergy, while the patient in turn supplies additional details pointedly aimed at discrediting her own report of an allergic reaction:

Clinician   **Uh, let me see what Dr. X said about that.**

Patient   I don't even think that Dr. X was here when I had that.

Dr. Y? Dr. Z? ... because that may be why you've been treated with all this other stuff.

But they, I remember I told them it did that to me, it might notta been that.

But it does say you're allergic to it.

That's 'cause I told him that.

I've never heard of anybody being allergic to it but it's ...

That's what I'm saying, it's ...

... certainly possible.

> Probably what happened was I broke out in hives in reaction to other things.

It is remarkable that the patient understands that the source of the data in question—or rather the interpretation in question—is herself ("'cause I told him that") and that she may not be the most reliable interpreter of the evidence. Perhaps, if she is the source of the original interpretation, she can also be the source of a new interpretation. In the end the clinician is persuaded—to some extent. Note the ensuing discussion in which various outcomes are valued and a decision is reached:

Clinician	**Well, I'll tell you what I want you to do. Since you have taken a lot of drugs because of all these urinary infections ...**
Patient	That might be why it's never left.
	Uh hum.
	So I'd rather take the Flagyl.
	Well, I'll tell you what I want you to do.
	It won't be your fault ...
	Well, I'm still the one that prescribes it. Let me tell you what I'd like you to do. I'd like you to take one pill as a test dose. OK? And if you have no reaction to it, then we will hope it is safe to take the rest, though we can't know for sure.
	Um hmm.
	Today, just one, see what happens. OK?
	OK.
	OK? So if you are allergic we'll know.
	Yeah, I'll get hives (ha ha).
	Well, let's just be on the safe side, let's use a test dose ... OK? Because *Trichomonas,* while it's uncomfortable, it can't kill you, so you know ...
	It can drive you mad.
	I know, but the point is that we don't want to do anything that would be harmful to your health.

Although there was a lot of back-and-forth maneuvering, the clinician takes ultimate responsibility for the decision ("I'm still the one that prescribes it"), but the decision is clearly influenced by the value the patient places on getting rid of the itch ("It can drive you mad"). The patient took the medication, had no reaction, and got rid of the itch. It is not difficult to imagine a different situation with a patient who, perhaps, had suffered more from hives. In that case, the negotiation would have resulted in a different outcome, such as prescribing a, perhaps, somewhat less effective therapy.

Negotiation Skills in the Clinical Interview, below, summarizes these concepts of negotiation, which are further demonstrated in our closing example of education and negotiation as they often coexist in everyday practice to influence patient behavior. The patient is a 46-year-old teacher, newly diagnosed with type 2 diabetes, who is being seen for a follow-up visit with his week-long food diary. He is a recovering alcoholic with a body mass index of 40, hypertension, hyperlipidemia, and obstructive sleep apnea.

WHAT TO SAY

Negotiation Skills in the Clinical Interview

- Begin with the core qualities of respect and empathy: "Let me make sure I understand your concerns."
- Provide the patient with enough information and opportunity to ask questions: "Do you have any questions?"
- Elicit the patient's perspective.
    - Goals
    "What would you like to happen?"
    "What do you think will happen?"
    - Suggestions
    "How do you think we should handle this?"
    "How do you think we should proceed?"
    - Preferences
    "Of the alternatives, which do you think will work best for you?"
    "Are there other alternatives, perhaps something you've read about, that we haven't discussed?"
- Help the patient weigh burdens and benefits, including trade-offs between quality and quantity of life: "Let's look at the pros and cons. We can even make a list."
- Consider your recommendations in light of the patient's beliefs and goals: "Given what you've told me about your concerns, here's what I would recommend."
- Modify your plan of action insofar as is possible to incorporate the patient's perspective: "Is this how you see it? Would you change anything?"
- Formulate an agreement with the patient on the nature of the problem and what should be done about it, always letting the patient have the last word. "Sounds like we agree on what the problem is and how to approach it.

I think we are on the same page. What do you think? Do you have any more questions or concerns?"

Patient   I remember you saying that this doctor, this diabetes expert, says that men over a certain waist size and weight will get diabetes. And now that's me. Here's my food diary for this past week.

Clinician   **[Clinician reviews written food diary.] You have a remarkable lack of vegetables here.**

That's true. I eat dinner at a restaurant and my only vegetable is the salad. And, of course, I load it with their blue cheese dressing.

Well, I want this conversation we are having today to be the beginning of a dialogue about how you can improve your health.

Tell me about that, what's that hemoglobin?

Right, it's the hemoglobin A-1-C. Your red blood cells, which have the hemoglobin, grab on to the sugar in your bloodstream. And your red blood cells circulate in your body for about 3 months. So this is a test for the sugar in the red blood cells which kinda gives us a read on what your sugar is over a 3-month period.

I think I understand.

And yours is definitely abnormal, which means you have diabetes, but it's not so high that I have to put you on medication right away.

I guess I knew this was coming. But eating is my addiction. The problem is you have to eat. When I gave up drinking and smoking it was complete. You don't drink AT ALL, you don't smoke AT ALL. But you have to eat, and there's where I lose control.

You were in the Ornish Program a few years ago, weren't you?

Yes. And it did work. But it's hard to sustain. Now when I buy cookies I eat the whole bag. I know I shouldn't, but I can't stop.

Are you aware that people are now having surgery for obesity?

Yes, what do you call that?

It has different names: gastric bypass or bariatric surgery.

I'm writing that down, how do you spell that, so I can look it up on the Web.

My job is to make sure that you can use that information and any additional information I can provide, so you can make a decision that's good for you. Given your history of addiction and problems with control, the surgery is a consideration. And

you would probably qualify under your insurance because of the diabetes and the sleep apnea and the high blood pressure and cholesterol.

Gee, I haven't really thought about this before.

Well, it's something to think about. I will want you to understand everything about it, including the possible complications.

Like?

Well, let's talk about this some more. As I said, we're just beginning this dialogue. Why don't you research it and we'll set up a follow-up visit in about six weeks. How does that sound?

It sounds good.

Note this clinician's respectful and empathic approach to this patient, her ability to provide information with clarity and precision, the opportunities for the patient to ask questions, the exploration of the patient's goals and preferences, and the weighing of the potential burdens and benefits of the various treatment options. The interview closes with an agreed-upon plan of action.

SUMMARY — Education and Negotiation

In this chapter we addressed the question of how you influence the patient's behavior and feelings through the clinical interview. We divided this influencing skill into components for the sake of discussion, although in practice they often flow together. The patient's understanding and recall of information must serve as a basis for any behavioral influence you might have. The patient cannot cooperate unless he or she knows what to do and how to do it. Moreover, the patient is not likely to be motivated to cooperate unless he or she knows why something is to be done and how it works. Finally, we discussed the role of negotiation in achieving an effective therapeutic outcome. Respect for the patient and knowledge of his or her beliefs helps you to influence the patient when you engage in a process of negotiation — the *give and take of ideas and feelings that allows you to arrive at a mutually agreed-upon plan of action.*

CHAPTER 19

The Medical Interview at Work

The Hunt Is On

Time after time I have gone out into my office in the evening feeling as if I couldn't keep my eyes open a moment longer.. . . But once I saw the patient all that would disappear. In a flash the details of the case would begin to formulate themselves into a recognizable outline, the diagnosis would unravel itself, or would refuse to make itself plain, and the hunt was on. Along with that, the patient himself would shape up into something that called for attention, his peculiarities, her reticences or candors. And though I might be attracted or repelled, the professional attitude which every physician must call on would steady me and dictate the terms on which I was to proceed.

William Carlos Williams, from *The Autobiography*

PUTTING YOUR SKILLS INTO PRACTICE

Throughout this text we maintain that most of the information you need to make appropriate diagnoses and to take care of your patients comes from the clinical encounter. For the sake of convenience and to create manageable pieces to learn, we have artificially dissected the interview into sequential parts as if the information presented itself in a linear fashion—chief complaint before patient profile, for example. In clinical practice, however, we interview persons, not cases or problems, and interviews—like persons—are rarely neat and linear. Interviews tend to be messy, with information coming at you in the opening moments that you may need to "file" in several places, perhaps in the present illness, family history, and other active problems, as for the patient who begins, "I'm a diabetic but I'm worried about this terrific headache I have because my father had a stroke when he was my age."

As you gain experience, you will be less distracted by what may, at first, seem like endless tangents that threaten to get you off track. Your mind is extremely busy not only following the flow of information, but also keeping track of how the patient's story is turning into a diagnosis, what questions you need to ask, what details need clarification, and whether you are developing rapport with the patient.

Figure 19–1 illustrates a way of conceptualizing the medical interview as a continual feedback loop of information, thinking, and technique that refines and remodels itself throughout the patient encounter. Elements of process or technique allow the clinician to obtain certain data (content), which are ultimately organized into the traditional sections of a medical history. Even in the earliest phases of the interview, however, the clinician formulates hypotheses that influence the continuing process of data collection. A central concern of clinical practice is differential diagnosis (i.e., formulating and ranking hypotheses about the nature of the patient's disease

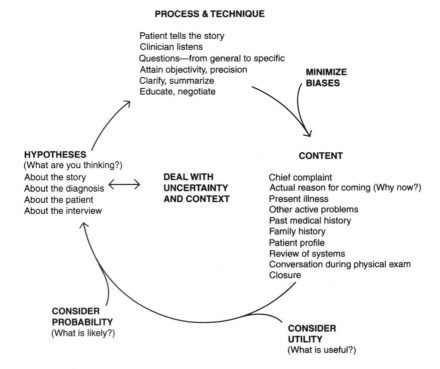

Figure 19–1 The Medical Interview at Work

process). However, the accuracy of differential diagnosis depends on a set of preliminary hypotheses about the quality of the story itself and about the patient as a person: Did X happen before or after Y? Is the narrative plausible? Does the patient exaggerate or minimize symptoms? The clinician generates hypotheses about the patient's personality and interactive style: What sort of coping style does he or she have? What might one expect in terms of adherence to treatment recommendations or behavioral change?

Finally, when problems arise in the interview, one must also consider hypotheses about the source of difficulty in the clinical encounter itself: What is going wrong here? Why do I feel so frustrated or uncomfortable? Why is the patient so angry? And because we often encounter patients who annoy us, or worry us, or confuse us, we must be aware of the need to minimize bias, consider utility (can the problem be fixed?) and probability (is the diagnosis likely?), and deal with uncertainty.

TRANSCRIPT

We close this text with a slightly altered transcript (to protect the patient's privacy and to shorten the length) taken from a real interview of a new patient by a medical resident. We have annotated the transcript to illustrate some of the skills and thought processes that have been presented throughout this book and summarized in Figure 19–1. We hope this interview provides opportunity for analysis and reflection as you develop your own style and techniques.

This 32-year-old woman comes into the clinic for a "checkup."

Transcript	Comments
It's good to meet you. I guess the best place to start is to ask you what brings you here today.	Greeting, opening.
Well, I haven't had a physical really since 5 years ago, since my son was born.	
I am going to be writing some things down on paper here, okay? Is there any particular reason why you chose *now* to come in?	Acknowledges note taking (an example of transparency). Open-ended question. Probe for iatrotropic stimulus, chief complaint.
I figured I kept putting it off and putting it off. I'd make appointments and put them off. There was no	

Transcript	Comments
particular reason. I just felt as though it was time, I suppose.	
Nothing is bothering you at this point?	Additional probe for actual reason for coming.
No, it's just that I am overweight, that's all. I go up and down, up and down.	
So that was your major concern, the weight problem?	Summary statement and interchangeable response. Agenda setting.
Yeah.	
Can you tell me about that?	Open-ended question.
Well, I've always been big. All the women in my family are big. It's never slowed me down or anything, but I would like to just like firm up, maybe my thighs and my stomach. From after having children I don't know, they say everything takes time, you don't put it on right away, but I guess I'm impatient.	Listening.
How much do you weigh right now?	The clinician inquires in detail about the symptom—what, how much, when, why?—developing accuracy and precision and hypotheses about the diagnosis and the patient.
I don't basically know. Last time I weighed myself I weighed 200 pounds and that was like about 2 months ago.	
Say a year ago, what did you weigh?	What happened first, what next?
A year ago I weighed about 230 pounds.	
230 pounds? So you have actually lost 30 pounds between then and now?	The clinician checks back with patient, confirming data.

Transcript	Comments
Yes.	
Have you been on a diet?	A closed-ended question, perhaps pursuing a hypothesis (e.g., could the patient have lost weight because she has become diabetic?)
No.	
How have you lost the weight?	
I don't know. In the last, I'd say the last 6 months or so to a year, I've been getting to the point I'd go all day without eating. I'm real active. I'm very active.	
Can you tell me about the activity?	Open-ended question with topic specified.
Well, I do a lot of tennis. I have dance class. It seems like I don't want to stop to fix anything when I'm working in the house. I won't stop to fix any-thing to eat. I'll just keep on going.	
Is that a conscious effort on your part, to try to lose weight?	Closed-ended and, perhaps, a leading question with a vague response.
Yeah, something like that.	
What did you used to consider your normal weight?	A series of closed questions, still dealing with the weight issue.
I always weighed about 140 pounds.	
How many years ago was that?	
When I was 18.	
When would you say that you had gained the majority of weight between then and now?	
When I had my second child.	
What do you think it was between then and now that's made you gain the weight?	Open-ended question with, per-haps, a surprising response regarding psychosocial issues.
Nerves made me do a lot of eating. Then a lot of marital problems.	

Transcript	Comments
Do you want to discuss that a little bit more?	Open-ended question, leading to further exploration of possible emotional causes for weight change. But leaving it up to the patient as to whether this topic is too intimate for her to discuss right now. Listening.
Oh, it was just a thing, me and my husband were—just like any other marriage, I guess—good times, bad times—but more bad times than good. I had gotten to the point that I felt as though, I got all these children, what am I worth? You know, that kind of depressed me a little bit and I started gaining all that weight. After I had my last child I don't know, something just hit me, and I came up out of that.	
When was that?	
Five years ago.	
So, how would you describe your general mood now?	Open-ended question, topic specified, taking advantage of the fact that the patient has raised the topic of mood.
Fine.	
You don't feel anything is wrong?	And not just taking "fine" for an answer.
No. I very seldom—last time I got depressed was one day about 2 months ago 'cause there wasn't no jobs and that's about it. But depression, I can't remember at all when I last felt depression. I feel good about myself, good about my surroundings, 'cause you know you are only doing the best you can.	Listening.
What do you think has brought about that change?	Probing for patient's beliefs.

Transcript

Well, after me and my husband had separated about 3 years ago I got to the point, well, the children have to depend on me now, because I was doing a lot of depending on him.

So since then you have generally felt better about yourself.

Yeah.

Can you describe your eating habits over the past several years?

Okay, well, I eat breakfast. I eat sometimes a large breakfast and during the midday I'll drink tea, eat some fruit, drink milk. I drink a lot of milk. I love milk. I might sit down and eat dinner about—lunch, I don't even worry about lunch 'cause I never see it. I eat dinner about 6 or 7 o'clock in the evening. In the last couple months I stopped snacking on a lot of sweets. Before I used to crave them at a certain period of the time, mostly when it was my menstrual period, I'd crave a lot of sweets. Lately I just don't even care for sweets too much. But I still drink a lot of milk, as long as it's cold, I'll drink a lot of milk.

So you eat basically two meals a day.

Yeah, sometimes one.

Comments

A summarization of the patient's statement and additive response.

Getting back to the chief complaint with an open-ended question, topic specified.
More specifics about dietary habits. Part of the history of the present illness even though most often part of the patient profile.
Listening to the details. Time for the interviewer to think and plan and "size up" the patient.

Checking back about important data, summary statement but also something the patient herself may not have realized and, therefore, an additive response.

Transcript	Comments
Now besides this weight problem, which seems to be improving, do you have any other complaints?	The clinician makes a transition to other active problems—perhaps an iatrotropic stimulus as yet unmentioned.
None whatsoever.	
None whatsoever?	With a mild confrontation (using a mirror or reflective response) the clinician elicits a new concern—edema.
Yeah—now, weird as it might sound, now my ankles—on my right leg, my ankle will not swell up, but my left leg swells up. And I was taking water pills there for a while from a doctor.	
How long has this been going on?	Beginning of specific, closed-ended questions defining and categorizing causes of edema. It might have been better for the interviewer to respond, "Tell me more about that."
I'd say for 3 months.	
When is the ankle swelling worse? Is it during the morning when you wake up?	
No, during the evening.	
As the day wears on?	
Yeah, as the day wears on.	
When you wake up in the morning, has it gone down?	
Yes.	
Have you been short of breath?	
No.	
How many pillows do you sleep on?	Now a series of questions that suggest the interviewer is working through some hypotheses about

Transcript	**Comments**
	what's causing the edema. Perhaps the interviewer should have introduced this section with a transitional statement such as "Now I'm going to ask you a series of questions about specific symptoms you might have had." Doing so would have been transparent.
One.	
Do you ever wake up in the middle of the night gasping for air?	
No.	
How many times do you go to the bathroom at night?	
About once.	
And that's your only other major complaint at this time?	Keep asking until you're sure there's nothing else.
Yes.	
Have you had any change in bowel habits?	Beginning of some review of systems (ROS)–type questions probing specifically for symptoms of thyroid disease, pursuing another hypothesis about the weight and edema.
No.	
Constipation? Diarrhea?	
No.	
Change in your voice?	
Yeah, my voice has gotten heavier.	Is it clear what the patient means by "heavier"? The clinician lets this pass.
How long has that gone on?	
I'd say in the about the last year and a half.	
Any change in your skin or your hair?	
No.	

Transcript

Comments

Do you ever feel hot in a room where everyone else is cold or cold whenever everyone else is hot?

I can't stand heat. I cannot stand heat at all. Summertime I stay in the house until the evenings. I've always been like that. Cold weather I love.

Okay. I'm going to ask you a lot of routine questions.
Do you have any drug allergies that you are aware of?

No.

Any medications that you are taking?

No. I'm allergic to penicillin.

What does penicillin do to you?

I broke out in hives.

Do you know of any medical problems that you have had in the past?

No. I have low blood. I'm anemic. I used to take iron pills there for awhile. That was about 10 years ago, then I just stopped because they made me feel tired.

How's your pep and energy been?

Fine.

Any other illness or operations that you remember?
No.

Transition to and beginning of past medical history with a transparent statement that orients the patient to the next phase of the interview.
Note the patient's "no" then "yes" that she does have a drug allergy.

Note the clarification—what does "allergy" mean?

Another "no" then "yes."

Some ROS-type questions as clinician appears to be ruling out another current active problem.

Transcript	Comments
You mentioned that you have children. Tell me about your family. [Patient describes her family and their health status.] So you have four children. Any problems with any of your pregnancies? [Patient describes.] Are you fortunate enough to have a job right now?	Transition to and beginning of the "social history," but notice how much you already know about this person from the manner in which the present illness inquiry is conducted. Notice how well this question is put (respect).
No, not right now.	
What's a typical day like for you?	
[Patient describes typical day.]	
What type of work did you do in the past?	
I've done various things. I drove a bus, did maintenance work, cashier in a store.	
How long have you been unemployed?	
For about 2 months now.	
Any prospects?	
No, just a lot of applications in. That's about it.	
How does that feel? You must be upset.	Occupational history question. Unsuccessful attempt at additive response. Patient has not yet revealed her feelings about this situation.
Not really. Something will come up. Something's bound to come up.	
So you are optimistic?	Successful interchangeable response, which corrects the clinician's prior misperception.
Yeah.	
Did you say you smoked cigarettes? How much do you smoke?	Transition to new topic.

Transcript	Comments
I smoke—a pack will last me about 2 days.	
How long have you smoked?	
I've been smoking since I was 16.	
Drink any alcohol?	
No.	
Have you ever?	
Yes, I stopped drinking when I was 18.	
Why was that?	
I was pregnant with my first child.	
Do you use any other type of drugs?	
No.	
I'm just going to run through a bunch of questions now. Have you had any headaches recently?	Transition to and beginning of formal ROS, clinician describing next phase of interview (transparency).
No.	
Trouble with your eyes or your vision?	
In one eye. This one jumps. It's the left one. That's been about 3 months now.	
What do you mean by jumps?	Attempt at establishing precise meaning.
It gets to quivering. I don't know whether it's nerves. I used to say something's going to happen.	
Do you ever see double out of that eye?	ROS-type questions continue.
No. Once in awhile when I come in from a different room area. Like this one will kind of dart and then it will clear up and my vision gets together.	

Transcript	Comments
Any difficulty hearing?	
No.	
Any bleeding through your nose, mouth, lips, and gums? Difficulty swallowing?	
No.	
I asked you about shortness of breath before. How about wheezing?	
Wheezing, yes, sometimes.	
When do you have the wheezing?	
At night when I sleep.	
Do you take anything for that?	
No, not really.	
Do you get up, or does it just go away?	
Sometimes I'll get up and drink some water and that's it.	
How often do you get that?	
Every night during the night.	
So every night you wake up feeling like you're wheezing and then you get up and have a drink of water?	Summary statement.
Yes, almost every night.	
Coughing any blood up at all?	
No.	
Any fever, chills, or sweats?	
No.	
Belly pain?	
No.	
Lumps or bumps anywhere in your breasts or under your arms?	
No. [Interruption at door.]	

Transcript	Comments
What was I asking you, about belly pains?	Clinician asks patient to help get back on track after an interruption.
Yes.	
No belly pains?	
No.	
Diarrhea or constipation?	
No.	
Any blood in your stools?	
No.	
Tell me about your menstrual periods.	
I guess they're normal, they come regular.	
Any pain or bleeding between periods? Are they heavy?	
No, nothing like that.	
Do you have any sexual problems or concerns about birth control?	
Well, I'm not doing anything right now.	
Okay, just a few more questions. Any swelling of any of your joints or joint pains? Anywhere on your body?	
Just my ankles.	
Okay, we already talked about that. Any rash?	
No.	
I think that's about all the questions I have for now. Do you have any questions for me? Is there anything else we need to cover?	Inviting the patient to have the last word.
No.	

Transcript	Comments
Well, we've gone over a lot of stuff. Let's do your physical exam and then we'll make a plan. I'll step out and I'll review your old records while you put this gown on. I'll be back in a few minutes. Does that sound okay?	Transition to physical exam and letting the patient know what to expect (orient to flow of visit, transparency).

The clinician went on to complete the evaluation of this patient, who turned out to have venous insufficiency as the cause of her pedal edema and reactive airway disease exacerbated by smoking. She did not have hypothyroidism or any other endocrine disorder. She and her clinician began working together on a program of weight loss and smoking cessation.

We wish you good listening and learning.

Resources

INTERVIEWING AS A CLINICAL SKILL

ACGME Outcome Project. Accreditation Council for Graduate Medical Education Web Site. Available at http://www.acgme.org (accessed May 2005).

Balint M. *The Doctor and His Patient and the Illness*. New York, International Universities Press, 1972.

Brown JB, Boles M, Mullooly JP, Levinson W. Effect of communication skills training on patient satisfaction. A randomized, controlled study. *Ann Intern Med* 1999; 131:822–829.

Cassell EJ. *Talking with Patients. Volume 1, The Theory of Doctor-Patient Communication.* Cambridge, MA, MIT Press, 1985.

Cassell EJ. *Talking with Patients. Volume 2, Clinical Techniques.* Cambridge, MA, MIT Press, 1985.

Coulehan JL. Being a physician. In: Mengel MB, Holleman W (Eds.). *Fundamentals of Clinical Practice. A Textbook on the Patient, Doctor, and Society.* New York, Plenum Medical Book Company, 2nd ed., 2002, pp. 73–98.

Feinstein AR. *Clinical Judgment.* Baltimore, Williams & Wilkins, 1967.

Frankel RM, Quill TE, McDaniel SH, eds. *The Biopsychosocial Approach: Past, Present, Future.* Rochester NY, University of Rochester Press, 2003.

Platt FW, McMath JC. Clinical hypocompetence: The interview. *Ann Intern Med* 1979; 91:898–902.

Rogers C. *On Becoming a Person.* Boston, Houghton Mifflin, 1961.

Rosenberg EE, Lussier MT, Beaudoin C. Lessons for clinicians from physician-patient communication literature. *Arch Fam Med* 1997; 6:279–283.

Sledge WH, Feinstein AR. A clinimetric approach to the components of the patient-physician relationship. *JAMA* 1997; 278:2043–2048.

Wall EM. The predictive value of selected components of medical history taking. *J Am Board Fam Pract* 1997; 10:66–67.

Yedidia MJ, Gillespie CC, Kachur E, Schwartz MD, Ockene J, Chepaitis AE, Snyder CW, Lazaea A, Lipkin M. Effect of communications training on medical student performance. *JAMA* 2003; 290:1157–1165.

RESPECT, GENUINENESS, AND EMPATHY

Balint M. *The Doctor and His Patient and the Illness.* New York, International Universities Press, 1972.

Cassell EJ. *Talking with Patients. Volume 1, The Theory of Doctor-Patient Communication.* Cambridge, MA, MIT Press, 1985.

Cassell EJ. *Talking with Patients. Volume 2, Clinical Techniques.* Cambridge, MA, MIT Press, 1985.

Charon R. Narrative medicine. A model for empathy, reflection, profession, and trust. *JAMA* 2001; 286:1897–1902.

Coulehan JL, Platt FW, Frankl R, Salazar W, Lown B, Fox L. Let me see if I have this right: Words that build empathy. *Ann Intern Med* 2001; 135:221–227.

Epstein RM. Mindful practice. *JAMA* 1999; 282:833–839.

Farber NJ, Novack DH, O'Brien MK. Love, boundaries, and the patient physician relationship. *Arch Intern Med* 1997; 157:2291–2294.

Frankel RM, Quill TE, McDaniel SH, eds. *The Biopsychosocial Approach: Past, Present, Future.* Rochester NY, University of Rochester Press, 2003.

Gross DA, Zyzanski SJ, Borawski EA, Cebul RD, Stange KC. Patient satisfaction with time spent with their physician. *J Fam Pract* 1998; 47:133–137.

Ivey AE, Authier J. *Microcounselling.* Springfield, IL, Charles C Thomas, 1978.

Novack DH, Suchman AL, Clark W, Epstein RM, Najberg E, Kaplan MD: Calibrating the physician. Personal awareness and effective patient care. *JAMA* 1997; 278:502–509.

Platt FW, McMath JC. Clinical hypocompetence: The interview. *Ann Intern Med* 1979; 91:898–902.

Realini T, Kalet A, Sparling J. Interruption in the medical interaction. *Arch Fam Med* 1995; 4:1028–1033.

Rosenberg EE, Lussier MT, Beaudoin C. Lessons for clinicians from physician-patient communication literature. *Arch Fam Med* 1997; 6:279–283.

Suchman AL, Markakis K, Beckman HB, Frankel R. A model of empathic communication in the medical interview. *JAMA* 1997; 277:678–682.

CHIEF COMPLAINT AND PRESENT ILLNESS

Adler HM. The history of the present illness as treatment. Who's listening and why does it matter? *J Am Board Fam Pract* 1997; 10:28–35.

Charon R. Narrative medicine. A model for empathy, reflection, profession, and trust. *JAMA* 2001; 286:1897–1902.

Feinstein AR. *Clinical Judgment.* Baltimore, Williams & Wilkins, 1967.

Haidet P, Paterniti DA. "Building" a history rather than "taking" one. *Arch Intern Med* 2003; 163:1134–1140.

Marvel MK, Epstein RM, Flowers K, Beckman HK. Soliciting the patient's agenda: Have we improved? *JAMA* 1999; 281:283–287.

Maynard DW. *Bad News, Good News: Conversational Order in Everyday Talk and Clinical Settings.* Chicago, University of Chicago Press, 2003.

Platt FW, Gaspar D, Coulehan JL, Fox L, Stewart M, Weston W, Smith RC, Adler A. Tell me about yourself: The patient-centered interview. *Ann Intern Med* 2001; 134:1079–1085.

White J, Levinson W, Roter D. "Oh, by the way ..." The closing moments of the medical visit. *J Gen Intern Med* 1994; 9:24–28.

Yedidia MJ, Gillespie CC, Kachur E, Schwartz MD, Ockene J, Chepaitis AE, Snyder CW, Lazaea A, Lipkin M. Effect of communications training on medical student performance. *JAMA* 2003; 290:1157–1165.

OTHER ACTIVE PROBLEMS, PAST MEDICAL HISTORY, AND FAMILY HISTORY

Boland BJ, Wollan PC, Silverstein MD. Review of systems, physical examination, and routine tests for case finding in ambulatory patients. *Am J Med Sci* 1995; 309:194–200.

Eisenberg L, Kleinman A. Clinical social science. In: Eisenberg L, Kleinman A. (Eds.) *The Relevance of Social Science to Medicine.* Dordrecht, Holland, D. Reidel, 1980.

Guttmacher AE, Collins FS, Carmona RH. The family history—more important than ever. *N Engl J Med* 2004; 351:2333–2336.

Haidet P, Paterniti DA. "Building" a history rather than "taking" one. *Arch Intern Med* 2003; 163:1134–1140.

Ramsey PG, Curtis JR, Paauw DS, Carline JD, Wenrich MD. History-taking and preventive medicine skills among primary care physicians: An assessment using standardized patients. *Am J Med* 1998; 104:152–158.

U.S. Surgeon General's Family History Initiative. Available at http://www.hhs.gov/familyhistory/resources.html (accessed May 2005).

Verdon ME, Siemensk K. Yield of review of systems in a self administered questionnaire. *J Am Board Fam Pract* 1997; 10:20–27.

Wall EM. The predictive value of selected components of medical history taking. *J Am Board Fam Pract* 1997; 10:66–67.

THE PATIENT PROFILE

Adams WL, Barry KL, Fleming MF. Screening for problem drinking in older primary care patients. *JAMA* 1996; 276:1964–1967.

Adler HM. The history of the present illness as treatment. Who's listening and why does it matter? *J Am Board Fam Pract* 1997; 10:28–35.

Astrow AB, Sulmasy DP. Spirituality and the patient-physician relationship. *JAMA* 2004; 291:2884.

Brown RL, Leonard T, Saunders LA, Papasouliotis O. A two-item conjoint screen for alcohol and other drug problems. *J Am Board Fam Pract* 2001; 14:95–106.

Eisenstat SA, Baucroft L. Domestic violence. *N Engl J Med* 1999; 341:886–892.

Elliot BA. Screening for family violence: Overcoming the barriers [editorial]. *J Fam Pract* 2000; 49:137–138.

Feldhaus KM, Koziol-McLain J, Amsbury HL, Norton IM, Lowenstein SR, Abbott JT. Accuracy of 3 brief screening questions for detecting partner violence in the Emergency Department. *JAMA* 1997; 277:1357–1361.

Frankel RM, Quill TE, McDaniel SH, eds. *The Biopsychosocial Approach: Past, Present, Future.* Rochester NY, University of Rochester Press, 2003.

Groopman J. God at the bedside. *N Engl J Med* 2004; 350:1176–1178.

Knight JR, Sherritt L, Gates EA, Harris SK. Should the CRAFT substance abuse screening test be shortened? *JCOM* 2004; 11:19–25.

Koenig HG. Taking a spiritual history. *JAMA* 2004; 291:2881.

Lo B, Ruston D, Kates LW, et al. Discussing religious and spiritual issues at the end of life: A practical guide for physicians. *JAMA* 2002; 287:749–754.

Maurice WL. *Sexual Medicine in Primary Care.* New York, Mosby-Year Book, 1999.

Miller TA. Diagnostic evaluation of erectile dysfunction. *Am Fam Physician* 2000; 61:95–104, 109–110.

Neufeld B. SAFE questions: Overcoming barriers to the detection of domestic violence. *Am Fam Physician* 1996; 53:2575–2580.

Newman LS. Occupational illness. *N Engl J Med* 1995; 333:1128–1134.

Pulchalski C, Romer AL. Taking a spiritual history allows clinicians to understand patients more fully. *J Pallia Med* 2000; 3:129–137.

Ramsey PG, Curtis JR, Paauw DS, Carline JD, Wenrich MD. History-taking and preventive medicine skills among primary care physicians: An assessment using standardized patients. *Am J Med* 1998; 104:152–158.

Rodriguez MA, Bauer HM, McLoughlin E, Gruneback K. Screening and intervention for intimate partner abuse: Practices and attitudes of primary care physicians. *JAMA* 1999; 282:468–474.

Rovi S, Mouton CP. Domestic violence education in family practice residencies. *Fam Med* 1999; 31(6):398–403.

Yedidia MJ, Gillespie CC, Kachur E, Schwartz MD, Ockene J, Chepaitis AE, Snyder CW, Lazaea A, Lipkin M. Effect of communications training on medical student performance. *JAMA* 2003; 290:1157–1165.

Zink T. Should children be in the room when the mother is screened for partner violence? *J Fam Pract* 2000; 49:130–136.

THE SEXUAL HISTORY

Maurice WL. *Sexual Medicine in Primary Care*. New York, Mosby-Year Book, 1999.

Miller TA. Diagnostic evaluation of erectile dysfunction. *Am Fam Physician* 2000; 61:95–104, 109–110.

Rhodes KV, Levinson W. Interventions for intimate partner violence against women: Clinical applications. *JAMA* 2003; 289:601–605.

Rodriguez MA, Bauer HM, McLoughlin E, Gruneback K. Screening and intervention for intimate partner abuse: Practices and attitudes of primary care physicians. *JAMA* 1999; 282:468–474.

Ross MW, Channon-Little LD, Rosser BRS. *Sexual Health Concerns: Interviewing and History Taking for Health Practitioners*. Philadelphia, FA Davis, 2000.

REVIEW OF SYSTEMS, PHYSICAL EXAMINATION, AND CLOSURE

Bergh KD. Time use and physicians' exploration of the reason for the office visit. *Fam Med* 1996; 28:264–270.

Boland BJ, Wollan PC, Silverstein MD. Review of systems, physical examination, and routine tests for case finding in ambulatory patients. *Am J Med Sci* 1995; 309:194–200.

Johnson KB, Feldman MJ. Medical informatics and pediatrics. Decision-support systems. *Arch Pediatr Adolesc Med* 1995; 149:1371–1380.

Mauksch LB, Hillenburg L, Robins L. The establishing focus protocol: Training for collaborative agenda setting and time management in the medical interview. *Fam Syst & Health* 2001; 19:147–157.

Verdon ME, Siemensk K. Yield of review of systems in a self administered questionnaire. *J Am Board Fam Pract* 1997; 10:20–27.

Wall EM. The predictive value of selected components of medical history taking. *J Am Board Fam Pract* 1997; 10:66–67.

White J, Levinson W, Roter D. "Oh by the way ..." The closing moments of the medical visit. *J Gen Intern Med* 1994; 9:24–28.

THE CLINICAL NARRATIVE

Charon R. Narrative medicine. A model for empathy, reflection, profession, and trust. *JAMA* 2001; 286:1897–1902.

Epstein RM. Mindful Practice. *JAMA* 1999; 282:833–839.

Frankel RM, Quill TE, McDaniel SH, eds. *The Biopsychosocial Approach: Past, Present, Future*. Rochester NY, University of Rochester Press, 2003.

Haidet P, Paterniti DA. "Building" a history rather than "taking" one. *Arch Intern Med* 2003; 163:1134–1140.

COMMUNICATION IN THE OFFICE SETTING

Bergh KD. Time use and physicians' exploration of the reason for the office visit. *Fam Med* 1996; 28:264–270.

Brody H. Transparency: Informed consent in primary care. *Hastings Cent Rep* 1989; 19:5–9.

Brown JB, Boles M, Mullooly JP, Levinson W. Effect of communication skills training on patient satisfaction. A randomized, controlled study. *Ann Intern Med* 1999; 131:822–829.

Cegala DJ, Marinelli T, Post D. The effects of patient communication skills training on compliance. *Arch Fam Med* 2000; 9:57–64.

Crigger BJ, Callahan M. Patients, physicians, and the Internet. *Seminars Med Pract* 2000; 3:9–16.

Delbanco T, Sands DZ. Electrons in flight—e-mail between doctors and patients. *N Engl J Med* 2004; 350:1705–1707.

Frankel RM, Quill TE, McDaniel SH, eds. *The Biopsychosocial Approach: Past, Present, Future*. Rochester NY, University of Rochester Press, 2003.

Gross DA, Zyzanski SJ, Borawski EA, Cebul RD, Stange KC. Patient satisfaction with time spent with their physician. *J Fam Pract* 1998; 47: 133–137.

Marvel MK, Epstein RM, Flowers K, Beckman HK. Soliciting the patient's agenda: Have we improved? *JAMA* 1999; 281:283–287.

Mauksch LB, Hillenburg L, Robins L. The establishing focus protocol: Training for collaborative agenda setting and time management in the medical interview. *Fam Syst & Health* 2001; 19:147–157.

Maynard DW. *Bad News, Good News: Conversational Order in Everyday Talk and Clinical Settings.* Chicago, University of Chicago Press, 2003.

Peltenburg M, Fischer JE, Bahrs O, et al. The unexpected in primary care: A multicenter study on the emergence of unvoiced patient agenda. *Ann Fam Med* 2004; 2:534–540.

Ramsey PG, Curtis JR, Paauw DS, Carline JD, Wenrich MD. History-taking and preventive medicine skills among primary care physicians: An assessment using standardized patients. *Am J Med* 1998; 104: 152–158.

Realini T, Kalet A, Sparling J. Interruption in the medical interaction. *Arch Fam Med* 1995; 4:1028–1033.

Seelert KR, Hill RD, Rigdon MA, Schwenzfeler E. Measuring patient distress in primary care. *Fam Med* 1999; 31:483–487.

White J, Levinson W, Roter D. "Oh by the way ..." The closing moments of the medical visit. *J Gen Intern Med* 1994; 9:24–28.

PEDIATRIC AND ADOLESCENT INTERVIEWING

Bennett HJ. Using humor in the office setting: A pediatric perspective. *J Fam Pract* 1996; 42:462–464.

Johnson KB, Feldman MJ. Medical informatics and pediatrics. Decision-support systems. *Arch Pediatr Adolesc Med* 1995; 149:1371–1380.

Steiner BD, Gest KL. Do adolescents want to hear preventive medicine counseling messages in outpatient settings? *J Fam Pract* 1996; 43:375–381.

Zink T. Should children be in the room when the mother is screened for partner violence? *J Fam Pract* 2000; 49:130–136.

INTERVIEWING THE GERIATRIC PATIENT

Adams WL, Barry KL, Fleming MF. Screening for problem drinking in older primary care patients. *JAMA* 1996; 276:1964–1967.

Bowie P, Branton T, Holmes J. Should the mini-mental state examination be used to monitor dementia treatment? *Lancet* 1999; 354: 1527–1528.

DeVore PA. Computerized geriatric assessment for geriatric care management. *Aging* 1995; 7:194–196.

Folstein MF, Folstein SE, McHugh PR. Mini-mental state: A practical method for grading the cognitive state of patients for the clinician. *J Psychiatry Res* 1975; 12:189–198.

Whooley MA, Avins AL, Miranda J, Browner WS. Case finding instruments for depression. *J Gen Intern Med* 1997; 12:439–445.

CULTURAL COMPETENCE IN THE INTERVIEW

ACGME Outcome Project. Accreditation Council for Graduate Medical Education Web Site. Available at http://www.acgme.org (accessed May 2005).

Assessing Cultural Competence in Health Care, U.S. Public Health service, Office of Minority Health, http://www.omhrc.gov/clas/ (accessed May 2005).

Barnett S. Clinical and cultural issues in caring for deaf people. *Fam Med* 1999; 31:17–22.

Carrillo JE, Green AR, Betancourt JR. Cross-cultural primary care: A patient-based approach. *Ann Intern Med* 1999; 130:829–834.

Cooper-Patrick L, Gallo JJ, Gonzales JJ, Vu HT, Powe NR, Nelson C, Ford DE. Race, gender, and partnership in the patient-physician relationship. *JAMA* 1999; 282:583–589.

Crawley L, Marshall P, Lo B, Koenig B. Strategies for culturally effective end-of-life care. *Ann Intern Med* 2002; 136(9):673–679.

Flores G. Culture and the patient-physician relationship: Achieving cultural competency in health care. *J Pediatr* 2000; 136:14–23.

Galanti GA. *Caring for Patients from Different Cultures: Case Studies from American Hospitals*. Philadelphia, University of Pennsylvania Press, 1997.

Kagawa-Singer M, Blackhall L. Negotiating cross-cultural issues at the end of life: "You got to go where he lives." *JAMA* 2001; 286:2899–3038.

Kelley M, Fitzsimons V, eds. *Understanding Cultural Diversity.* Sudbury, MA, Jones and Bartlett, 2000.

Like RC, Steiner RP, Rubel AJ. Recommended core curriculum guidelines on culturally sensitive and competent health care. *Fam Med* 1996; 28:291–297.

Morris DB. *Illness and Culture in the Postmodern Age.* Berkeley, University of California Press, 1998.

Rhian FL et al. Educating medical students for work in culturally diverse societies. *JAMA* 1999; 282:1–11.

Rothschild SK. Cross-cultural issues in primary care medicine. *Disease-a-Month.* 1998; 44:293–319.

Shapiro J, Lenahan P. Family medicine in a culturally diverse world: A solution-oriented approach to common cross-cultural problems in medical encounters. *Fam Med* 1996; 28:249–255.

DIFFICULT PATIENT-CLINICIAN INTERACTIONS

American Psychiatric Association. Somatoform disorders. In: *Diagnostic and Statistical Manual of Mental Disorders* (Text Revision), 4th ed. Washington DC, American Psychiatric Association, 2000, pp. 445–469.

Balint M. *The Doctor, His Patient and the Illness*. New York, International Universities Press, 1972.

Barsky AJ. The patient with hypochondriasis. *N Engl J Med* 2001; 345:1395–1399.

Groves JE. Taking care of the hateful patient. *N Engl J Med* 1978; 398:883–887.

Kahana RJ, Bibring GL. Personality types in medical management. In: Zinberg NE (Ed.), *Psychiatry and Medical Practice in a General Hospital*. New York, International Universities Press, 1964, pp. 108–123.

Keeley R, Smith M, Miller J. Somatoform symptoms and treatment non-adherence in depressed family medicine outpatients. *Arch Fam Med* 2000; 9:46–54.

Novack DH, Suchman AL, Clark W, Epstein RM, Najberg E, Kaplan MD. Calibrating the physician. Personal awareness and effective patient care. *JAMA* 1997; 278:502–509.

Rosenberg EE, Lussier MT, Beaudoin C. Lessons for clinicians from physician-patient communication literature. *Arch Fam Med* 1997; 6:279–283.

Schafer S, Newlis DP. Personality disorders among difficult patients. *Arch Fam Med* 1998; 7:126–129.

Servan-Schreiber D, Kolb NR, Tabas G. Somatizing patients. Part I. Practical diagnosis. *Am Fam Physician* 2000; 61:1073–1078.

Simon GE, VonKorff M, Piccinelli M, Fullerton C, Ormel J. An international study of the relation between somatic symptoms and depression. *N Engl J Med* 1999; 341:1329–1335.

Whooley MA, Avins AL, Miranda J, Browner WS. Case finding instruments for depression. *J Gen Intern Med* 1997; 12:439–445.

TELLING BAD NEWS

Ambuel B, Mazzone MF. Breaking bad news and discussing death. *Prim Care* 2001; 28(2):249–267.

Block SD. Psychological considerations, growth, and transcendence at the end of life: The art of the possible. *JAMA* 2001; 285:2898–2905.

Campbell ML. Breaking bad news to patients. *JAMA* 1994; 271:1052.

Chochinov HM. Dignity-conserving care—a new model for palliative care. *JAMA* 2002; 287:2253–2260.

Christakis, NA, Clipp, EC, McIntyre, L, McNeilly, M, Steinhauser, KE, Tulsky, JA. Factors considered important at the end of life by patients, family, physicians, and other care providers. *JAMA* 2000; 284 (19):2476–2482.

Crawley L, Marshall P, Lo B, Koenig B. Strategies for culturally effective end-of-life care. *Ann Int Med* 2002; 136(9):673–679.

Lo B, Quill T, Tulsky J. Discussing palliative care with patients. *Ann Intern Med* 1999; 130:744–749.

Maynard DW. *Bad News, Good News: Conversational Order in Everyday Talk and Clinical Settings.* Chicago, University of Chicago Press, 2003.

Miranda J, Brody RV. Communicating bad news. *West J Med* 1992; 156: 83–85.

Poulson J. Bitter pills to swallow. *N Engl J Med* 1998; 338:1844–1846.

Ptacek JT, Eberhardt TL. Breaking bad news. A review of the literature. *JAMA* 1996; 276:496–502.

Quill T. Initiating end-of-life discussions with seriously ill patients: Addressing "the elephant in the room." *JAMA* 2000; 284:2502–2507.

Tulsky JA, Fischer GS, Rose MR, Arnold RM. Opening the black box: How do physicians communicate about advance directives? *Ann Intern Med* 1998; 129:441–449.

Vandekieft GK. Breaking bad news. *Am Fam Physician* 2001; 164: 1975–1978.

TALKING WITH PATIENTS ABOUT COMPLEMENTARY AND ALTERNATIVE MEDICINE

ACGME Outcome Project. Accreditation Council for Graduate Medical Education Web Site. Available at http://www.acgme.org (accessed May 2005).

Astin JA. Why patients use alternative medicine. Results of a national study. *JAMA* 1998; 279:1548–1553.

Druss BG, Rosenheck RA. Association between use of unconventional therapies and conventional medical services. *JAMA* 1999; 282:651–656.

Eisenberg DM, Kessler RC, Foster C, Norlock FE, Calkins DR, Delbanco TL. Unconventional medicine in the United States. Prevalence, costs, and patterns of use. *N Engl J Med* 1993; 328:246–252.

Elder NC, Gillcrist A, Minz R. Use of alternative health care by family practice patients. *Arch Fam Med* 1997; 6:181–184.

Kaptchuk TJ, Eisenberg DM. The persuasive appeal of alternative medicine. *Ann Intern Med* 1998; 129:1061–1064.

Kaptchuk TJ, Eisenberg DM. Varieties of healing. 1: Medical pluralism in the United States. *Ann Intern Med* 2001; 135(3):189–195.

Kaptchuk TJ, Eisenberg DM. Varieties of healing. 2: A taxonomy of unconventional healing practices. *Ann Intern Med* 2001; 135(3):196–204.

Lazar JS, O'Connor BB. Talking with patients about their use of alternative therapies. *Prim Care* 1997; 24:699–711.

Miller FG, Emanuel EJ, Rosenstein DL, Strauss SE. Ethical issues concerning research in complementary and alternative medicine. *JAMA* 2004; 291:599–604.

Rao JK, Mihaliak K, Kroenke K, Bradley J, Tierney WM, Weinberger M. Use of complementary therapies for arthritis among patients of rheumatologists. *Ann Intern Med* 1999; 131:409–415.

Sierpina VS. *Integrative Health Care: Complementary and Alternative Therapies for the Whole Person.* Philadelphia, FA Davis, 2001.

ETHICS AND THE LAW

ACGME Outcome Project. Accreditation Council for Graduate Medical Education Web Site. Available at http://www.acgme.org (accessed May 2005).

American Medical Association, Council on Ethical and Judicial Affairs. *Code of Medical Ethics.* Chicago, AMA, 1996.

Beauchamp TL, Childress JF. *Principles of Biomedical Ethics*, 5th ed. New York, Oxford University Press, 2001.

Brody H. Transparency: Informed consent in primary care. *Hastings Cent Rep* 1989; 19:5–9.

Department of Health and Human Services, Office for Civil Rights. Medical Privacy—National Standards to Protect the Privacy of Personal Health Information (HIPAA), http://www.hhs.gov/ocr/hipaa/ (accessed May 2005).

Katz J. *The Silent World of Doctor and Patient.* New York, The Free Press, 1984.

Mazor KM, Simon SR, Yood RA, et al. Health plan members' views about disclosure of medical errors. *Ann Intern Med* 2004; 140:409–418.

McNutt RA. Shared medical decision making: problems, process, progress. *JAMA* 2004; 292:2516–2518.

Thurman AE. Institutional responses to medical mistakes: Ethical and legal perspectives. *Kennedy Inst Ethics J* 2001; 11:147–156.

MALPRACTICE AND THE CLINICAL INTERVIEW

Bogardus ST, Holmboe E, Jekel JF. Perils, pitfalls, and possibilities in talking about medical risk. *JAMA* 1999; 281:1037–1041.

Brody H. Transparency: Informed consent in primary care. *Hastings Cent Rep* 1989; 19:5–9.

Katz J. *The Silent World of Doctor and Patient.* New York, The Free Press, 1984.

Levinson W, Roter DL, Mullooly JP, Dull VT, Frankel RM. Physician-patient communication. The relationship with malpractice claims among primary care physicians and surgeons. *JAMA* 1997; 277:553–559.

Lichtstein DM, Materson BJ, Spicer DW. Reducing the risk of malpractice claims. *Hosp Pract* 1999 (July 15); 34:69–72, 75–76, 79.

EDUCATION AND NEGOTIATION

Balint M. *The Doctor and His Patient and the Illness.* New York, International Universities Press, 1972.

Beckman HB, Frankel RM. The effect of physician behavior on the collection of data. *Ann Intern Med* 1984; 101:692–696.

Buetow S. Four strategies for negotiated care. *JR Soc Med* 1998; 91:199–201.

Cegala DJ, Marinelli T, Post D. The effects of patient communication skills training on compliance. *Arch Fam Med* 2000; 9:57–64.

Fins JJ. Approximation and negotiation: Clinical pragmatism and difference. *Camb Q Healthc Ethics* 1998; 7:68–76.

Krueter MW, Chheda SG, Bull FC. How does physician advice influence patient behavior? Evidence for a priming effect. *Arch Fam Med* 2000; 9:426–433.

O'Mara K. Communication and conflict resolution in emergency medicine. *Emerg Med Clin North Am* 1999; 17:451–459.

THE MEDICAL INTERVIEW AT WORK

Epstein RM. Mindful Practice. *JAMA* 1999; 282:833–839.

Sledge WH, Feinstein AR. A clinimetric approach to the components of the patient-physician relationship. *JAMA* 1997; 278:2043–2048.

INDEX

Note: Page numbers followed by "f" and "t" indicate figures and tables, respectively.